HUMAN
STRUCTURE

HUMAN STRUCTURE

- Matt Cartmill

- William L. Hylander

- James Shafland

Harvard University Press
Cambridge, Massachusetts,
and London, England

Library of Congress Cataloging-in-Publication Data
Cartmill, Matt.
  Human structure.

  Includes index.
    1. Anatomy, Human.   2. Human evolution.   3. Anatomy,
Comparative.   I. Hylander, William L.   II. Shafland,
James.   III. Title.   [DNLM: 1. Anatomy.   QS 4 C327h]
QM23.2.C36   1987   611   86-11982
ISBN 0-674-41805-0 (alk. paper)

Contents

PART IV   THE LIMBS

Preface

Why study human anatomy? Like other brute facts, the facts of anatomy are not very interesting in themselves. After mere curiosity has been satisfied and the horrid fascination of dissecting a human cadaver has worn off, the study of anatomical facts as an end in itself soon becomes sterile and pedantic. Apart from the purely practical sort of interest that drives artists and surgeons to learn anatomy, there are two chief reasons why the mind is drawn to the scientific study of the body. The first is a wish to understand the body's functioning. The second is a desire to understand why the facts of anatomy should be as they are—that is, to explain human structure.

The two questions are closely related. To understand function is to explain a lot, because there are functional reasons for most anatomical facts. Ears are evidently built to receive sounds, and feet seem to be made for walking on. This sort of straightforward functional explanation was good enough for early scientific anatomists, whose demonstrations of the detailed correspondences between form and function in animal bodies provided theologians with compelling arguments for the existence and wisdom of a divine Creator.

But as knowledge of anatomy and understanding of function accumulated, it became painfully evident that some facts could not be explained in functional terms. It was all very well to invoke the infinite wisdom of the Creator in accounting for the marvelous intricacies of the human hand or eye; but there were other situations where form and function were less perfectly matched, and it seemed inappropriate to blame these on Providence. Some differences between species of animals are apparently just plain arbitrary; for instance, birds have their aorta on the right side and mammals have theirs on the left, but there is no corresponding difference in function. Some organs have no apparent function at all—for example, the little muscles of the external ear in man, which can make the ear twitch slightly in some people, but not in others, and serve no useful purpose in either case. Finally, and worst of all from the standpoint of natural theology, some organs appear to be downright ill-designed. There is no evident reason, for instance, why the human testicle could not develop in the scrotum; but as a matter of fact it develops just below the diaphragm in the embryo and then creeps down the inside of the belly muscles to slip out into the scrotum, dragging its blood vessels and ducts along with it. As a result of this peculiar arrangement, human males are prone to a variety of painful and occasionally fatal maladies, including inguinal hernia and varicose testicular veins. It is not very satisfying from either a scientific or a religious standpoint to explain this questionable contrivance as the handiwork of God. Evidently, anatomy is subject to constraints of some sort beyond the mere requirements of good design.

As we understand them today, these constraints are those imposed by history, of two sorts: the history of the individual and the history of the individual's ancestors. Neither can be understood without some knowledge of the other. We may think of any organism as a pattern of organization through which matter is continually passing, like an enormously complicated wave or vortex. Eventually such patterns develop instabilities and collapse—waves break, tornados disintegrate, and people die. Simple physical patterns like waves and tornados are endlessly being brought into existence by the forces of nature, but animals and plants are too complicated for that. The long-term survival of a biological pattern of organization depends on that pattern's capacity to incorporate more and more matter into new duplicates of itself. This duplication, or reproduction, is inexact. Random changes accumulate through many duplications. Usually these changes render the altered pattern less stable, so they and their possessors vanish from the scene. When they do not—when hereditary changes persist and spread—the result is long-term historical change: biological evolution.

The evolutionary history, or phylogeny, of a species is the sum of changes in its pattern of ontogeny (the anatomical history of a typical individual) from generation to generation. Because every individual's ontogeny is on the whole like those of its ancestors (with modifications), a developing organism goes through phases and develops organs that it has no use for itself but that were important to its ancestors.

For example, the shoddy design of the human testicle becomes understandable when we know something about its ontogeny and phylogeny. In early fishes, the testis was an appendage of a kidneylike organ, the mesonephros, which filtered wastes from the blood and dribbled the resulting urine into a long hollow duct leading to the anal end of the gut. The testis lay alongside the mesonephros and ejected its sperm into the same duct. When the ancestors of land-dwelling vertebrates gave up life in the water, they needed a more efficient, water-conserving urinary organ. Eventually an improved auxiliary kidney with its own separate duct evolved. In time, this new kidney replaced the mesonephros. But the mesonephros could not be given up altogether, because its duct was needed by the testis. The mesonephros in a human embryo develops alongside the backbone just below the liver (as it would in a fish or a salamander), stays around long enough for its duct to hook up with the testis, and then regresses and disappears. This leaves the testes sitting up under the liver. In a lizard or a turtle, they would stay in that spot. But the high body temperatures of mammals prevent sperm from maturing; so the testes of fetal mammals must be relocated to a cooler, more external position. In human beings, they descend before birth into the scrotum alongside the penis, drawing their ducts and blood vessels along with them—and creating a line of weakness along which herniating loops of intestine can push their way into the scrotum, too. The testes develop in the abdomen for reasons of ontogenetic necessity, dictated by phylogenetic history. Their descent into the scrotum is a makeshift demanded for physiological reasons, not the best anatomical arrangement that could be imagined. To understand the anatomical facts, one must understand all these factors.

Unfortunately, standard textbooks of human anatomy offer a lot of description and very little explanation. What little explanation they provide is mostly functional, though some textbooks add a smattering of embryology. The phylogenetic aspect of anatomy is almost wholly ignored. This deficiency is not exactly a flaw in the standard textbooks; they are just presupposing a traditional educational background that can no longer be taken for granted. The enormous growth in biological knowledge at the cellular and molecular levels during the last thirty years or so has tended to oust the traditional mudpuppy-and-fetal-pig sort of comparative and developmental anatomy from the preprofessional curriculum in the health sciences. There is nothing wrong with this trend in principle, but it has meant in practice that students increasingly lack the background in comparative anatomy and embryology that they need to digest a fact-crammed textbook of human gross anatomy.

This book is intended as an aperitif to promote such digestion. It is the product of fifteen years of experience in teaching an abbreviated "core course" in gross anatomy to medical and allied health students at Duke University. Compelled by curriculum reforms to teach human anatomy in one-quarter the time previously allotted to that subject, we hit upon the plan of presenting the anatomical facts as a series of regional variations from a schematic vertebrate ground plan—the typical body segment—in an idealized primitive fish or human embryo.

We begin this book with an exposition of the segmental organization characteristic of vertebrates. We then undertake a description of the most obviously segmented parts of the human body: the bones, muscles, vessels, and nerves of the trunk between the neck and the pelvis. From this, we progress through regions where the basic plan has undergone more and more radical modifications, and we end the book with the ancient and extreme specializations found in the head. At each step, we show how these modifications have been imposed, ontogenetically or phylogenetically, upon simpler precursors. We hope that this kind of analysis will help our readers to grasp the logic of the human body from the outset and to fit each new fact they encounter into a single explanatory picture, so that rote memorization can be reduced to a minimum.

We have found in our teaching experience that some students find thinking more painful than memorizing. Such students shrink from explanations, which for them represent only an additional strain on the memory. This book is intended not for them but only for those students of anatomy who, like the book's authors, welcome any expedient that reduces the number of unexplained brute facts that need to be hammered into memory. We think that most students who approach the study of anatomy in this way not only will find it easier and more enjoyable to assimilate the facts of human anatomy but also will come to understand the fascination that anatomy holds for scientific investigators. That fascination lies, not in the facts of anatomy, but in the interpretation of those facts as a transient stage in a historical process of great beauty and unparalleled complexity.

Acknowledgments

Our first and most fundamental indebtedness is to our own professors. We want to acknowledge in particular Drs. Albert Dahlberg, Charles Oxnard, Ronald Singer, Russell Tuttle, David Wake, and the late Dr. Leonard Radinsky, all of whom we were fortunate to have as teachers during our years as graduate students. We continue to remember them as examples to be emulated, both for their knowledge of the facts and for their skill in communicating that knowledge to others.

We have learned almost as much from our professional colleagues at our own and other universities. We thank especially those who have taught alongside us in the gross anatomy laboratory: Drs. Richard F. Kay, Ross D. E. MacPhee, and Kathleen Smith at Duke University; Dr. Timothy Strickler, of Grand Valley State College; and Drs. Bruce Bogart, Douglas Cramer, and David Howard, of New York University. All the chapters that follow draw liberally upon their vision and understanding. For information, criticism, and advice during the writing of this book, we are grateful to them and to Drs. William Jungers and Jack Stern, of the State University of New York at Stony Brook; Drs. Nell Cant and Sheila Counce, of Duke University; Dr. Mary Ellen Morbeck, of the University of Arizona; and Dr. Malcolm Johnston, of the University of North Carolina.

This version of *Human Structure* is the much-changed descendant of a preliminary draft first distributed to Duke medical students in August 1970. For their help and support in producing that draft and its successors, we are indebted to Dr. J. David Robertson, Chairman of the Department of Anatomy, and to many of our other present and former co-workers at Duke University. Special thanks are due to Dr. John Buettner-Janusch for his long-standing helpfulness and kindness; to Susan Padilla, for overseeing and expediting the production of those early versions with characteristic energy, generosity, and good humor; to Wayne Williams, Mary White, and other artists whose illustrations for those early versions provided models for many of the figures in this volume; and to Marlene Johnson, Pat Thompson, Alice Wheeler, and Barbara McPartland, who undertook the huge job of typing and retyping successive drafts of the manuscript. Dr. David Sabatini, Chairman of the Department of Cell Biology at New York University, has also been very supportive of our work in developing this book.

The great majority of the illustrations in this book are the work of scientific illustrator Dorothy L. Norton. We are thoroughly indebted to her for executing hundreds of complex drawings with unfailing artistry, intelligence, and good humor in the face of a demanding and erratic schedule. Whatever value this book has for its readers has been greatly enhanced by the elegance and clarity of her work. Figures 1-3, 1-4, 1-6, 1-7C, 1-8, 6-1 through 6-8, 7-1 through 7-10, and 7-12 are from the accomplished pen of Margaret L. Estey, whom we thank for her valuable contribution. Figures 2-4 and 7-11, drawn by Dorothy Norton and the senior author respectively, derive from draft versions by Ms. Estey. The senior author is also responsible for Figures 14-14, 15-1, 17-8, and the labeling of all the figures. Figures 1-7, 9-4, and 10-2 were redrawn after figures in *Medical Embryology* by J. Langman, copyright © 1963; by permission of Williams & Wilkins Company, Baltimore. Figures 5-1, 5-9A, 8-3, 8-9, 10-7, and 19-11 were redrawn after figures in *Grant's Method of Anatomy,* 10th ed., by J. V. Basmajian, copyright © 1980; by permission of Williams & Wilkins Company, Baltimore, and J. V. Basmajian. Figures 6-2, 10-1, 13-12, 19-7, 19-8, and 21-1B were redrawn after figures in *The Vertebrate Body,* 5th ed., by Alfred Sherwood Romer and Thomas S. Parsons; copyright © 1977 by W. B. Saunders Company; by permission of CBS College Publishing. Figure 7-12 was redrawn after a figure in *A New System of Anatomy,* 2nd ed., by Lord Zuckerman, copyright © 1981; by permission of Oxford University Press. Figure 9-16 was redrawn after a figure in *Primary Anatomy,* 7th ed., by J. V. Basmajian, copyright © 1982; by permission of Williams & Wilkins Company, Baltimore, and J. V. Basmajian. Figure 22-5 was redrawn after a figure in *Cunningham's Manual of Practical Anatomy,* 12th ed., by G. J. Romanes, copyright © 1976; by permission of Oxford University Press.

The artwork and text would not have come together or made it into print without the guidance and encouragement that we have received from the editorial staff of Harvard University Press. We are grateful to William Patrick for initiating and promoting this project, and to Howard Boyer for seeing it through to completion. We thank Marianne Perlak for her praiseworthy design of the book. Special thanks are due to our editor Jodi Simpson, whose enthusiasm, sympathetic understanding, and critical intelligence have improved every page of *Human Structure* and helped to make the task of preparing it for publication a rewarding and often enjoyable experience.

But our deepest gratitude for making this book a reality belongs to Dr. Kaye Brown. During the five long years that went by between the signing of a contract and the final delivery of copy, she selflessly and unflaggingly dedicated herself to providing the determination, ingenuity, energy, and insight that we lacked and needed to finish the job. In a research-oriented university setting, completing a book of this kind comes near the bottom of the list of institutional priorities; and it would have remained dead last on ours if she had not ceaselessly broken through our resistance to remind us where our real priorities and best aspirations lay. For all her care and enterprise and for helping us to rearrange our lives and calendars to provide the time and space needed for completing this task, we are profoundly grateful to her. In a very real sense, this is her book.

VERTEBRATE ANATOMY
AND THE
SEGMENTED TRUNK

PART I

The
Vertebrate
Body

All living things on this planet, from the higher plants and animals down to bacteria and viruses, have a common ancestry in the distant past, perhaps around four billion years ago. Your great-great-to-the-*n*th-power grandparents were also the progenitors of the plants and animals you ate for lunch yesterday. So many changes have accumulated over billions of years in the various branches of this immense fratricidal family that the family resemblance can be seen only at the molecular level of organization. It is still a literal family resemblance: the relationship between you and your brothers and sisters differs only in degree from the relationship between you and a pineapple.

Some organisms are so closely related to each other that we can still see the family resemblance in their anatomy. When you look at a dog, you have no trouble matching up the parts of your body with the dog's and identifying them as eyes, teeth, kidneys, ears, and so on. These similarities are inherited from the last common ancestor of people and dogs. In more distant relatives, inherited resemblances like these, called **homologies,** become fewer and harder to pick out. We have no trouble identifying the eyes and teeth on a tuna fish, but finding the equivalents of lungs and shoulder blades is much harder, and ears and toenails are nowhere to be found. Still more distant relatives share no anatomical homologies at all. Cockroaches have legs of a sort; but their legs are not homologous with ours, because the last ancestor that people and cockroaches had in common was legless. (Talking about the "legs" of a cockroach involves the use of a metaphor, like talking about the "jaws" of a power shovel.)

The largest collection of organisms in which we can still see a clear anatomical family resemblance is called a **phylum.** There are about twenty phyla of many-celled animals. The one to which man belongs is the phylum **Chordata,** or chordates. The family resemblance that unites the members of a phylum is more easily seen in some members

Inherited resemblances between different organisms are called homologies.

of that phylum than in others. The earlier and more primitive members of a phylum are usually simpler in their anatomy. Later, more specialized members have added some parts, lost some, and changed others almost beyond recognition. It is generally easiest to understand the morphological ground plan of a phylum by looking at its most primitive members.

That ground plan is also usually easier to make out in embryos or larvae than it is in the adult stages of the same animals. The things that make a chordate a chordate show up during the first few days of embryonic development; the features that tell you whether it is going to wind up as an alligator or a mudhen or a platypus become apparent only later. Because the identifying peculiarities of a animal tend to show up late in its development, researchers once held that "ontogeny recapitulates phylogeny"—that is, that the embryonic development (ontogeny) of the individual retraces the evolutionary history (phylogeny) of all the generations of its ancestors.

This principle of recapitulation is not strictly true. We all had umbilical cords as fetuses, but people did not evolve from animals that ran around as adults trailing umbilical cords. Still, the principle of recapitulation is true in the sense that human ontogeny and phylogeny both start from rather similar fishlike beginnings and end up producing a human adult. Naturally, the two sets of changes show many parallels, and knowing both makes it easier to grasp the anatomical logic of the adult body. The rest of this chapter will be devoted to sketching the basic chordate ground plan found in *Homo sapiens*. Throughout this book, we will use this ground plan as a starting point for studying the anatomy of various regions and systems.

▪ *Branchiostoma:* A Primitive Chordate

Most chordates are fish, and most of the rest (including ourselves) are specialized fish out of water; but there are a few living chordates that are too primitive to merit the title of fish at all. The most familiar of these is the lancelet or amphioxus, *Branchiostoma*, a small and rather wormlike creature that inhabits shallow sea bottoms. *Branchiostoma* looks like a simplified sketch of a fish with the bones, eyes, jaws, and fins left off (Fig. 1-1). It lives with its tail buried in the mud and its head sticking out, sucking in water and squirting it out through slits

Fig. 1-1 *Branchiostoma*. A. Section through a larval animal (simplified). B. An adult in its usual feeding position, buried in mud with its mouth protruding.

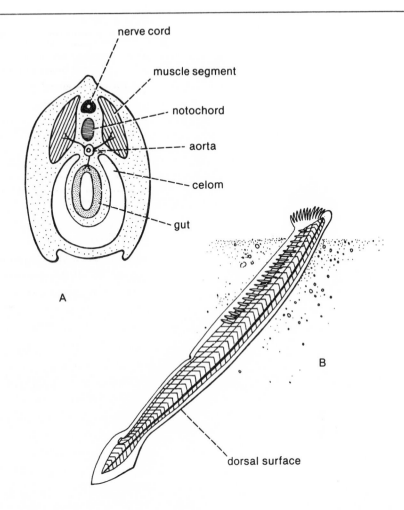

in the sides of its "throat." In this way, it strains out suspended organic debris, which it swallows.

When a lancelet is disturbed, muscles running along the sides of the animal contract rhythmically to wriggle its body from side to side, propelling it through the water. To produce this sinuous motion, some of the muscles on one side of the body must contract while those directly opposite relax. This coordination is facilitated by the division of the musculature on each side into a series of separate blocks or **segments** that can contract individually. A **dorsal nerve cord** running down the middle of the lancelet's back sends a **segmental** nerve into each muscle segment. Impulses passing along this nerve make the muscle contract. The nerve cord keeps the contractions of all the segments coordinated so that the wriggling motion is smooth and efficient. Underneath the nerve cord lies the **notochord,** a stiff rod of connective tissue that keeps the animal's body length constant and thus forces the contracting muscle segments to bend the body rather than shorten it.

The segmental arrangement of the lancelet's muscles and nerves is mimicked by other systems of the body. As a result, a lancelet is made up of little repeating units like a string of identical beads. Each body segment includes right and left muscle blocks, segmental nerves, and reproductive and sensory organs. The segments on each side are separated by intersegmental blood vessels branching from a bigger blood vessel, the **dorsal aorta,** that runs the length of the body under the notochord.

The unsegmented "string" running through this chain of beads is the gut, which connects the jawless mouth with the anus. The gut tube does not run the whole length of the animal, however. It ends at the anal opening, about five-sixths of the way down the lancelet's belly; the notochord, nerve cord, aorta, and muscle segments extend beyond this to form a short postanal tail. The lancelet's gut is partially surrounded by a fluid-filled cavity in the body tissues, the **celom,** which is U-shaped in cross section. The dorsal side of the gut stays attached by nerves and vessels to the aorta and dorsal nerve cord (Fig. 1-1).

The anatomical arrangements in *Branchiostoma* are part of the basic morphological pattern of the phylum Chordata. The same pattern is seen in all chordate bodies, including our own. The segmental organization of the human body has been blurred and obscured by half a billion years of reworking various segments to serve different special functions. What started off as a simple string of identical beads has gradually become something more like a charm bracelet. But each segment of the human body is still composed of comparable elements connected in essentially the same way.

■ Vertebrates and Their Development

The lancelet is a chordate, but not a vertebrate. Most chordates (including ourselves) are vertebrates. Vertebrates differ from nonvertebrate chordates in having an internal skeleton of bone or cartilage, which supplements or replaces the notochord. Vertebrates also have a more elaborate head region than lower chordates have. In vertebrates, the head end of the dorsal nerve cord swells and wrinkles up to produce a brain with two eyes sticking out of it. Parts of the body surface overlying the brain sink into the head to become paired sense organs of smell and balance: the nose and the inner ear.

Primitive vertebrates were fishes. They lived in water and laid their eggs there. At first, land-dwelling vertebrates returned to the water to lay their eggs, just as frogs and other amphibians do today. The eggs of frogs hatch into fishlike larvae that are able to swim and procure their own food while they work up a set of legs and lungs. In higher vertebrates (reptiles, birds, and mammals), this larval stage has been eliminated, and the embryo stays inside the egg until its legs and lungs are in working order.

Getting rid of the larval stage meant that the egg could be laid directly on land, thereby freeing the adults from their attachment to aquatic sex. This change was a tremendous evolutionary success. It led to an explosive evolutionary radiation of the early reptiles and of their furred and feathered descendants, and reduced the amphibians to a few remnants lingering around the edges of ponds and streams. But it involved extensive changes in the anatomy of the egg.

The egg of a fish or frog is squirted out of the mother's body directly into the water, where it is fertilized. The developing embryo finds itself in relatively congenial surroundings. It can absorb the water and oxygen it needs from the surrounding medium, and the wastes it produces as it grows can be excreted directly into the water around it. When it hatches as a tadpole, it can find its own food; the egg needs to contain only enough food to support the embryo until it is able to wiggle its tail and swim. The chief threat it faces from its environment is a host of predators with a taste for caviar or tadpoles. This predator pressure may have been one of the things that favored the "invention" of an egg that could be laid out of the water.

Although it may have fewer predators, an egg laid out of water is exposed to a harsher environment. It must be watertight and must contain all the water needed for growth and excretion. Space must be provided inside the egg for storing the embryo's solid and liquid wastes—and because water must be conserved, liquid wastes must be kept to an absolute minimum. There must be some mechanism for absorbing oxygen and getting rid of CO_2 without losing any water to the air; and the embryo must be cushioned in some way against mechanical shock. All the supplies and gadgets the egg needs to contain make it too big to support its own weight out of water, so it needs a stiff skeleton of some sort to maintain its shape.

This last problem was met by enclosing the egg in a hard shell. The others were solved by elaborating parts of the embryo's surface into membranous bags, the **extraembryonic membranes** (Fig. 1-2). There are four of these: the yolk sac, allantois, amnion, and chorion. The **yolk sac**, a bag hanging off the embryonic gut and containing stored food for the embryo, was an old chordate feature that needed only to be made larger. The **allantois**, another outpouching of the gut, serves the embryo as a combination lung and cesspool; in the shelled eggs laid by reptiles and birds, the allantois stores the embryo's excretions, and its surface absorbs and releases gases through the eggshell. The **amnion** serves as a cushioning "water jacket" for the embryo, and the **chorion** encloses the other contents of the egg and acts as a barrier to water loss. Most mammals no longer lay shelled eggs; the egg is retained inside the mother's body, and the extraembryonic membranes have different functions. Nevertheless, the same membranes are present in all birds, reptiles, and mammals. These higher vertebrates are called **amniotes**, after the amnion.

Fig. 1-2 Extraembryonic membranes of bird (A) and human (B) embryos. The human allantois and yolk sac are vestigial. Schematic midline sections, seen from the left.

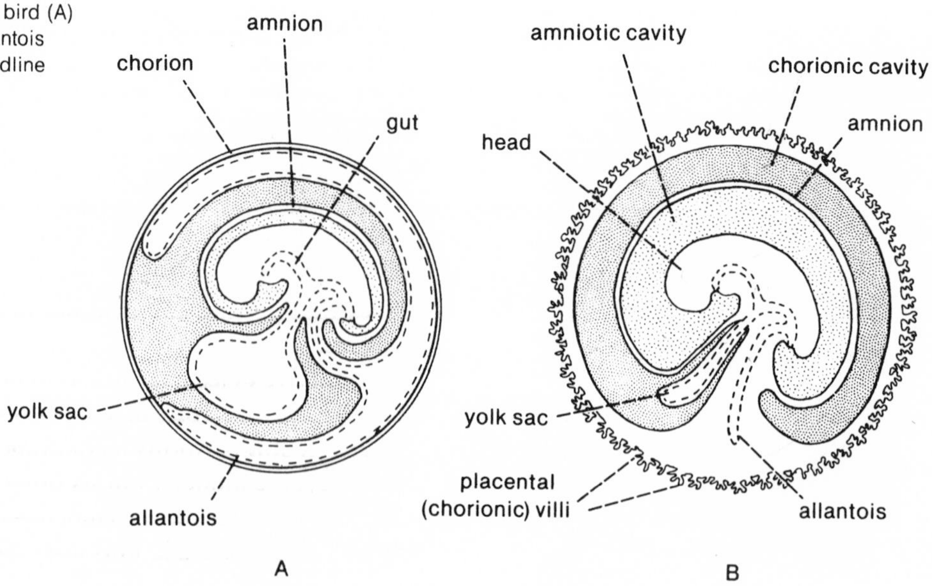

■ Placentation

Three species of living mammals—the echidnas and platypus of Australia and New Guinea—still lay eggs much like those of an alligator or a chicken. All other mammals today retain the developing embryo inside the mother's body until it can survive outside the protecting extraembryonic membranes. This arrangement furnishes the embryo with a safer and more constant environment, but it also poses new problems that have necessitated further reworking of the amniote egg. There is not much fresh air inside a uterus, so the growing embryo is forced to tap into the mother's bloodstream for oxygen. The embryonic mammal has also seized the opportunity to parasitize the mother's blood for its other needs, including food and water. Therefore the eggs of mammals (other than platypuses and echidnas) are small and naked, with little or no yolk—and no shell to wall off the embryo from the mother's tissues.

Because the embryo and the mother are different individuals, the mother can develop antibodies to the embryo and try to reject it as though it were an unsuccessful organ transplant. To survive, the mammalian embryo must suppress or avoid its mother's immunological assault. **Marsupials**—opossums, kangaroos, and other pouched mammals—have chosen a strategy of avoidance. Most marsupial embryos develop only a fleeting contact with the inside of the uterus, and they get out the instant they have enough coordination and strength to climb into the mother's pouch and latch onto a nipple. This strategy has not been very successful; marsupials have generally been outcompeted in the world's faunas by the **placentals,** the other group of live-bearing mammals. Placental embryos have somehow learned the trick of staying in prolonged and intimate contact with the inside of the uterus without triggering an immune reaction in the mother. This contact is maintained and policed by the organ from which these animals take their name, the **placenta** (Latin, "cake"). The embryonic tissues that go into the placenta develop from the chorion and the allantois.

In primitive placentals, just as in birds and reptiles, the allantois is a richly vascularized bag that spreads out between the embryo and the chorion. It still performs its old function of storing the excretions of the embryonic kidneys, but its other reptilian function—providing a respiratory surface for the embryo—has been much altered. The outside of a placental's allantois fuses with the inside of the chorion, and the blood vessels of the allantois grow out into the chorion to absorb oxygen and nutrients diffusing inward from the mother's tissues.

In higher primates, including ourselves, the surface of the chorion is elaborated into **placental villi** (Fig. 1-2), which invade the maternal tissues and induce a localized breakdown of the uterine wall. As a result, the primate embryo sinks into the wall of the uterus and becomes surrounded with little pools or lakes of the mother's blood, which lie in direct contact with the surface of the chorion. Further differentiation of maternal and embryonic tissues soon results in the formation of a disk-shaped placenta, which mediates and regulates the transfer of food and oxygen out of the mother's bloodstream into that of the developing baby. The embryo's metabolic wastes are eliminated through the placenta into the mother's blood and excreted in her urine. The allantoic cavity is thus no longer needed as an embryonic urine dump, and it has become reduced to a mere vestige (Fig. 1-2). The arteries of the allantois are still the vessels that carry the blood to the placenta, but they are renamed **umbilical** arteries in the human embryo.

■ Early Development in *Homo*

By the fifth day after conception, the fertilized human egg has developed into a hollow sphere of cells, the **trophoblast,** with an inner cell mass at one end (Fig. 1-3). The inner cell mass thickens and differentiates into two layers, an outer one and an inner one. Cells from the inner layer of this mass spread out and coat the inside of the hollow trophoblastic sphere, thereby turning it into a two-layered ball. A second hollow, the amniotic cavity, forms within the outer layer of the inner cell mass. The embryo at this stage resembles a two-layered disk forming a partition between two hollow bubbles: the amniotic cavity and the primary yolk sac (Fig. 1-3C).

The development of the human embryo (or of any other chordate embryo) is usually described in terms of three so-called germ layers: ectoderm, mesoderm, and endoderm (Greek for "outer skin," "middle skin," and "inner skin"). Two of these layers are now visible in the embryonic disk. The cells facing into the yolk-sac bubble constitute the **endoderm,** which will develop into the lining of the gut all the way from mouth to anus. The other (amniotic) surface of the embryonic disk is the **ectoderm,** which will become the outer surface of the body. The embryo at this stage can be thought of as a tiny sandwich

Fig. 1-3 Early embryonic development in *Homo*. Diagrammatic sections through embryos 5 days (A), 8 days (B), and 12 days (C) after conception.

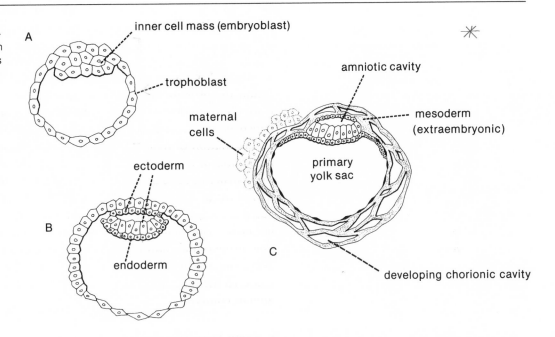

A — inner cell mass (embryoblast)

trophoblast

maternal cells

amniotic cavity

mesoderm (extraembryonic)

primary yolk sac

ectoderm

endoderm

B

C

developing chorionic cavity

(0.2 mm across) with no filling: a disk of skin lying on top of a disk of gut lining, with nothing much in between.

What eventually goes in between these two layers is the third germ layer, the **mesoderm.** Most of the tissues of the adult body—muscles, skeleton, blood vessels, and connective tissue of all sorts—develop from mesoderm. The formation of the mesoderm is complex. Mesoderm inside the embryonic disk—the filling of the aforementioned sandwich—proliferates from ectodermal cells that migrate toward the midline of the embryo's "back," sink in, and spread out in all directions between endoderm and ectoderm. The line along which they sink in is called the **primitive streak.** It soon becomes a groove, and its head end forms a distinct dimple, the **primitive pit.** The mesodermal cells that sink in via this pit organize themselves into a notochord (like that of *Branchiostoma*). This rudimentary predecessor of the vertebral column elongates, growing away from the primitive streak but in line with it (Fig. 1-4):

The three-layered embryonic disk now has left and right halves, a head end (toward which the notochord points), and a tail end. It has a back surface that is covered with ectoderm and a belly surface that is

Fig. 1-4 Mesoderm formation. A. Section through a 13-day embryo, showing extraémbryonic mesoderm (*stippled*). B. Ectodermal cells on the embryo's dorsal surface stream toward the midline (*arrows*) and sink in to become intraembryonic mesoderm. The notochord forms as a condensation in this mesoderm and grows toward the head end of the embryonic disk.

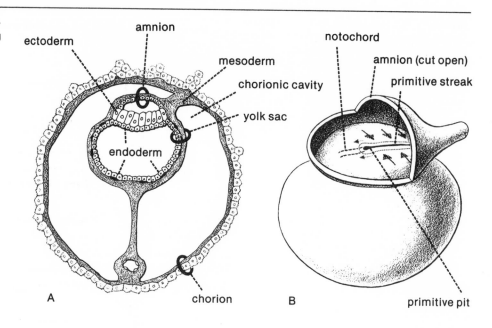

covered with endoderm and faces into the cavity of the yolk sac. We can now start to describe the embryo and its parts using the standard anatomical terms. The most important of these are **ventral,** meaning "of or toward the belly side" (L. *venter,* "belly"), and its antonym **dorsal,** "of or toward the back" (L. *dorsum,* "back"). The corresponding adjectives for head and tail are **cranial** and **caudal.**

Each of the three germ layers in the embryonic disk has its representative outside the embryo, in the extraembryonic membranes. The sheet of ectodermal cells on the dorsal surface of the embryo is folded back around beyond the edges of the embryonic disk to form the lining of the amniotic cavity; this part of the sheet is usually referred to as **extraembryonic ectoderm.** Similarly, the lining of the yolk sac is **extraembryonic endoderm. Extraembryonic mesoderm** has an origin separate from that of the mesoderm in the embryonic disk—in fact, it forms while the disk itself is still two-layered (Fig. 1-3C). Extraembryonic mesoderm seems to develop from the inner surface of the trophoblast. The extraembryonic mesoderm soon splits into two layers separated by a fluid-filled space, the **chorionic cavity** (Fig. 1-4). The formation and splitting of extraembryonic mesoderm converts chorion, yolk sac, and amnion into two-layered bags (Fig. 1-4). The

Fig. 1-5 Schematic cross section of embryos 21 days (A) and 22 days (B) after conception, showing formation of neural tube (*upper arrows,* A) and continuity of celom with chorionic cavity (*lower arrows,* A).

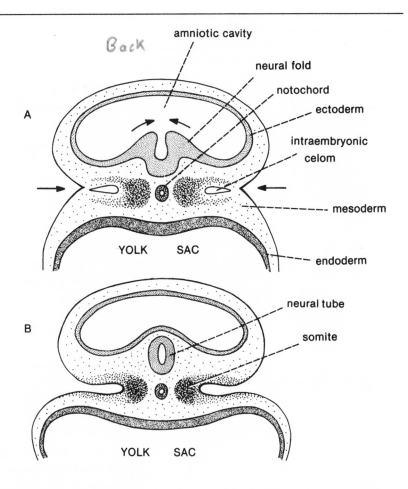

mesoderm on the inside of the chorion and that on the outside of the yolk sac are separated by the chorionic cavity, but they remain connected at one point, near the tail end of the embryonic disk. This connection, the **body stalk,** will become the umbilical cord.

While all this activity is going on in the mesoderm, the embryonic ectoderm is differentiating, too. As the notochord grows forward, the ectodermal "skin" over it thickens and humps itself up into right and left **neural folds** separated by a midline cleft (Fig. 1-5). The two folds lean toward each other, touch, and fuse to form a hollow tube of ectoderm. This tube, the **neural tube** or **dorsal nerve cord,** lies in the midline below the skin of the back, just dorsal to the notochord—

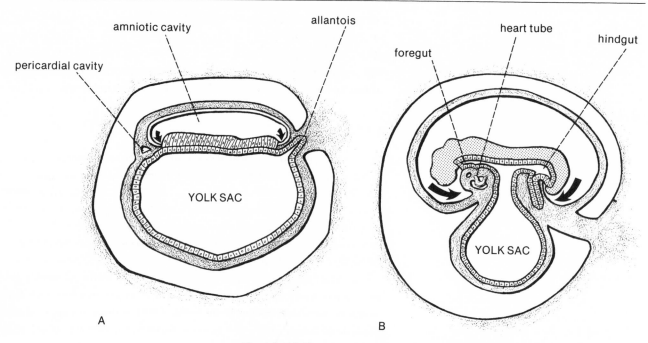

Fig. 1-6 Midline sections through two successive embryonic stages. The flat embryonic disk (A) curls under on all sides (*arrows*), pinching off the gut from the yolk sac (B).

exactly as in *Branchiostoma* (Fig. 1-1). It will develop into the spinal cord and brain of the human adult.

Like the extraembryonic mesoderm, the mesoderm *inside* the embryonic disk soon starts to split into two layers separated by a fluid-filled cavity. The split begins near the edges of the disk and spreads outward; eventually the cavities inside the embryo reach the disk's edges and open into the chorionic cavity (Fig. 1-5). The mesoderm-enclosed cavities on either side of the embryo are the rudiments of the celom—and so the chorionic cavity is sometimes called the **extraembryonic celom,** because it is continuous with the celom proper during early development.

While the celom has been opening up, the ectodermal back surface of the embryonic disk has been growing faster than the ventral or endodermal surface. As a result, the edges of the disk curl under on all sides (Fig. 1-6). The yolk sac is gradually pinched off from the endoderm inside the embryo proper; this intraembryonic endoderm becomes constricted into a tubular gut. Before the mouth of the yolk sac begins to narrow, a small outpouching of endoderm, the allantois, grows out a short distance into the body stalk. Its arteries keep growing beyond it, out through the body stalk into the mesodermal lining of the chorion, and become the arteries of the placenta.

■ The Somites and Their Derivatives

The formation of the notochord in a chordate embryo starts the process of segmentation. The mesoderm on either side of the notochord soon condenses into a series of blocks known as **somites** (Fig. 1-5B). In primitive chordates like *Branchiostoma,* these develop into the muscle segments that wiggle the body from side to side in swimming. The somites of vertebrate embryos also give rise to muscle segments; but part of each somite develops into bone as well.

Primitive chordates have no bones. Their only skeleton is the notochord. In the early vertebrates, bone of two sorts evolved: **dermal bone** and **cartilage-replacement bone.** Dermal bone forms in sheets of connective tissue under the skin. It provided a sort of armor plating for the primitive fishes and was concentrated in the vulnerable head region. Parts of the human skull are made-over remnants of this bony armor.

Cartilage-replacement bone is preformed in cartilage; a cartilaginous model of the bone condenses out of mesoderm early in development, and the cartilage is gradually replaced by bone as development progresses. In early vertebrates, a long chain of bones of this sort formed around the notochord, lending it added stiffness; and each bone sent processes up to wrap protectively around the dorsal side of the nerve cord. The bones in this chain are the **vertebrae,** after which vertebrates are named. In most living vertebrates, the column of vertebrae has completely replaced the notochord as the central skeletal support for the adult body.

Shortly after the somites begin to form in the human embryo—during the fourth week after conception—each somite divides into two masses of tissue: a dorsolateral **myotome** (Gk., "muscle slice") and a ventromedial **sclerotome** (Gk., "hard slice"). These masses develop into the segmented muscles and the segmented vertebral column, respectively.

We might expect the left and right sclerotomes of each body seg-

Fig. 1-7 Ontogeny of verte-brae. A. Dorsal view, four-week embryo. Each body segment contains a left (*vertical hachure*) and a right sclerotome. B. Later stage. Each vertebral rudiment forms intersegmentally—and so incorporates parts of four sclerotomes. C. Schematic ventral view of adult.

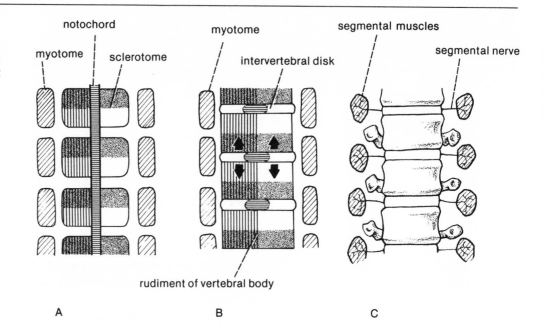

notochord

myotome   myotome   segmental muscles

sclerotome   intervertebral disk   segmental nerve

rudiment of vertebral body

A   B   C

ment to give rise to one vertebra. But if the muscle segments are going to be able to move the vertebral column, each segment must attach to two vertebrae: one in front of it and one in back of it. (If both ends of a muscle are attached to the same bone, the bone will not move when the muscle contracts.) Each vertebrae is therefore formed from parts of *two* body segments—or four sclerotomes (two rights and two lefts). Before any bone or even cartilage forms, each sclerotome divides into a cranial half and a caudal half, and the caudal half fuses with the cranial half of the sclerotome just behind it. This fused mass develops into the left or right side of a vertebra (Fig. 1-7). Because the vertebrae are intersegmental, each muscle segment can produce movement at the joint between two vertebrae.

The cartilaginous vertebral primordia on either side of the notochord fuse across the midline to form the main part of the verte-bra, the **vertebral body** (Fig. 1-8). In the process, the notochord is almost obliterated; all that remains of it are lens-shaped, gelatinous remnants between adjacent vertebrae. A dorsal projection grows out of the vertebral body on each side; these outgrowths push upward toward the back, wrap around the dorsal nerve cord, and fuse, thereby producing a complete ring or **vertebral arch** through which

Fig. 1-8 Vertebra of a newborn baby. The arch ossifies in two pieces (Fig. 2-4), which at birth are still separated from the vertebral body and each other by cartilage (*cross-hatching*). The three bones fuse together during childhood.

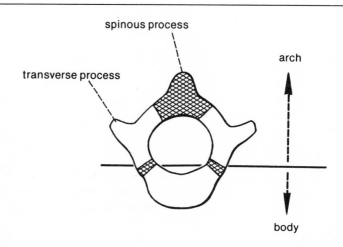

the dorsal nerve cord passes. In the adult human being, the spinal cord is almost completely enclosed in bone. A gap remains between the bases of the arches of each pair of adjoining vertebrae. Through these **intervertebral foramina** (L. *foramen,* "hole"), **spinal nerves** emerge from the spinal cord to innervate the corresponding body segments.

Several more bony projections grow out from each vertebra's arch. One of these projections is the **transverse process** (Fig. 1-8). From the left and right sides of each vertebral arch, a transverse process pushes laterally into the developing myotome lying alongside and splits the myotome into two masses of muscle tissue (Fig. 1-9): **epaxial** musculature dorsal to the transverse process and **hypaxial** musculature more ventrally (Gk. *epi-* and *hypo-,* "above" and "below"). The spinal nerves have separate dorsal and ventral branches that correspond to this dorsal–ventral division in the segmental muscles. In fishes, the epaxial division of the myotome is the larger of the two; but in land-dwelling vertebrates, the hypaxial division is larger and more important because the paired limbs develop from this part of the myotome.

▪ Unsegmented Mesoderm

We have seen how the mesoderm closest to the spinal cord and notochord becomes segmented into somites, which develop into the vertebrae and the muscles that move them. The more ventral sheets of mesoderm, those surrounding the fluid-filled celom (Fig. 1-9), remain

Fig. 1-9   Cross sections of successive (A, B, C) prenatal stages. Differentiation and growth of the hypaxial muscles encloses the celom inside a muscular body wall.

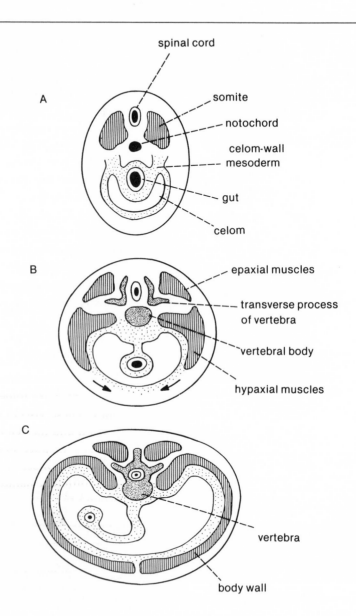

unsegmented. This unsegmented mesoderm of the celom wall develops very differently from the mesoderm of the somites. Three important generalizations can be made about the development of celom-wall mesoderm:

1. The celom-wall mesoderm does not give rise to bones; it gives rise only to muscles, glands, blood vessels, and connective tissue.

2. The muscles that form from celom-wall mesoderm are smooth muscles and cardiac (heart) muscles. They are histologically and physiologically different from the striated muscles that develop from the myotomes.

3. Unlike the striated muscles, the glands and muscles that develop from celom-wall mesoderm are not under direct control from the cortical part of the brain; hence we cannot control them voluntarily. They are controlled by a distinct, semi-independent system of nerves called the **autonomic nervous system.**

The innermost layer of the celom-wall mesoderm develops into the definitive lining of the celomic cavity. In the embryo, the celom is a single cavity that hugs the ventral surface of the developing intestines and other viscera (Fig. 1-9). As development proceeds, this body cavity becomes partitioned into several closed and flattened bags or sacs, which are folded intimately around the heart, lungs, and intestines. These viscera expand, contract, and slide around in a living person, and the celomic bags wrapped around them provide lubrication and support for their movements. The lining of each bag secretes a thin film of serous fluid that acts as a lubricant. The visceral bags have different names; **pleura** around the lungs, **serous pericardium** around the heart, **peritoneum** around the intestines.

The lining of the gut is derived from endoderm, but most of the substance of the adult's gut tube is formed by unsegmented mesoderm that condenses into concentric layers of smooth muscle surrounding the gut lining. These smooth muscles form the walls of the adult stomach and intestines. Contraction of the gut muscles changes the shape of the stomach and intestines and pushes the gut contents along by peristaltic action. Other viscera—the lungs, the liver, the pancreas—form as branching, treelike outgrowths from the endodermal lining of the gut tube. Unsegmented mesoderm condenses around these budding endodermal trees and forms much of the substance of the organs—connective tissue, blood vessels, and so on.

Another set of viscera forms in the dorsal wall of the celom, ventral

Fig. 1-10 Cross section of a 26-day embryo. Mesoderm ventral to the somites condenses to form nephrotomes, which give rise to urogenital organs.

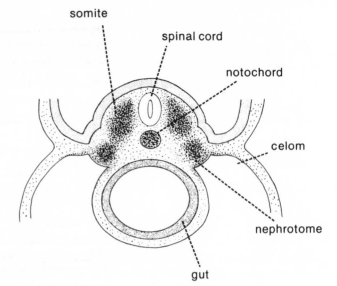

to the somites (Fig. 1-10). This region of the unsegmented mesoderm, called the **nephrotome,** is in closer contact with the segmented part of the body than other parts of the celom wall are, and it also is more or less segmented in very early developmental stages. The nephrotomes in all the segments fuse together to form a pair of ridges that run the length of the dorsal celom wall and give rise to most of the tissues of the kidneys and gonads. (The genital and urinary systems are closely tied up with each other in human ontogeny, for complex phylogenetic reasons sketched in the Preface; cf. Chapter 10.) Peculiarly enough, the gametes—eggs or sperm—develop from cells that originate in the wall of the embryonic gut and migrate laterally and dorsally into the developing gonad.

The celom-wall mesoderm also gives rise to blood vessels, which soon grow out from the celom wall into the segmented parts of the body. Like other muscles that form from celom-wall mesoderm, the muscles in the walls of the blood vessels are smooth and involuntary. The first vestiges of the heart form outside the embryo, just in front of the head end of the embryonic disk. The heart is folded into the body as the edges of the disk curl under and the mouth of the yolk sac narrows (Fig. 1-6).

■ The Growth of the Hypaxial Muscles

The vertebral column is surrounded by the segmented muscles that originally evolved as swimming muscles in primitive chordates like *Branchiostoma*. In vertebrates, each muscle segment is divided into epaxial and hypaxial parts, which lie respectively above and below the transverse processes of the vertebrae. The epaxial muscles stay put during development, becoming the deep muscles of the back in the human adult.

The hypaxial part of the myotome has a larger territory to cover, and it spreads out during development. Some hypaxial muscles remain closely apposed to the vertebral column. Others form a sheet that spreads outward and downward to enclose the viscera. This hypaxial muscle sheet grows down ventrally around the lateral wall of the celom, eventually meeting its fellow of the opposite side to form a complete, muscular **body wall** (Fig. 1-9). In a human adult, the body wall includes the belly muscles, the muscles in between the ribs, and the voluntary muscles around the anal and genital openings.

Another set of vertebral processes, the **costal processes,** grow out into the body wall. In a fish, all the costal processes form long **ribs;** so the rib cage extends from the neck to the base of the tail. In the human body, most of the costal processes are mere bumps. Although our heart, lungs, and liver are protected by the rib cage, the lower abdominal viscera are protected only by a boneless sheet of hypaxial muscle. Mammals, unlike fish or many reptiles, have a broad, soft underbelly.

Why have mammals lost the protection of their abdominal ribs? Mammals have evolved a muscular diaphragm that stretches across the rib cage underneath the lungs. They breathe by forcing the diaphragmatic "floor" of the thorax tailward, thus increasing the volume of the thorax and sucking air into it. When a mammal inhales, it pushes its stomach, liver, and intestines caudally; and the abdomen has to stretch to accommodate them. The boneless abdominal body wall stretches more easily than it would if it were supported by bony ribs. (In placental mammals, the abdominal wall also has to stretch a lot during pregnancy.) The abdominal ribs of mammals are therefore vestigial. The absence of supporting ribs in the belly and flanks means that an upright mammal like *Homo sapiens* is apt to develop a paunch.

The hypaxial mesoderm also gives rise to the bones and muscles of the limbs. In a fish, the **limb girdles**—shoulder blades and hipbones—are thin plates of bone embedded in the body wall. The fin itself is a cluster of small bones wrapped in hypaxial muscle and covered with skin: a specialized flap of the body wall that sticks out sideways. These paired flaps function as steering organs in swimming.

In the late Devonian period, about 370 million years ago, several groups of fishes developed adaptations for surviving out of water for short lengths of time. Certain species in one of these groups gained the ability to flounder from puddle to puddle by pushing themselves along the ground with enlarged, muscular fins. Terrestrial vertebrates evolved from these puddle-hopping Devonian fishes.

Walking around on land involved sweeping changes in almost all the systems and parts of the body. The fins enlarged from small steering vanes into huge propulsive and supporting structures. These hypertrophied fins, our arms and legs, account for about half the weight of an adult human body. Such ponderous organs could no longer be anchored simply by being attached to the body-wall muscles; they needed to be tied down to the vertebral column. The hipbones developed a direct attachment to the adjacent ribs; and the whole complex—ribs, their vertebrae, and both hipbones—became bound together to form a solid, bony ring, the **pelvis**, encircling the body just in front of the anal opening. The forelimb girdle remained more mobile. Ventrally, the shoulder blade developed an indirect attachment to the rib cage via the **clavicle**, or collarbone, which was originally part of the back edge of the head's dermal armor. Body-wall muscles attached to the shoulder blade spread dorsally over the epaxial back muscles to reach the **spinous processes** projecting from the vertebral arches in the midline (Fig. 1-8). The entire front end of the trunk of land-dwelling vertebrates is thus wrapped in a cloak of hypaxial forelimb muscles that anchor, steady, and move the bones at the base of the limb. The muscles just under the skin of the human back are therefore limb muscles, not part of the true (epaxial) back musculature.

▪ The Nervous System in Primitive Chordates

The chordate nervous system is divisible into two parts: the dorsal nerve cord, or **central nervous system** (CNS), and the various nerve fibers and cells that lie outside the cord and constitute the **peripheral**

nervous system. Nerve cells, or **neurons,** typically consist of a cell body trailing one or more elongated "transmission cables," or **axons.** The cell body may also sport one or more short **dendrites,** which receive impulses to be transmitted along the axons. The neurons of the CNS have a variety of complicated shapes, but the neurons that lie in (or stick out into) the peripheral nervous system mostly have a single, long axon. The axon's tip lies in close contact with another neuron or with the cells of some muscle or gland. This point of contact is called the **synapse.** Impulses that arrive at the synapse pass across a short gap and stimulate activity in the neighboring cell: contraction in a muscle, secretion in a gland, or initiation of a new nerve impulse in another neuron.

Nerve impulses can move along the axon in either direction, but they can only be transmitted from the synapse end of the axon. Thus neurons are usually unidirectional; they "point" in a particular direction. For this reason, it is convenient to divide them into three categories: afferent, efferent, and internuncial. **Afferent** (L. *ad,* "toward," + *ferentes,* "carrying") neurons are triggered by stimuli in the peripheral tissues of the body, outside the CNS. They carry sensory input—touch, pain, and so on—into the brain and spinal cord; hence they can be described as **sensory** neurons. **Efferent** (L. *ex,* "out of," + *ferentes*) neurons carry impulses leaving the CNS. Efferent nerve impulses induce a response in some peripheral organ—the contraction of a muscle, say, or the secretion of a gland. Efferent neurons are also known as **motor** neurons. Within the CNS itself, we find **internuncial** neurons, which pass impulses along from one neuron to another. The human CNS (our spinal cord and brain) is made up largely of internuncial cells.

In the primitive chordate *Branchiostoma,* both the sensory neurons and the motor neurons have their cell bodies inside the dorsal nerve cord. Their arrangement is simple and straightforward. A bundle of motor-nerve axons emerges from the ventral surface of the cord in every segment and passes into the adjoining myotome, supplying the muscle segment with the motor fibers that make it contract. Sensory fibers from the various structures in each segment of the body come together and form bundles that enter the dorsal surface of the cord. The sensory bundles going in dorsally are called **dorsal roots;** the motor bundles that emerge ventrally from the cord are known as **ventral roots.**

▪ Nerves to the Viscera

Branchiostoma has no motor nerves to its viscera. Its gut contents are moved along from mouth to anus by cilia (microscopic, whiplike projections from the cells lining its gut) instead of being squeezed tailward by waves of gut-muscle contraction (peristalsis) as our own gut contents are. In fact, *Branchiostoma* does not have any gut muscles. Its heart and other blood vessels are muscular, but they have their own built-in rhythm of pulsation—so they have no motor nerves, either.

In vertebrates, heartbeat, gut movement, and other visceral responses are elaborated and brought under effective central control by the appearance of an **autonomic nervous system.** The modern lamprey—a jawless, finless fish that is probably the most primitive living vertebrate—gives us some idea of the original arrangement of the autonomic nervous system. Like a lancelet, a lamprey has segmental nerves of two types: dorsal roots carrying sensation back to the CNS and ventral roots carrying motor commands to the muscle segments. But some new motor components have been added to take care of the lamprey's gut muscles, which *Branchiostoma* lacks.

The new motor fibers to the gut mostly emerge through the lamprey's dorsal roots, in the same bundle with the sensory nerves but traveling in the opposite direction, away from the CNS. The head end of the lamprey's CNS is expanded to form a small **brain** (another vertebrate peculiarity not seen in lancelets). In lampreys and other vertebrates, the dorsal and ventral roots that emerge from the brain are called **cranial** nerves; the others, which come out of the spinal cord (the nonbrain part of the CNS), are called **spinal** nerves. Most of the new motor fibers to the lamprey's gut muscles emerge via cranial sensory nerves—that is, through dorsal roots attached to the brain. The tail end of the gut is not supplied by cranial nerves; it receives a separate motor innervation, via dorsal roots of the neighboring spinal nerves. These two regions of motor-nerve outflow to the muscles (and glands) of the gut constitute the rudiments of the **parasympathetic** half of the autonomic nervous system. The spinal nerves lying in between these two regions also have motor fibers in their dorsal roots, but these fibers do not reach the lamprey's gut. Instead, they supply other smooth muscles and glands—for instance, the genital and urinary organs, the heart and other blood vessels, and the glands of the skin. These non-gut-related fibers represent the other, **sympathetic** half of the autonomic nervous system. The parasympathetics get their name from the fact that they come out from the head and tail regions, beyond either end of the region of sympathetic outflow (Gk. *para,* "alongside, beyond").

From what we see in lampreys, we can conclude that there was originally no functional opposition between these two autonomic components. Practically no regions of a lamprey's body receive both sympathetic and parasympathetic fibers. (In the lamprey's heart, where the two systems do overlap, they have the same effect; they make the heart beat faster.) But the two systems naturally tend to operate in different situations. The head-and-tail-end fibers supplying the gut govern digestion and peristalsis, which go on mainly during periods of relaxation and safety. Organs controlled by the intermediate, sympathetic fibers—the heart and reproductive organs—are most active during stress or excitement.

During vertebrate evolution, each of these two systems has tended to spread into the other's territory. (This is especially true of the sympathetic system, which sends fibers to all parts of our own bodies.) In higher vertebrates, the two systems produce opposite responses wherever they overlap. This antagonism is managed by a chemical difference between the two types of nerves. When any nerve impulse arrives at a synapse, it is transmitted across to the next cell by a chemical released from the end of the axon. Parasympathetic fibers that synapse on glands or smooth muscles release the chemical **acetylcholine;** sympathetic fibers that reach the same organs release the chemical **norepinephrine.** Those organs that receive both kinds of nerves generally respond in opposite ways to the two chemicals. For example, acetylcholine makes most gut muscles contract, whereas norepinephrine relaxes them.

The sympathetic system in mammals produces responses that are appropriate in situations of danger or excitement. The whole set of these responses is known as the "fight-or-flight" reaction. The blood vessels of our skin and gut shrink under sympathetic stimulation, thereby channeling more blood into the limb muscles and heart (and incidentally making the skin look paler). The sphincters along the gut close and peristalsis ceases. The heart speeds up. The little smooth Arrector Pili muscles (Fig. 5-1) at the bases of our hairs contract, making the hairs stand on end—a vestigial response left over from our hairier ancestors, whose bristling fur could discourage or misdirect the bite of an enemy. All the responses we associate with fear or anger—a dry mouth, a cramped gut, rapid heartbeat, pallor, sweaty palms, gooseflesh—are mediated by sympathetic nerves.

The parasympathetic system of mammals produces responses appropriate to situations of serenity and relaxation. These responses include slowing of the heart and stimulation of all the involuntary processes associated with digestion: salivation, peristalsis, secretion of stomach juices, and so on. The parasympathetic system is still largely a gut-related system. Apart from the heart, most of our organs that receive parasympathetic innervation are derivatives of the gut tube.

Almost all of the parasympathetic fibers that emerge from our brain still come out through dorsal (sensory) roots, just as they do in a lamprey. But the rest of our autonomic outflow—the tail-end parasympathetics and all of the sympathetics—comes out of the CNS through *ventral* roots, along with the motor nerves to the myotome-derived muscles. It is not clear why this shift from dorsal to ventral roots took place, or why it occurred only in spinal nerves, but it goes back a long way. Even in lampreys, a few fibers of the spinal-cord autonomics emerge through ventral roots; in sharks, most of them do so; and in bony fish and their descendants (including us), all of them do. Thus the dorsal roots of our *spinal* nerves are wholly sensory—just as they are in a lancelet.

▪ The Gill Muscles and Their Nerves

The gut muscles innervated by the autonomic nervous system are involuntary. You cannot stop peristalsis at will or command your stomach to dump its contents into the small intestine at the count of three. But the muscles surrounding the head end of the gut are voluntary. They need to be voluntary because we need to use our brains about what we eat. If the muscles surrounding the head end of the gut were typical gut muscles, anything that got into our mouths—forks, toothbrushes, our fingers—would automatically be bitten off, chewed up, and swallowed. Although our fishy ancestors had neither forks nor fingers to worry about, their tiny brains still had to make decisions about swallowing or spitting out dubious food items. As a result, the muscles surrounding the head end of the gut had to be under direct control of the brain.

We can see a rudiment of this musculature even in a lancelet, which has a strip of voluntary, or at least striated, muscle (no organ in a brainless animal can really be called voluntary) that runs along underneath its pharynx (the expanded head end of the gut). Ordinarily, a feeding lancelet sucks water into its mouth, expels the water through holes in the sides of the pharynx, and allows anything left over to be driven down into its intestines by cilia. But if the leftovers prove to be too prickly or toxic, they are spat out by a reflex contraction of the muscle under the pharynx. This strip of muscle, unlike any of the lancelet's other muscles, is innervated by motor-nerve fibers that emerge from the CNS through the *dorsal* roots of the segmental nerves.

The vertebrate pharynx is surrounded by similar muscles, similarly innervated by dorsal roots—from the cranial nerves. Vertebrates, too, have holes in the sides of their pharynx. In most fishes, the tissues surrounding these holes are elaborated to form **gills** (to increase the surface available for absorbing oxygen from the water), and the holes themselves are called **gill slits.** The fleshy bars in between the slits are called **gill arches.** They contain little bones (Fig. 19-7) that make it possible to open and close the slits. The voluntary muscles surrounding the vertebrate pharynx attach to these gill-arch bones, so we refer to them collectively as **gill muscles** (Fig. 21-1). In most air-breathing vertebrates, the gill slits never open up to form real slits, but they are represented in the embryo by a series of little outpocketings from the inside of the pharynx and matching dimples in the overlying skin. (Even in human beings, an outpocketing will occasionally open up into a dimple, producing a vestigial gill slit that causes its possessor to drool saliva onto the inside of his collar until a surgeon repairs the defect.)

Most textbooks describe the gill muscles as specialized gut musculature. Recent experiments indicate, however, that the gill muscles are in fact derived from myotomes in the head region, even though they—unlike all other such muscles—are innervated via dorsal roots. The similarly wired pharynx muscles in lancelets suggest that this departure from the typical pattern is exceedingly old. The head end of the vertebrate body is anciently specialized. The general patterns that help us to understand the logic of the rest of the human body are only dimly traceable in the head, and most anatomical generalizations have an exception somewhere in the head and neck. Our gut is surrounded by smooth muscles derived from celom-wall mesoderm—except in the head and neck, where the gut is wrapped in striated muscles derived from myotomes. The body's muscles and bones develop from mesoderm—except in the head, where some of them develop from ectoderm. The head contains organs like the eye and the nose that have no counterparts in the typical body segment, and none of the rules apply to these organs.

The ancestral vertebrates had six gill arches. The hindmost three of the six (arches 4, 5, and 6) were all supplied by a single cranial nerve. This same nerve also carried all the parasympathetic fibers running out of the brain to innervate the gut muscles proper. We preserve this arrangement (minus the gill slits) in our own bodies. The nerve that does all these jobs is the tenth of our twelve cranial nerves. Because it covers so much territory, it is named the **vagus** (L., "wandering") nerve.

▪ Peripheral Ganglia and the Neural Crest

In a lancelet, all the motor neurons and most of the sensory ones have their cell bodies inside the dorsal nerve cord, with just the axons sticking out. In people and other vertebrates, there are clusters of nerve cell bodies outside the CNS; such clusters are called **ganglia**. Two important generalizations can be made about the ganglia in the human body:

1. All sensory (afferent) neurons have their cell bodies in ganglia.
2. All autonomic motor pathways synapse in a ganglion.

Although the cell bodies of sensory neurons are outside the human CNS, they are not far from it. Each body segment contains a left and a right sensory ganglion, lying alongside the spinal cord. The axons of these sensory neurons pass from the ganglion into the dorsal surface of the spinal cord, forming a dorsal root like those of a lancelet—and so the sensory ganglia are called **dorsal-root ganglia**.

All sensory pathways leading back to the CNS involve only one nerve cell, even if that cell has to be a meter or more long (say, to reach the big toe). Voluntary motor pathways also involve only one neuron. However, all autonomic motor pathways in mammals involve *two* neurons. The cell body of the first neuron along an autonomic pathway lies in the CNS; that of the second neuron lies in an autonomic ganglion somewhere. The first neuron's axon stretches from the CNS to the ganglion, where the impulse is passed across a synapse to the second cell in the chain. The axon of the second neuron—a **postganglionic** or **postsynaptic** axon—carries the impulse

Fig. 1-11 Formation of peripheral ganglia. Neural-crest cells migrate ventrally in the embryo and develop into sensory and autonomic-motor ganglia.

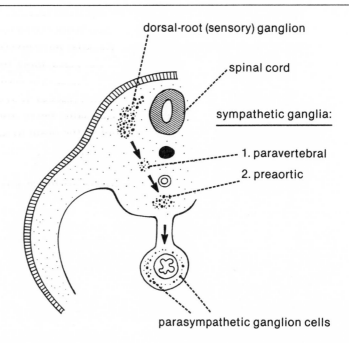

dorsal-root (sensory) ganglion

spinal cord

sympathetic ganglia:

1. paravertebral

2. preaortic

parasympathetic ganglion cells

the rest of the way to the target organ. The ganglia of the sympathetic nervous system lie some distance from the target, but parasympathetic ganglion cells (except for those in the head) are actually embedded *in* their target organs; so their postganglionic axons are extremely short.

Ganglion cells are not derived from the ectoderm that invaginates to form the dorsal nerve cord. They develop from a strip of ectoderm that lies more laterally, on either side of the invaginating cord—a strip called the **neural crest**. Before the embryo's mesoderm has finished sorting itself out into myotomes, sclerotomes, nephrotomes, and so on, ectodermal cells from the neural crest plunge into the mesoderm and stream down toward the gut. Some of them come to rest just alongside the spinal cord, and develop into sensory (dorsal-root) ganglia. Others come to rest lateral or ventral to the developing vertebral column; these will become the peripheral (postsynaptic) neurons of the **sympathetic** nervous system. Yet others reach the gut tube and heart, and bury themselves right in the walls of these organs. These will become postsynaptic neurons of the **parasympathetic** nervous system (Fig. 1-11).

A single axon can pass thru several nerve bundles.

■ The Typical Spinal Nerve

One major difference between the spinal nerves of a lamprey and those of a human being is that all our spinal motor fibers emerge through *ventral* roots. A second major difference is that the dorsal and ventral nerve roots in each segment of the human body run into each other and fuse, forming a single spinal nerve on each side. All our spinal nerves (and their main branches) are *mixed* nerves, containing both sensory and motor axons. Afferent and efferent impulses are of course carried by different neurons inside the nerve. Nerves are just named bundles of nerve-cell axons. The names they have been given were invented long ago by dissectors who had never heard of cells, neurons, or synapses; and these names do not correspond to the actual neurological "wiring." A single sympathetic axon running from the spinal cord to the ganglia around the stomach passes through six bundles with different names (ventral root, mixed spinal nerve, ventral ramus, white ramus communicans, sympathetic trunk, and greater splanchnic nerve), described in Chapter 3. Several named "nerves" are involved, but one neuron carries a single impulse through all of them.

Each of our spinal nerves passes out through its segment's intervertebral foramen and immediately divides into a **dorsal ramus** (L. *ramus,* "branch") and a **ventral ramus.** The dorsal ramus goes to the epaxial muscles and the overlying skin; the ventral ramus supplies the rest of that body segment. All the sympathetic fibers (if any) in the nerve's ventral root pass into its ventral ramus, on the first stage of their journey toward a peripheral ganglion (Fig. 3-2).

Less than half of our spinal nerves carry preganglionic sympathetic fibers in their ventral roots. Only the twelve thoracic nerves (lying below each of the twelve ribs), plus the first two nerves below those twelve, ordinarily carry sympathetic outflow. But *all* the body's segments need sympathetic innervation. How do the segments with no sympathetic outflow of their own get some? The answer is that every body segment contains sympathetic *ganglia*. From each segment's ganglia, postganglionic axons—axons of the second neuron in the two-neuron chain—spread out to supply that segment. If a segment's own nerve contains no *pre*ganglionic fibers, such fibers reach the ganglia of that segment by running up or down from ganglia in other segments. These ascending and descending preganglionic fibers spread sympathetic impulses throughout the body and tie the sympa-

Fig. 1-12 The typical body segment.

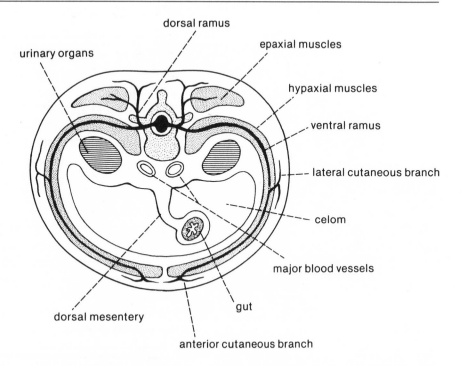

thetic ganglia together into several lumpy, longitudinal bundles, which form accessory spinal cords of a sort for the sympathetic nervous system.

■ **Summary: The Typical Body Segment**

The human body is segmented, like that of a lancelet or an earthworm. The typical body segment centers around the spinal cord and vertebral column, which are much-modified equivalents of the dorsal nerve cord and notochord of *Branchiostoma*. Columns of epaxial and hypaxial muscle run along the vertebral column and control its movements, and the hypaxial muscles also extend down around the celom to form a body wall. Spinal nerves emerge through the gaps between vertebrae and divide into dorsal and ventral rami. The dorsal rami supply motor fibers to epaxial musculature; their branches (Fig. 1-12) also transmit sensation from the skin of the back. The ventral ramus similarly supplies the hypaxial region. (It also carries sympathetic fibers passing to and from the sympathetic ganglia.) Urogenital organs and the major blood vessels lie in the dorsal wall of the celom. The gut hangs in the middle of the celom, connected to the rest of the body by a double fold of celomic lining (the **dorsal mesentery**) that encloses the gut's vessels and nerves. A tangle of parasympathetic nerves, derived from the vagus, surrounds the gut and relays impulses to the little postsynaptic neurons buried in the gut wall.

This picture adds up to a generalized cross section of the human body: the **typical body segment** (Fig. 1-12). No segment of the body really matches it in all details, although the upper part of the abdomen comes close. The rest of this book will present the actual regional anatomy of the body as a series of increasingly radical deviations from this typical plan.

2

The Vertebral Column

Branchiostoma is segmented from one end to the other, with myotomes extending down to the end of the tail and up through almost all of the head. In a lamprey, the head end has become specialized, and the series of myotomes in the cranial region is distorted and obscured by outpocketings of the pharynx and nerve cord. More advanced fishes have paired fins, and the ventral rami that supply those fins swap fibers back and forth to produce multisegmental nerves. The more advanced or specialized the vertebrate we look at, the more regional distortions of the basic segmental pattern we see. This principle—that evolution leads to reduction in number and specialization in function of the parts of an organism—is sometimes called Williston's law. Like all "laws" governing historical processes, it has many exceptions.

Williston's law holds for *Homo sapiens,* however. This vertebrate has an extremely specialized head region, large limbs innervated by many segmental nerves, and a relatively short vertebral column. There are about forty segments in the adult human body. (The uncertainty reflects the fact that segmentation in the head region is vestigial.) Of these forty-odd segments, only those that make up the rib cage and the upper part of the abdomen have remained fairly discrete and unspecialized. We therefore shall begin our study of the human body with the segmented trunk; and our study of the segmented trunk will begin with the vertebral column because the vertebrae show less regional specialization than do the muscles, nerves, or blood vessels.

▪ The Numbers and Kinds of Vertebrae

Because a vertebra forms by fusion of parts from two adjoining segments (Fig. 1-7), it follows that vertebral levels and segmental levels are not the same. Each muscle segment extends across the joint between two vertebrae. Each segmental (spinal) nerve emerges from the

33

Fig. 2-1 A thoracic vertebra, seen from above (A) and from the right side (B).

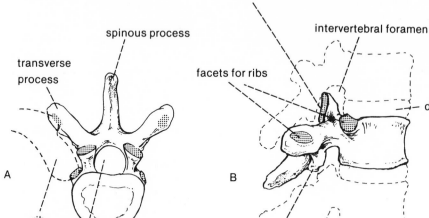

spinal cord through an intervertebral foramen between two adjacent vertebrae (Fig. 2-1).

In the human body, there are usually thirty-one pairs of spinal nerves and thirty-three vertebrae. Why are there more vertebrae than spinal nerves? Because not every vertebra in a mammal's tail is provided with a spinal nerve of its own. The vestigial human tail still retains four vertebrae, but the spinal nerves that should come out below the last three coccygeal (tail) vertebrae ordinarily do not develop.

The vertebral column can be divided into five regions. The function and shape of the vertebrae differ in each region (Fig. 2-2). At the top, the skull rests on a flexible column of seven **cervical** (neck) vertebrae. Below these, the twelve **thoracic** (chest) vertebrae and their ribs form a relatively inflexible bony cage for the lungs and heart. Five **lumbar** (lower back) vertebrae constitute another flexible section for the column, allowing flexion (bending forward) and extension (straightening out) of the column between pelvis and thorax. The five **sacral** vertebrae are fused together to form an immobile, wedge-shaped bone, the **sacrum**, which provides attachment to the hipbone on either side. The four **coccygeal** vertebrae serve merely to anchor certain pelvic muscles and ligaments.

Fig. 2-2 The five regions of the vertebral column, illustrating regional differences in the numbers and shapes of vertebrae. The right ribs and hipbone have been removed to expose the thoracic vertebrae and sacrum. Sample vertebrae from each region are seen from the cranial aspect.

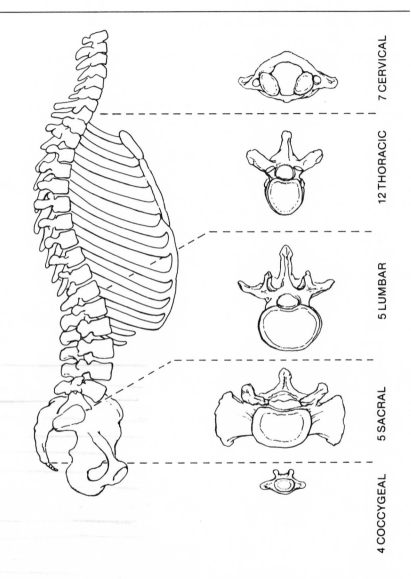

7 CERVICAL

12 THORACIC

5 LUMBAR

5 SACRAL

4 COCCYGEAL

The cervical and lumbar regions of the column are concave on the dorsal aspect; the other regions of the column are convex dorsally. The two dorsal concavities permit the erect posture characteristic of our species. If the column were a single uniform curve, there would be a tendency to topple forward onto our hands when we tried to stand upright.

The vertebrae of the various parts of the column are all very similar

Fig. 2-3   Serial homology in (A) cervical, (B) thoracic, (C) lumbar, and (D) sacral vertebrae, showing correspondence between central (*light tone*) and costal (*dark tone*) elements.

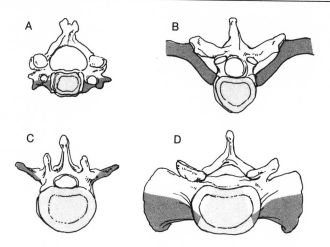

in early developmental stages, and the parts of a vertebra from any region of the column show a one-to-one correspondence with those of vertebrae from all other regions. This kind of correspondence between equivalent parts of different body segments is called **serial homology.** The vertebrae of the human body are all serially homologous (Fig. 2-3). The most striking variation involves the ribs, although there are regional variations in all the other features of the vertebrae.

▪ The Parts of a Vertebra

A vertebra forms by fusion of a **vertebral body** with a **vertebral arch** (Fig. 1-8). The vertebral body forms around the notochord and gradually replaces it; the arch forms around the back of the spinal cord and protects its originally exposed dorsal surface (Fig. 2-4). The hole enclosed by the fused-together vertebral arch and body is called the **vertebral foramen.** The spinal cord runs through these holes like the string through a line of beads. The whole series of vertebral foramina, through which the fetal spinal cord runs from the head to the vestigial tail, is called the **vertebral canal** (Fig. 2-1).

The body is the weight-bearing part of the vertebra. Most of the vertebral bodies are spool-shaped in human adults, with flat tops and bottoms and a slight waisting in between. Because we are upright

Fig. 2-4 Formation of cartilage and bone in a developing vertebra. Schematic cross sections of two successive fetal stages (A, B). Compare with Fig. 1-8 (newborn).

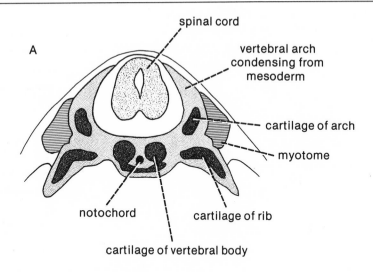

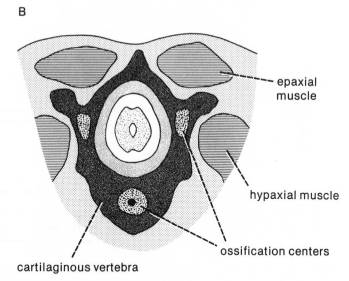

animals, walking around with our vertebral columns held vertically, each vertebra has to carry more of the body's weight than the one above it. Accordingly, each vertebra is slightly larger than the one above it, from the cervical region down to the upper end of the sacrum. From the upper sacral vertebrae, the body's weight is transferred to the bony pelvis; so the remaining vertebrae dwindle in size from the lower sacrum down to the last coccygeal vertebra.

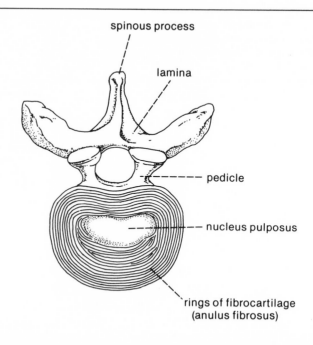

Fig. 2-5 An intervertebral disk, sitting atop the underlying (thoracic) vertebra, as seen from above.

spinous process

lamina

pedicle

nucleus pulposus

rings of fibrocartilage
(anulus fibrosus)

The vertebral arch (like the vertebral body) forms as a cartilaginous mass and later ossifies. The left and right halves of the arch ossify separately; the **spinous process** connecting them in the midline is still cartilaginous at birth. Three more bony processes (Fig. 2-1) grow out of each half of the arch, near its junction with the vertebral body: the **transverse process** (which separates epaxial from hypaxial muscles and furnishes them with a lever arm for moving the vertebra) and the upper and lower **articular processes** (through which each arch articulates with its fellows directly above and below). The parts of the arch that lack projecting processes also have special names: the **pedicles** are the stout bases of the arch that fuse with the vertebral body, and the **laminae** are the thinner bony plates stretching between spinous and transverse processes (Fig. 2-5). Note that the intervertebral foramen is simply the space between pedicles of adjacent vertebrae.

■ Intervertebral Joints and Movements

There are two kinds of joints between adjacent vertebrae. One is the **cartilaginous joint** between the vertebral bodies. Each pair of adjacent bodies is separated by an **intervertebral disk,** which is made up of concentric rings of extremely fibrous cartilage (Fig. 2-5). These

Fig. 2-6   Section through a typical synovial joint.

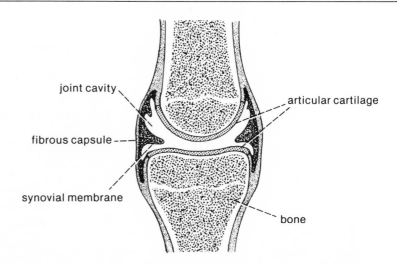

fibrocartilaginous disks transmit almost all of the weight borne by the vertebral column. They also absorb jolts and jars transmitted along the column and contribute to the distinctive curvatures of the column. In children and younger adults, the center of each disk is a jellylike mass, the **nucleus pulposus,** which is the only important derivative of the notochord that survives into adult life (Fig. 1-7). This gelatinous blob can herniate through the fibrous rings surrounding it. If the herniated nucleus pulposus pops out into the vertebral canal, it can press on the spinal cord or spinal-nerve roots and cause pain or paralysis. Such an injury is commonly but misleadingly called a "slipped disk."

The second kind of intervertebral joint is the **synovial joint** between each pair of articular processes. In a synovial joint, the two articulating bones are covered with wear-resistant cartilage on their bearing, or articular, surfaces (Fig. 2-6). When the joint moves, the articular cartilages slide across each other. A tube-shaped sleeve of strong, inelastic connective tissue, the **fibrous capsule,** encloses the joint. The two openings of this tube attach all around the edges of the matching articular surfaces of both bones, thus defining and enclosing a sealed-off **joint cavity** between the two bones. Motion at the joint is limited and guided by the fibrous capsule: the tighter the capsule, the less mobile the joint.

The fibrous capsule is lined with a delicate layer of highly vascular connective tissue, the **synovial membrane.** This membrane secretes a slippery, slightly yellowish **synovial fluid** resembling egg white. A thin film of this fluid lubricates all the articular surfaces. Synovial fluid also contains nutrients for the cells of the articular cartilages (which lack a blood supply of their own) and white blood cells (which remove bacteria and dead tissue).

Both kinds of intervertebral joints—the synovial joints between the arches, and the disks between adjacent vertebral bodies—limit the movements that can occur between adjoining vertebrae. The joints and the movements they permit differ from region to region in the vertebral column. The fused-together sacral vertebrae are of course immobile, and the synovial joints between them are lost. (The sacral intervertebral disks linger on as soft nodules in the surrounding bone, but they have no function.) The coccygeal vertebrae that form our vestigial tail also tend to fuse together into a bony lump, which may fuse with the sacrum late in life.

The rest of the column is more flexible. The most flexible part is the neck, where the vertebral bodies are small and the disks are thick. These features permit the cervical vertebrae to bend and twist in all directions. The facets of their synovial joints are roughly horizontal, and the joint capsules are loose, so the cervical vertebral arches can slide across each other as the column bends this way and that. The disks of the thoracic vertebrae are much thinner, and their synovial facets lie in a plane more or less parallel to the skin of the back. This arrangement restricts flexion and extension. Side-to-side bending in the thoracic region is also severely limited (by the ribs' bumping into each other). However, the thoracic vertebrae can twist more freely around a vertical axis. In the lumbar part of the column the disks are thick again, and the synovial-joint facets lie parallel to the body's midline plane. This arrangement permits a lot of flexion and extension, and some side-to-side bending, but no twisting.

Longitudinal ligaments run along the vertebral column, binding the entire column together. The **anterior longitudinal** ligament runs along the anterior (ventral) sides of the vertebral bodies, and the **posterior longitudinal** ligament runs along their posterior sides, inside the vertebral canal (Fig. 2-7). These ligaments tie each vertebral body to its neighbors (and to the intervening disk) in front and back. The spinous processes of the vertebral arches are bound together by **interspinous** and **supraspinous** ligaments. All these ligaments limit the flexibility of the column by becoming taut in flexion or extension. Yellowish, elastic ligaments (**ligamenta flava**) stretch between the arches of adjacent

Fig. 2-7 Midline section through the vertebral column, showing the intervertebral ligaments.

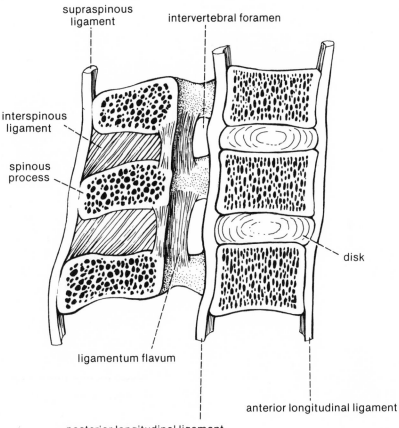

vertebrae. When the column flexes, these ligaments stretch as the arches move apart—until flexion is checked by the supraspinous ligaments, the posterior longitudinal ligaments, and the tension of the back muscles. Try palpating the spinous processes of your own vertebrae in various parts of the column as you bend over and straighten up, noting how they move toward and away from each other. You may have trouble finding the cervical spinous processes; they are short, deeply buried in neck muscle, and surmounted by an enlarged interspinous ligament, here called the **ligamentum nuchae** (L., "neck ligament"). The second and seventh cervical spinous processes may be palpable; it depends on how fat or muscular you are and what your sex is.

Fig. 2-8 Adult sternum and costal cartilages (*stippled*). Anterior view. Dashed lines indicate boundaries between fused sternebrae. The attached ribs (ribs 1 to 10) are shown on the right side only.

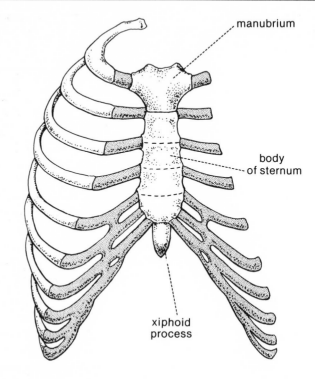

▪ The Ribs and the Sternum

All the vertebrae (except the coccygeal ones) have ribs—or, more properly, **costal** (rib) **processes** (Fig. 2-3)—but only the twelve thoracic ribs become long bony extensions that curve around to the ventral side of the body. The upper seven pairs of thoracic ribs extend all the way around the ventral midline of the body and articulate with the breastbone, or **sternum** (Fig. 2-8). The sternum acts like an accessory ventral vertebral column. It originally ossifies as a series of **sternebrae,** each of which corresponds roughly to a segment of the body wall. These later fuse together, and the definitive sternum has only three pieces, called **manubrium, body,** and **xiphoid process.** The xiphoid process usually fuses to the body of the sternum after puberty, and the manubrium and body may fuse in old age.

The ribs, like the other parts of the vertebrae, are initially cartilaginous. The ventral end of each rib never ossifies but remains as a **costal cartilage** that articulates with the sternum. The costal cartilages of ribs 8, 9, and 10 end, not in the sternum, but in the costal cartilage of the next highest rib; the cartilages of the last two (or three) ribs do not attach to anything but the muscles of the body wall. The number of ribs is variable; there may be 13 or 11, there may be a rib on the last cervical vertebra (C.7), and any rib may be bifurcated or partly fused with its neighbor. The five sacral "ribs" are fused together at their extremities. The upper three of these "ribs" are stout, weight-bearing structures that articulate with the pelvis. The smaller cervical and lumbar "rib" processes (Fig. 2-3) serve only as sites for muscle attachment.

The thoracic ribs and the sternum form a bony basket, the rib cage, enclosing the heart and lungs. This basket provides some protection to those vital organs (and also to the liver, kidneys, and other abdominal viscera that stick up under its lower edge). But its most important function is in respiration; the muscles attached to the ribs can change the volume of the thorax by swinging the ribs in and out (Chapter 8). These movements force air in and out of the thorax and the enclosed lungs. The rib cage thus serves the same purpose in breathing that the hinged wooden frame serves in pumping a bellows. It also provides a rigid frame for the muscular diaphragm, which likewise sucks air into the thorax (by shoving the abdominal viscera tailward) when it contracts. Paralysis of the respiratory muscles attached to the ribs—say, from polio—naturally results in death from asphyxiation unless the patient is attached to a mechanical respirator.

▪ The Atlas and Axis

The two uppermost vertebrae of the neck are anciently and peculiarly specialized. The first cervical vertebra (C.1) holds up the skull; it is called the **atlas,** after the Titan of Greek mythology who supported the sky on his shoulders. Unlike all the other vertebrae, it lacks a vertebral body and so has no articular disks above or below it. It articulates with the skull above and with C.2 below through its synovial joints alone.

In primitive reptiles, the joint between the skull and the body of the atlas was a ball-and-socket joint; the ball on the skull fitted into a socket on the body of C.1. The joint had three axes of movement—nodding, side-to-side wagging, and rotation (around a head-to-tail axis). In the carnivorous reptiles from which mammals evolved, the "ball" split into two, forming left and right **occipital condyles** on the

Fig. 2-9 Human atlas and axis (A), compared with a typical vertebra in a newborn baby (B). The atlas and axis are viewed dorsally and swung apart from each other to show their opposing surfaces. The anterior arch and transverse ligament of the atlas form a socket for the reception of the dens (*black arrow*).

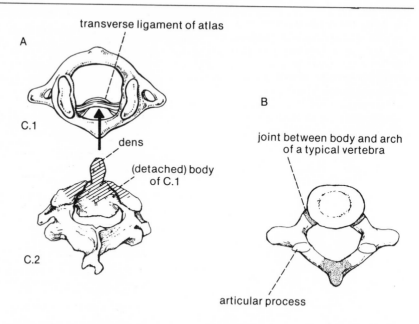

skull. (The matching concavity on the body of C.1 of course divided in the same way.) This may have improved the stability of the head on the neck (an important consideration in a meat-eater that kills with its teeth). As the skull's condyles (and their sockets on C.1) moved further and further apart, two things happened: (1) rotation of the head on C.1 became impossible; and (2) the condyles' sockets on C.1 gradually shifted so far laterally that they moved entirely off the vertebral body and onto the vertebral arch on either side. As a result, the C.1 vertebral body lost its articulation with the skull.

Although the loss of a midline ball-and-socket joint prevented the skull from rotating on the atlas, some rotation was still possible, because the right and left halves of the C.1 vertebral arch had never fused to the C.1 body. It was possible for the skull and the attached neural arches of C.1 to move a bit as a unit on the detached body of C.1. As reptiles evolved into mammals, these movements were refined and freed up, thereby restoring something close to the old rotatory mobility. The right and left halves of the C.1 arch fused to each other ventrally (and dorsally) and formed a solid bony ring around the spinal cord. The old C.1 body, still attached to the body of C.2, developed an extension that stuck up inside this ring and acted as a pivot around which the ring could turn (Fig. 2-9A). In mammals this

Fig. 2-10 The ligaments of the atlas and axis. A. Midline section viewed from the right. B. Cruciform and alar ligaments seen from behind with the arch of C.1 removed. Note that the so-called posterior atlantooccipital membrane (posterior AOM) is equivalent to the ligamenta flava, not to the posterior longitudinal ligament.

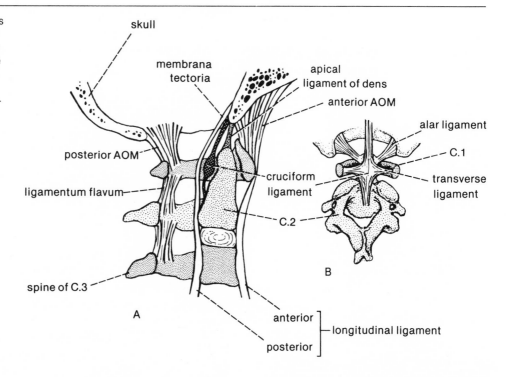

projecting pivot is called the **dens** (L., "tooth"). The old C.1 body, including the projecting dens, is now fused solidly to the body of C.2; the disk between them has been lost. When we turn our head from left to right, the skull and the attached C.1 ring rotate as a unit around the stationary C.2-and-dens complex—which is called the **axis,** for obvious reasons. The whole axis is regarded as our second cervical vertebra, although it incorporates elements that belong developmentally to C.1.

The paired synovial joints between our atlas and axis are not like typical intervertebral joints. Their abnormal position (partly ventral instead of wholly dorsal to the transverse processes) suggests a serial homology with the transitory cartilaginous joints seen between the body and arch of a typical vertebra in a newborn baby (Fig. 2-9B).

Two more synovial atlantoaxial joints form in the midline, enclosing the dens of the axis. The dens is held snugly against the ventral arch of the atlas by the **transverse ligament of the atlas,** which stretches across from one side of the atlas ring to the other. This transverse ligament divides the central hole in the ring-shaped atlas into two compartments: a big one in back for the spinal cord and a smaller ventral compartment for the dens. A flattened sac of synovial membrane lubricates the movement of the dens against the ligament, and another synovial joint is formed between dens and atlas in front. The atlas and its transverse ligament together form such a tight socket for the dens that nodding movements between C.1 and C.2 are impossible. (Those movements occur between the skull and the atlas, just as in mammal-like reptiles.) The atlantoaxial joint is purely rotatory.

In addition to the usual longitudinal ligaments and ligamenta flava (which take on special names where they extend from the vertebral column to the skull; Fig. 2-10), there are some peculiar ligaments that bind the dens and skull together. The **alar** ligaments are two strong cords that run sideways from the tip of the dens to attach to the occipital condyles. They limit the rotatory movement of the skull-and-atlas unit around the dens of the axis and also help to restrict flexion between skull and atlas. In the midline, a wispy little **apical ligament of the dens** connects the tip of the dens to the skull base just above it, in front of the spinal cord. It has no known function, but it is embryologically interesting, because it is a remnant of the notochord. Because the human atlas is a detached vertebral arch with no body, the posterior longitudinal ligament has no attachment to it (which is why that ligament assumes a different name, **membrana tectoria**, between C.2 and the skull). Its absence is partly made up for by thin longitudinal bands running up and down from the transverse ligament encircling the dens. These bands convert the transverse ligament into a cross-shaped structure, the **cruciform** ligament (Fig. 2-10).

The Spinal Cord
and the
Spinal Nerves

3

■ Numbering the Body's Segments

The segments of the human body are intervertebral; each vertebra is composed of parts of two adjacent segments (Fig. 1-7). From the neck down, the segments and their nerves are numbered with reference to the adjacent vertebrae (Fig. 3-1). Although the back of the skull is also segmentally arranged during development, the fused segments incorporated into the skull are not numbered—so the so-called first body segment is the one lying between the skull and the first cervical vertebra. It is labeled C.1, meaning "first cervical." The next segment (between vertebrae C.1 and C.2) is labeled C.2, and so on down through segment C.7. The segment between vertebrae C.7 and T.1 (first thoracic) ought, by the same rule, to be numbered T.1. Instead, this segment and its nerve are numbered C.8. (Thus, there are eight cervical *nerves*, but only seven cervical *vertebrae*.) The next nerve, whose ventral ramus runs between the first two ribs, is called the first thoracic nerve (T.1)—and so on down the vertebral column. From T.1 on, each segment (and nerve) is named for the vertebra directly above.

■ The Typical Spinal Nerve and the Sympathetic Trunk

Every segment of the body contains a pair of segmental nerves, each of which is formed by the union of a dorsal (sensory) and ventral (motor) root. The dorsal and ventral roots unite as they emerge from the vertebral canal and form the trunk of the segmental nerve. That trunk, the **mixed spinal** nerve, is very short; it divides almost immediately into dorsal and ventral rami. The dorsal ramus plunges directly back into the epaxial musculature (Fig. 1-12). The ventral ramus enters the hypaxial musculature and runs around the body wall toward the ventral midline of the body, giving off a sizable

47

Fig. 3-1 Numbering scheme for cervical nerves (right side only shown) and vertebrae. Schematic dorsal view.

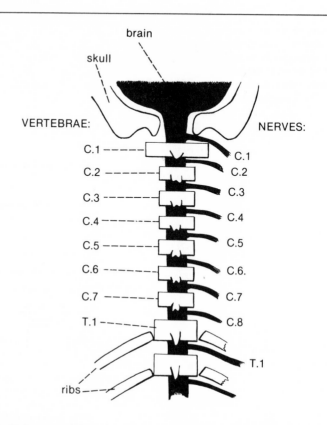

lateral cutaneous branch halfway around and a small **anterior cutaneous** branch near the midline.

The typical spinal nerve also contains sympathetic motor fibers, which innervate the segment's smooth muscles and glands. These fibers leave the spinal cord via the ventral root (like all spinal motor fibers) and pass into the ventral ramus (like the fibers to the hypaxial muscles). But the sympathetic fibers do not simply stream out to their target organs with the ventral ramus's branches; they have to pass their nerve impulses on to a second sympathetic neuron located in some peripheral ganglion. Accordingly, the sympathetic fibers from the spinal cord leave the ventral ramus almost at once and run medially along the inside of the body wall in back, heading toward a ganglion in which they can synapse.

In most of the body's segments, paired sympathetic ganglia are located on the sides of the bodies of the vertebrae. These **paraverte-**

Fig. 3-2 Spinal-cord sections at cervical (*top*) and thoracic (*bottom*) levels, showing sympathetic pathways in the attached nerves. Cervical segmental nerves get their sympathetic component from thoracic nerves via the sympathetic trunk. The lower lumbar and sacral nerves have similar connections with the sympathetic trunk. You can picture these by turning the figure upside down. The second (postsynaptic) neuron in each sympathetic pathway is shown in black.

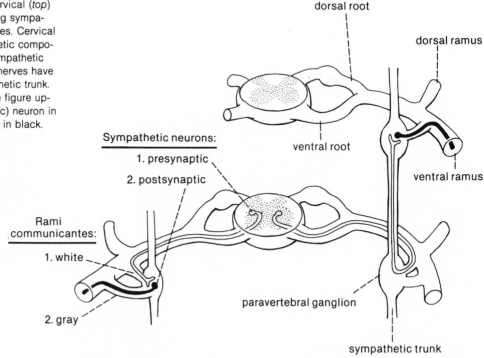

bral ganglia are pinkish gray lumps, ranging in size and shape from that of a half-peanut to that of a flattened BB shot. A second, midline (unpaired) series of sympathetic ganglia occurs in front of the abdominal part of the aorta (Fig. 1-11). Postsynaptic fibers from these ganglia supply the intestines and other abdominal viscera. The rest of the body's glands and smooth muscles get their sympathetic innervation from neurons whose cell bodies lie in the paravertebral ganglia.

In the typical spinal-nerve arrangement (Fig. 3-2), presynaptic sympathetics leave the ventral ramus, enter a paravertebral ganglion, and synapse. Some postsynaptic fibers run *medially* from the ganglion to supply viscera (in the thorax and pelvis). The rest of the postsynaptic sympathetic fibers run back *laterally* and reenter the ventral ramus. Most of them get distributed with the ventral ramus's branches. A few run back to the mixed nerve and enter the *dorsal* ramus, to be distributed to skin glands and smooth muscles throughout the epaxial region.

Because presynaptic sympathetic fibers are wrapped in a fatty "insulation" of myelin, they are whitish in color; the wrappings of the postsynaptic fibers are nonmyelinated and grayish. In theory, the two fiber types form two sorts of bundles connecting each paravertebral ganglion to the neighboring ventral ramus: a **white ramus communicans** (L., "communicating branch") carrying presynaptic fibers *to* the ganglion, and a **gray ramus communicans** bringing postsynaptic fibers back *from* it. (In reality, various mixed types of rami communicantes occur.)

All body segments contain structures that need sympathetic innervation (for example, the smooth muscles in arterial walls)—and therefore *all ventral rami receive gray (postsynaptic) fibers from the paravertebral ganglia.* But not all ventral rami supply white (presynaptic) fibers *to* those ganglia. Only spinal nerves T.1 through L.2 (second lumbar) or thereabouts carry sympathetic outflow from the spinal cord and contribute white rami communicantes. The other spinal nerves get their sympathetic component indirectly, via fibers that run up or down from one paravertebral ganglion to another. Such fibers innervate segments above or below the one where they came out of the spinal cord (Fig. 3-2). These ascending and descending fiber tracts tie the whole series of paravertebral ganglia together into a lumpy, ganglionated chain on each side, extending from the upper neck to the lower end of the sacrum. The chain is called the **sympathetic trunk.** All the presynaptic sympathetic fibers enter it through white rami communicantes. Most of them synapse in the ganglia of the trunk. But some pass through the trunk without synapsing and continue on medially down into the abdomen. There they end by synapsing on neurons in the preaortic ganglia instead—or else on cells in the suprarenal medulla (see Chapter 10).

▪ Regional Variation in the Spinal Nerves

At several places in the body, branches of two or more segmental nerves commingle to form **nerve plexuses.** The most important of these plexuses supply the limbs. The ventral rami of spinal nerves C.5 through T.1 supply the upper limb, and those of nerves L.2 through S.4 (fourth sacral) supply the lower limb. As these ventral rami approach the base of the limb they innervate, they swap fiber tracts back and forth, thus producing a plaited plexus whose terminal branches carry fibers from more than one segmental nerve (Fig. 13-3). These ventral rami that go into the limb plexuses are exceptionally large, and most of the spinal cord at these segmental levels is given over to innervating the limbs. In the segments at the midpoint of each plexus—nerves C.7 and C.8 in the upper-limb plexus, and L.4 and L.5 in that of the lower limb—the spinal cord is so preoccupied with the limbs and ventral rami that the dorsal rami lack cutaneous branches. The resulting gaps in sensory innervation of the back are filled in by the dorsal rami of adjacent segmental nerves. Ventral rami of the upper cervical region also get woven together into a smaller and simpler plexus that supplies the discontinuous "body-wall" muscles of the neck (Fig. 22-5).

The dorsal rami of the spinal nerves are not involved with the limbs and thus show far less regional variation than the ventral rami do. The dorsal ramus of C.1 ordinarily does not reach the skin, and it may even lack a dorsal (sensory) root altogether. The dorsal rami of the next two nerves (C.2 and C.3) fill in for it, sending cutaneous branches upward to supply the back of the scalp (Fig. 4-2). The first three or four dorsal rami are often joined to one another by little nerve loops running through the epaxial muscles. Similar loops on the back of the sacrum connect each sacral dorsal ramus to its neighbors above and below; branches from these loops supply the overlying skin. These dorsal-ramus loops are simple nerve plexuses, although nobody calls them that.

■ The Spinal Cord

Until the third month after conception, the fetal spinal cord extends all the way to the coccygeal end of the vertebral canal. From then on, it increases in length more slowly than the vertebral column; so the tail end of the cord gradually gets pulled away from the coccyx. In an adult, the tail end of the spinal cord is nowhere near the coccyx; usually, it lies near the disk between vertebra L.1 and L.2. Therefore, the roots of a segmental nerve emerge from the spinal cord at a point higher than that nerve's intervertebral foramen (through which the nerve leaves the vertebral canal). This discrepancy is most marked for the coccygeal, sacral, and lumbar nerves and less so for those nerves closer to the head (Fig. 3-3). The roots of the spinal nerves below L.2 have to run downward beyond the end of the spinal cord to reach their respective intervertebral foramina. They form a bundle called the **cauda equina** (L., "horse tail") inside the tail end of the vertebral canal (Fig. 3-6).

Fig. 3-3 In fetal life (A) the spinal cord (*white*) extends all the way down the vertebral column. In an adult (B) the column has grown past the end of the cord, and the lower nerve roots must run tailward to reach their intervertebral foramina. Note that the cord's cervical and lumbar segments are enlarged to handle the innervation of the limbs.

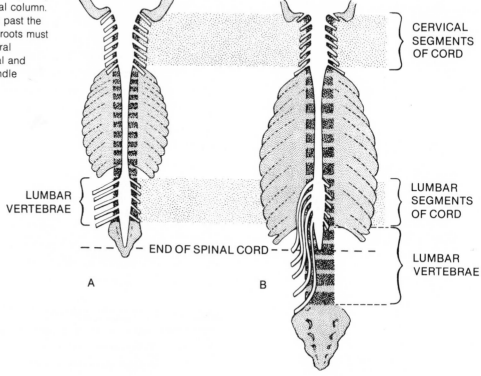

CERVICAL
SEGMENTS
OF CORD

LUMBAR
VERTEBRAE

LUMBAR
SEGMENTS
OF CORD

LUMBAR
VERTEBRAE

END OF SPINAL CORD

A

B

The spinal cord itself is composed of neurons and their processes, intermingled with a variety of other cell types that have various supporting functions and are collectively called **neuroglia.** The embryonic spinal cord develops as a hollow tube, but the central canal in the adult is tiny and may not even be patent. Figure 3-4 shows a cross-section of the cord. The central canal is surrounded by a grayish mass of nerve-cell bodies. This central **gray matter** looks like a butterfly in cross section. The butterfly is surrounded by **white matter**—myelinated axons ascending and descending in the superficial layers of the cord. The butterfly's two ventral wings contain the cell bodies of motor neurons supplying voluntary muscles (that is, those derived from somites), and the dorsal wings contain the cell bodies of internuncial neurons. The autonomic motor neurons that carry impulses from the spinal cord out to peripheral ganglia are clustered on either side of the central canal, forming paired **intermediolateral columns** of

Fig. 3-4 Cross section through a thoracic segment of the spinal cord, showing gray matter (*stippled*) and the roots of a segmental nerve. ILC, intermediolateral column.

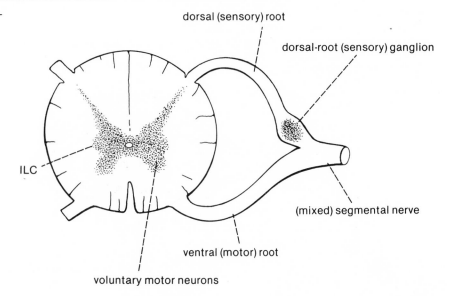

dorsal (sensory) root

dorsal-root (sensory) ganglion

ILC

(mixed) segmental nerve

ventral (motor) root

voluntary motor neurons

gray matter. In the sacral segments (S.2–S.4), these columns contain *parasympathetic* neurons; in the thorax and upper lumbar segments (T.1–L.2), *sympathetic* neurons; and in the brain, extensions of these columns contain *parasympathetic* neurons again. Thus, voluntary muscles and involuntary muscles are innervated from different columns of gray matter, from one end of the body to the other. In the cervical segments and in segments L.3–S.1, which go almost wholly into the limb plexuses, there is no intermediolateral column at all.

■ The Meninges

The dorsal nerve cord of a human embryo is surrounded by a membranous wrapping that condenses out of neural-crest cells and the surrounding mesoderm. By the time of birth, this wrapper has differentiated into three concentric layers called **meninges** (Fig. 3-5). The outermost meninx, the **dura mater** (L., "tough mother"), is a strong, fibrous jacket tailored to fit loosely around the brain and spinal cord. The innermost meninx, the **pia mater** (L., "tender mother") forms a tight-fitting "skin" around the central nervous system, dipping into every little cleft and convolution in is surface.

The remaining meninx is the **arachnoid mater,** which lies in be-

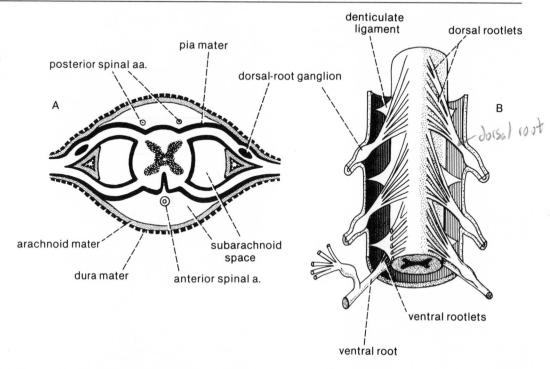

Fig. 3-5 The meninges.
A. Diagrammatic cross section through the spinal cord, showing the three meninges.
B. Dorsal view of the cord, nerve roots, and denticulate ligaments inside the vertebral canal.

tween the outer "jacket" and the inner "skin" like a suit of long underwear. The arachnoid starts out in the embryo as a layer of cells on the outer surface of the pia, but the two soon become separated by fluid-filled cavities that merge to form a single **subarachnoid space** (Fig. 3-6). The fluid filling this space—a clear, watery filtrate of blood plasma known as **cerebrospinal fluid**—is secreted by special vascular patches inside the brain's enlarged central canal. It percolates through holes in the brain stem into the subarachnoid space. The cerebrospinal fluid serves as a flotation bath for the brain and spinal cord, ensuring that their soft, mushy tissues do not get crushed against the surrounding bone by their own weight.

The brain and spinal cord have to be held in place inside their subarachnoid bath, to keep them from bumping into its walls when the head is moved abruptly. They are anchored by strands of tissue that persisted between the pia and the arachnoid when the two split apart. Inside the braincase, these strands are fine and dense, forming a sort of loose, wet felt that cushions the brain against sudden impacts.

Fig. 3-6 Cauda equina and filum terminale inside the tail end of the dural sac. Nerve roots have been removed on the right. Schematic dorsal view.

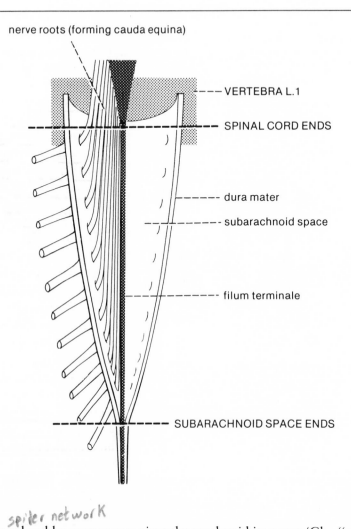

nerve roots (forming cauda equina)

VERTEBRA L.1

SPINAL CORD ENDS

dura mater

subarachnoid space

filum terminale

SUBARACHNOID SPACE ENDS

spider network

Their cobwebby appearance gives the arachnoid its name (Gk., "cobwebby"). There are few such strands surrounding the spinal cord, which is anchored instead by a fold of thickened pia sticking out on each side between the dorsal and ventral roots of the spinal nerves. This fold is tacked down at intervals to the surrounding arachnoid and dura, thus forming a series of taut **denticulate** ligaments (Fig. 3-5). These ligaments prevent the cord from banging around inside the subarachnoid space.

The tail end of the cord is held in place by a final thread of pia, the **filum terminale,** which stretches down to the back of the coccyx.

(This attachment marks the original position of the tip of the embryonic spinal cord; the filum terminale was pulled out into a thread as the vertebral column grew out beyond the end of the spinal cord.) The dura and arachnoid also attach to the coccyx and are similarly drawn out into the filum terminale in the adult, but they do not dwindle to mere threads until they reach vertebra S.2 or thereabouts. Therefore, from L.2 to S.2, the vertebral canal is filled by a dural sac that contains the filum terminale and cauda equina but no spinal cord (Fig. 3-6). A hypodermic needle can be thrust into the big subarachnoid space here to draw off a sample of cerebrospinal fluid without running any risk of stabbing the spinal cord. Below S.2 the vertebral canal encloses only the filum terminale and the dura-wrapped spinal-nerve roots (for the segments from S.3 down).

The meninges also contain the blood vessels that supply the brain and spinal cord. The principal *arteries* of the central nervous system (Fig. 3-5) lie within the subarachnoid space, from which they send pia-enclosed branches into the brain and spinal cord. The principal *veins* lie within the substance of the dura mater. Those of the spinal cord drain into larger veins that lie surrounded by fat on the outer surface of the dural sac. Inside the braincase, the dura is attached directly to bone, so there are no extradural veins or fat. Blood from the brain drains off exclusively through a few big veins lying in the dura mater.

All the spinal nerves give off delicate **meningeal branches,** which arise from the trunk of the mixed nerve and run back into the vertebral canal to furnish sensory innervation to the meninges and surrounding tissues. The brain's meninges are innervated mostly by cranial nerves, but also partly by meningeal branches from spinal nerves C.1–C.3. Because no sensory fibers extend into the central nervous system itself, our brain and spinal cord are as devoid of feeling as our hair or fingernails. The pain produced by injury or disease of the brain results from inflammatory pressure on the sensitive meninges.

4

The Epaxial Muscles

The epaxial muscles are deep muscles of the back, innervated by dorsal rami. They form a strip of musculature down the middle of the back, attaching to the vertebral arches from the sacrum all the way up to the base of the skull.

A four-footed mammal's epaxial muscles are important in locomotion. In a galloping dog or cat, they rhythmically extend the flexed vertebral column, thus adding length and force to each stride. Our own epaxial muscles also extend or arch the back. But because our forelegs do not touch the ground when we run, straightening out the vertebral column contributes nothing to our locomotion. Human epaxial muscles have three general functions: (1) they hold the vertebral column upright when we walk or stand; (2) they straighten the back when we arise from a stooped-over posture; and (3) they control the speed of back flexion when we bend over.

It is obvious that we use our epaxial muscles to straighten the back, but it may seem paradoxical that we need them also in bending over. Most of the weight of our head, neck, arms, and thorax lies ventral to the vertebral column when we stand—so the column has a natural tendency to flex, and gravity does the work when we bend over. The epaxial muscles are nevertheless needed to slow the flexion and keep it under control, like a man lowering a weight on a rope. This sort of "lengthening contraction" or "antigravity" action can be easily demonstrated in a limb muscle, the large **Deltoideus** (Fig. 13-11) that passes across the top of the shoulder joint. Place your elbow on a shelf at shoulder height, and palpate the relaxed Deltoideus with your opposite hand. In this position, lean away from the shelf. You will find that as your elbow nears the edge, the Deltoideus suddenly contracts—preparing not to raise the elbow but to slow its imminent descent. When the elbow reaches the bottom of its swing, the Deltoideus relaxes. Similarly, the epaxial muscles are only slightly active in the upright posture, highly active in bending forward, and more or less inactive in complete flexion. In the slouched-over sitting posture so detested by parents and schoolteachers, the intervertebral ligaments become taut, thus checking vertebral flexion and allowing the epaxial muscles to relax completely.

▪ Divisions of the Epaxial Musculature

Most of the body's named muscles are discrete chunks of flesh that you can cut out and lay on a table. This is not generally true of the epaxial muscles. In this region, the names of muscles label *patterns of attachment,* not individual muscular bundles. For example, small epaxial muscle slips arise from the tips of the vertebral transverse processes and slope medially up to insert into spinous processes two or three vertebrae up the column. The entire complex of these slips, extending from the sacrum up to the spine of C.2, is called the **Multifidus** muscle. It is a *layer* of little muscles that are serial homologs of each other, not a separate and distinct lump of muscle tissue like Deltoideus.

The epaxial muscles consist of many layers of this sort. Their attachments are so complex, and their functions so similar, that learning all their origins and insertions is a waste of time for most purposes. They can be divided into three groups: superficial, intermediate, and deep. The more superficial the epaxial muscle, the more intervertebral joints it crosses. The epaxial muscle slips of the superficial layer mostly run laterally as they approach the head; deeper epaxial muscles run medially. The following outline presents a more detailed but still oversimplified picture of the epaxial muscles.

SUPERFICIAL LAYER
The two muscles in this layer, **Erector Spinae** and **Splenius,** originate near the midline and run laterally toward the head end of the body (Fig. 4-1A). Their fibers span many body segments between origin and insertion.

Erector Spinae The lowest slips of the composite muscle Erector Spinae arise from a strong tendinous sheet attached to the sacrum and the neighboring part of the hipbone's edge. From that origin, three columns of long, thin muscle slips fan out to insert into the ribs (**Iliocostalis**), the transverse processes (**Longissimus**), and the spinous

Fig. 4-1 Epaxial musculature. A. Superficial layer. Black arrows on the left show the attachment patterns of the three divisions of Erector Spinae. B. Intermediate layer of muscles (Multifidus, Semispinalis) and their attachment patterns (*black arrows*). The Levatores Costarum (B) represent the deepest, single-segment layer of epaxial muscles.

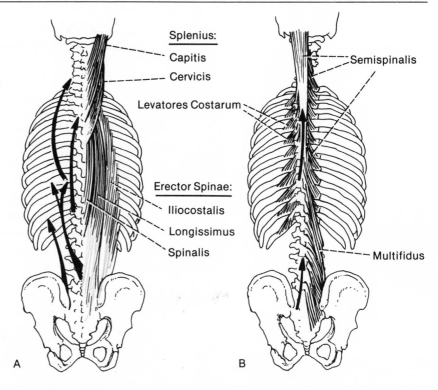

Splenius:
- Capitis
- Cervicis

Levatores Costarum

Semispinalis

Erector Spinae:
- Iliocostalis
- Longissimus
- Spinalis

Multifidus

A

B

processes (**Spinalis**). These three divisions of Erector Spinae are further subdivided into lumbar, thoracic, and cervical portions, which are named accordingly (Iliocostalis Lumborum, Longissimus Thoracis, Spinalis Cervicis, and so on). The Longissimus series is the longest of the three, as its name implies; it extends from the sacrum all the way to the back of the skull. (The part that inserts on the skull receives a special name, Longissimus Capitis.) No single slip of Longissimus spans this whole distance, however; the fibers that attach to neck vertebrae and skull originate from thoracic transverse processes.

Splenius The slips of Splenius arise from the ligamentum nuchae and the upper thoracic spinous processes. They wrap laterally around Longissimus (L. *splenius,* "bandage") to insert on cervical transverse processes (Splenius **Cervicis**) and on the surface of the skull in back of the ears (Splenius **Capitis**).

INTERMEDIATE LAYER

The two muscle complexes in this layer run *medially* as they approach the head (Fig. 4-1B); their individual slips cross fewer segments than those of the superficial layer do. The intermediate layer includes two muscles: **Multifidus,** described earlier, and the more superficial **Semispinalis.**

Semispinalis has the same pattern of origin and insertion that Multifidus has, but its individual slips cross more vertebrae—six or seven—between origin and insertion. Its highest slips form a stout muscle (**Semispinalis Capitis**) that attaches to the back of the skull near the midline on either side of the ligamentum nuchae. The cervical portion, **Semispinalis Cervicis,** arises from the upper five or six thoracic transverse processes and inserts into the spines of the cervical vertebrae—especially into the big spinous process of C.2 (Fig. 4-2). The lowest slips of Semispinalis, known as Semispinalis Thoracis, are feeble and unimportant.

INTERVERTEBRAL (DEEP) LAYER

The deepest epaxial muscles are short slips that connect adjacent vertebrae. They include four named complexes: Rotatores, Levatores Costarum, Interspinales, and Intertransversarii.

Rotatores   Each Rotator runs medially from a transverse process up to the spinous process of the vertebra immediately above. When it contracts, it pulls medially on the transverse process (and laterally on the spinous process), thus rotating the intervertebral joint. The Rotatores are best developed in the thorax, where the joint surfaces and ligaments permit a fair amount of intervertebral rotation.

Levatores Costarum (L., "rib lifters")   Each Levator passes obliquely downward and laterally from a thoracic transverse process to the external face of the rib just below (Fig. 4-1B). The Levatores probably do what their name implies, thus helping to expand the rib cage when drawing in breath.

Interspinales   The Interspinales connect adjacent spinous processes. They probably help to extend the vertebral column (or to control flexion).

Fig. 4-2 Suboccipital region, viewed from behind, with overlying muscles (Trapezius, Splenius, Semispinalis Capitis) removed. The C.2 and C.3 dorsal rami are shown on the right. R.C.P., Rectus Capitis Posterior.

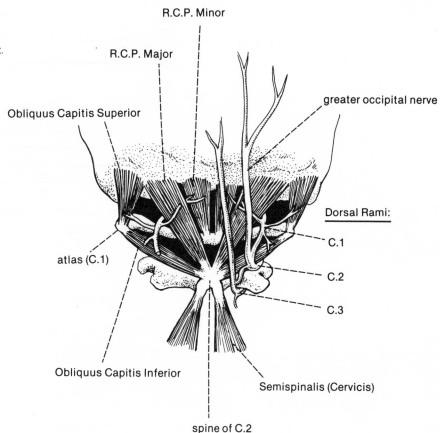

Intertransversarii The Intertransversarii connect adjacent transverse processes and presumably aid in producing and controlling side-to-side bending of the vertebral column. (As might be expected from this, they are best developed in the neck, where side-to-side bending is freest.) The epaxial Intertransversarii are supplemented by hypaxial ones (Fig. 22-3), innervated (of course) by ventral rami.

▪ The Suboccipital Muscles

The projecting back of the skull is called the **occiput,** and the part of the neck that it overhangs is the **suboccipital** region. Four deep epaxial muscles here have become specialized for producing the special movements between the first two vertebrae and the skull. Two of them are **Rectus** (L., "straight") **Capitis Posterior** (R.C.P.) muscles that run from the spines of these vertebrae to the skull: R.C.P. **Major** from C.2 and the shorter R.C.P. **Minor** from C.1. They rock the skull backward on the atlas. The other two suboccipital muscles are **Oblique** muscles that attach to the long transverse process of the atlas. **Obliquus Capitis Inferior,** which runs medially down to the spine of the axis, pulls that spine toward its own side, thus rotating the atlas and skull to left or right around the dens of the axis. **Obliquus Capitis Superior,** sloping up medially from C.1 to the skull, helps the Recti in rocking the skull backward.

The two Obliqui and the Rectus Major form a little scalene triangle, called the **suboccipital triangle** (Fig. 4-2). The dorsal ramus of the first cervical nerve (C.1) emerges in the middle of this triangle and innervates all four suboccipital muscles.

The
Body
Wall

5

■ The Layers of the Body Wall

The outer wall of the celom is surrounded by a body wall made up of concentric layers of skin, hypaxial muscle, and connective tissues. The human body wall, like that of any other vertebrate, protects the viscera from injury. It also includes structures involved in reproduction (the mammary glands), respiration (the intercostal and diaphragmatic muscles), and excretory functions (the superficial sphincters of the anus and urethra) and plays an important role in locomotion.

A surgeon opening up the celomic cavity in the abdomen must cut through five successive layers of body-wall tissue: (1) skin; (2) superficial fascia (and fat); (3) muscle (or associated tendons); (4) abdominal fascia (and fat); and (5) celomic lining (peritoneum). To understand the functions served by these layers of the body wall, we need to comprehend the roles they play in the body as a whole.

■ The Skin

There are two layers in the skin: the epidermis, which is superficial, and the dermis, which is deeper and more complex (Fig. 5-1). The **epidermis** is derived from embryonic ectoderm. The adult's epidermis consists mostly of dead tissue shed by a thin germinal layer of living cells that are constantly dividing and constantly dying. The dead cells become tiny scales or flakes of a hornlike substance on the skin's surface. This horny material is continually being worn off and replenished from underneath. **Hairs** and **nails** are specialized horny structures growing from folds of the germinal layer that penetrate deeply into the underlying dermis. Glands of the skin form as similar invaginations. These invaginations differentiate into **sebaceous** glands, which secrete oils; **sweat** glands, which secrete a saline fluid and play an excretory and thermoregulatory role; and **mammary** glands, which secrete milk. The epidermis includes nerves but no blood ves-

fascia = connective tissue

63

Fig. 5-1 Skin as seen through a microscope. Diagrammatic cross section.

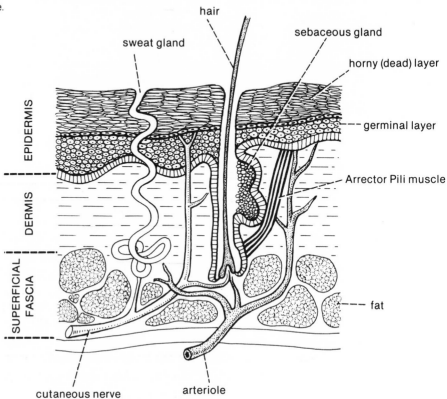

sels. Its outer layer is dead; but the germinal layer, which contains sensory nerve fibers and receives oxygen and nutrients by diffusion from the dermis, is metabolically active.

The **dermis** is the vascular part of the skin. The skin structures that need a direct blood supply—smooth muscles, glands, hair follicles—are embedded in it. The dermis is principally composed of connective-tissue fibers, which give the skin its elasticity and strength.

▪ Fascia

Almost any sheet of connective tissue can be referred to as a **fascia;** the term is not a very precise one in anatomical nomenclature. Most of the tissues called fascia belong to two classes: (1) **areolar tissue,** which is elastic and extremely weak, and (2) **deep fascia,** which is inelastic and strong. Their characteristics reflect the percentage of inelastic collagen fibers they include. Some deep fascia is almost wholly collagenous; such fascia differs in no significant way from an **aponeurosis,** which is a muscle tendon that takes the form of a flat sheet. Ligament, tendon, deep fascia, areolar tissue, and fatty tissue differ principally in the proportions of their constituents, and they grade into one another with no clear boundaries. Indeed, all connective tissue in the body is continuous with all other connective tissue.

A layer of areolar tissue called **superficial fascia** lies deep to the dermis (Fig. 5-1). Observe how freely the skin on the back of your hand moves over the underlying bones and muscles. This mobility is due to the elasticity of the superficial fascia, which contains fat that is liquid at body temperature and does not interfere with the mobility of the skin. On the soles of the feet, the skin is much less mobile; collagenous fibers anchor the dermis directly to the deep fascia, immobilizing the skin so that we do not slide around on our own skin when we walk. The same arrangement is found in the palms of the hands, for similar reasons.

Another layer of elastic fascia lies deep to the body-wall muscles, separating them from the peritoneum. This **abdominal fascia** is known by a bewildering variety of different names in different parts of the body: transversalis fascia, psoas fascia, iliacus fascia, internal spermatic fascia, and so on. It is all an indivisible sheet of connective tissue. Fat is deposited on its inner surface—especially on the dorsal side, near the kidneys. In the pelvis, this fatty extra-peritoneal layer is specialized to form a variety of sheets or ligaments that help to support the rectum and uterus and prevent them from prolapsing out through their orifices.

Deep fascia invests muscles. In most muscles, some muscle fibers originate from the inner surface of the enclosing deep fascia. Some muscles originate from or insert into the deep fascia surrounding other muscles. The deep fascia of a muscle is continuous with the periosteum of the bones to which the muscle attaches and also with the connective-tissue septa that separate the bundles of muscle fibers within a single muscle. Accordingly, changing an in*tra*muscular fascial sheet into an in*ter*muscular sheet involves a relatively small developmental change, and it is not uncommon to find two muscles fused into one or a single muscle divided into two.

Deep fascia is best-developed in the limbs. Because it is inelastic, it is poorly developed over the thorax and abdomen, which must expand and contract in breathing. (Wrapped around your rib cage, a dense sheet of deep fascia would have about the same effect as an anaconda.)

■ The Body-Wall Muscles

The hypaxial muscles constitute most of the muscle tissue in the adult human body. There are three divisions of the hypaxial muscles. (1) Most of the embryo's hypaxial mesoderm spreads downward in a sheet around the outer wall of the celom (Fig. 1-9). This mesoderm develops into the **muscles of the body wall.** (2) An outer, or superficial, lamina of the body wall splits off and develops into the bones and **muscles of the limbs.** (3) Part of the hypaxial mesoderm stays put near the vertebrae and develops into **prevertebral** muscles. These run along the ventral surfaces of the vertebrae and act to flex the vertebral column. In most segments of the human body, the prevertebral muscles are poorly developed.

The body wall is composed of four layers of muscles: a **rectus series,** which runs longitudinally along the middle of the belly, and three concentric layers on each side. In primitive vertebrates, the rectus series extends all the way from the pelvis to the lower jaw; but in mammals and other vertebrates with a well-developed sternum the thoracic part of the rectus musculature atrophies. What is left is a **Rectus Abdominis** running from pelvis to rib cage and a "rectus cervicis" complex in the neck (Fig. 5-2).

The three *lateral* layers of body-wall muscle are best developed in the abdomen. In the thorax, ribs are interposed between the muscle segments; hence the lateral body-wall muscle sheets are split into a series of **Intercostal** muscles that run from one rib to the next. The celom does not extend into the neck, and the lateral part of the body wall is incomplete there. Nothing is left of it but a series of three **Scalene** muscles (Scalenus Anterior, S. Medius, and S. Posterior). The Scaleni run from cervical transverse processes to the first two ribs and help to lift the whole series of ribs when we inhale. Another part of the cervical body-wall musculature is even more important in breathing: it migrates into the thorax during fetal life and develops into the muscles of the **diaphragm** (Chapter 8).

Fig. 5-2 Rectus series of hypaxial muscles: Rectus Abdominis below the thorax and three "rectus cervicis" muscles (Geniohyoid, Omohyoid, Sternohyoid) above it. The two deeper "rectus cervicis" muscles (attached to the larynx) are omitted; the little Pyramidalis is shown only on the left.

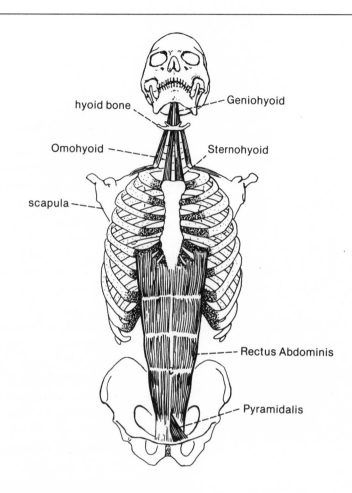

▪ The Abdominal Muscles

The layers of body-wall muscle are most clearly seen in the abdominal part of the body wall. The rectus element, **Rectus Abdominis**, arises by a flat and narrow tendon from the front of the pelvis, just above the external genitals; it runs up and attaches onto the outside of the rib cage as far up as the fifth costal cartilage (Fig. 5-2).

The attachments of the three lateral body-wall layers are more complicated. It is convenient to start with the second or middle layer, the **Internal Oblique** muscle (Obliquus Internus Abdominis; Fig. 5-3). Most of its fibers arise from the flaring lateral brim of the pelvis and

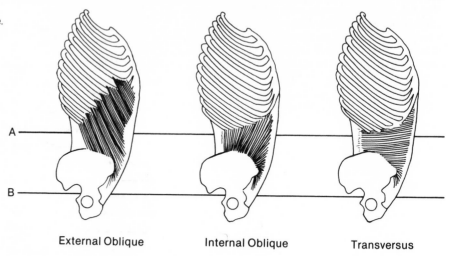

Fig. 5-3 The three layers of the lateral body wall in the abdomen, seen from the right side. Compare with Fig. 5-4.

External Oblique   Internal Oblique   Transversus

slant headward around toward the midline of the belly. The fibers that come off the pelvis furthest back run into the lower edge of the rib cage and attach to it, but the more ventral fibers reach the edge of Rectus Abdominis. As they near it, they become aponeurotic, and this aponeurosis then splits to enclose the Rectus in a tendinous tube called the **rectus sheath** (Fig. 5-4). At the midline the two layers of the aponeurosis fuse again and attach to their mirror-image counterparts from the opposite side. The tendinous band thus formed in the midline is called the **linea alba** (L., "white line"). It separates the left and right Rectus Abdominis muscles throughout their length, from the sternum all the way to the pubic region. Because the lowest fibers of the Internal Oblique have to run ventrally downward to reach this pubic attachment, the whole muscle forms a fleshy fan radiating ventrally from the flaring pelvic brim.

The other two lateral abdominal muscles (Fig. 5-3) also become aponeurotic in front, and their aponeuroses fuse with the rectus sheath. The innermost, **Transversus Abdominis,** originates in back by another aponeurosis that attaches to the transverse processes of the lumbar vertebrae. From this tendinous sheet (and from the lower edge of the rib cage and the upper edge of the pelvis), fleshy fibers arise, run horizontally around the abdomen toward the rectus sheath, and fuse with the sheath's deep surface (behind Rectus Abdominis). The

Fig. 5-4 Cross sections through abdominal muscles at the two levels (A,B) indicated in Fig. 5-3. At the lower level (B) the aponeuroses of all three lateral muscles pass ventral to Rectus Abdominis (RA).

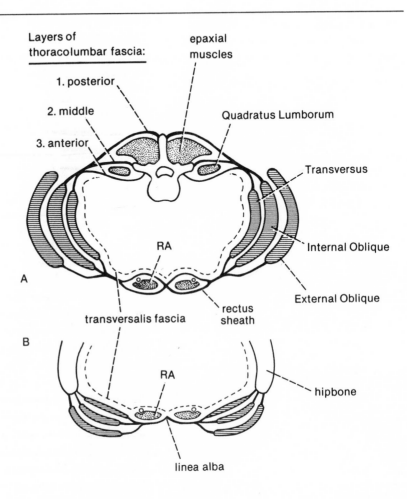

Transversus thus forms a contractile tube like a rubber girdle around the whole abdominal celom.

The third and outermost of the three abdominal muscles is the **External Oblique** (Obliquus Externus Abdominis). It arises by fleshy slips from the sides of the lower eight ribs. The eight slips run slantwise downward toward the front of the belly, blend into a single sheet of muscle, and end as an aponeurosis that fuses to the *front* of the rectus sheath.

Two smaller muscles of the abdominal body wall deserve mention. The stout **Quadratus Lumborum** (Figs. 5-4 and 15-7) connects the last rib to the lumbar transverse processes and the dorsal edge of the pelvic rim. When it contracts, it flexes the lumbar vertebral column toward its own side. The more trivial **Pyramidalis** (Fig. 5-2) is a superficial triangular slip running up from the front edge of the pelvis to insert into the linea alba a few inches higher. Often absent, it is the vestigial remnant of a second, superficial rectus layer in reptiles.

Just as the aponeurosis of the Internal Oblique divides to form a sheath for the Rectus Abdominis in front, so the dorsal aponeurosis of Transversus Abdominis divides to wrap around longitudinal muscles in back. As it approaches the lumbar transverse processes, this aponeurosis splits into three parallel sheets of deep fascia: a superficial one that wraps around the epaxial muscles to attach to the spines of the lumbar vertebrae, a deep one that encloses the ventral surface of the Quadratus Lumborum, and an intermediate one that goes between these two muscle masses and attaches to the transverse processes (Fig. 5-4). The three aponeurotic sheets thus form two muscle sheaths between them. These sheets are known as the **anterior** (ventral), **middle,** and **posterior** (dorsal) **layers** of the **thoracolumbar fascia**—not the best terminology imaginable, but we are stuck with it. The posterior layer also provides a surface of origin for some of the hypaxial muscles of the forelimb, and the fascia covering it has a couple of variable and trivial little hypaxial muscle slips in it (Serratus Posterior Superior and Inferior).

The back (dorsal) layer of the rectus sheath ends about two-thirds of the way down Rectus Abdominis. Below this point, the aponeurotic fibers of the lateral body-wall muscles all pass in front of the Rectus; so the lower third of Rectus has nothing behind it but abdominal fascia (here known as **transversalis fascia,** after the Transversus Abdominis). Arteries (described later) enter the rectus sheath through this posterior defect and supply the muscle. The curved upper edge of the defect is called the **arcuate line** (Fig. 5-5).

At the beginning of this chapter, we noted that an abdominal incison would pierce skin, superficial fascia, hypaxial muscle, abdominal fascia, and peritoneum, in that order. The muscles that must be incised and pulled apart vary depending on the site of the incision. An incision near the midline must pierce the rectus sheath and Rectus Abdominis. If the incision extends above the arcuate line, the surgeon must cut through an aponeurosis on the front and back sides of Rectus Abdominis; below that line the scalpel encounters aponeurosis only in front of Rectus and only abdominal fascia behind it. An

Fig. 5-5 Posterior (dorsal) surface of rectus sheath and Rectus Abdominis, showing epigastric arteries (*left side*) and arcuate line.

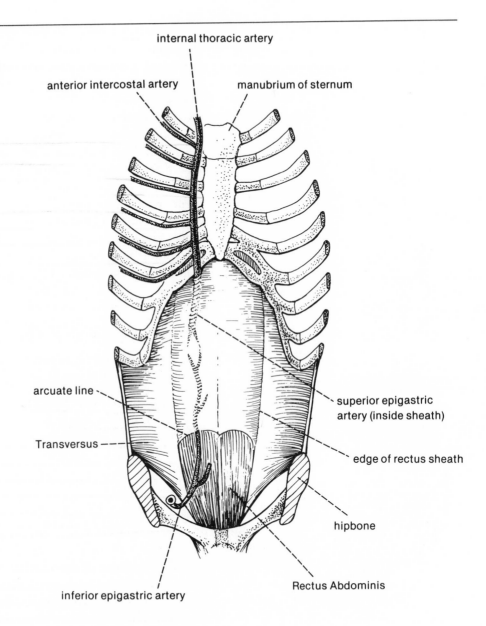

internal thoracic artery

anterior intercostal artery

manubrium of sternum

arcuate line

Transversus

superior epigastric artery (inside sheath)

edge of rectus sheath

hipbone

Rectus Abdominis

inferior epigastric artery

incision made further laterally must pass through the three lateral body-wall muscles—each of which must be incised and pulled apart separately, because their fibers run in different directions (Fig. 5-3).

During development, the gonads of male mammals slide down from a position near the kidneys to a point at the tail end of the belly, just above the edge of the pelvis in front. Here, the layers of the abdominal body wall balloon outward to form pouches into which the gonads slip. The body wall's two outermost layers—the skin and superficial fascia—form an outer pouch called the **scrotum.** Within this shared, external pouch, each testis lies surrounded by a separate, deeper pouch of its own, derived from the Oblique muscles and transversalis fascia. Extensions of these deeper body-wall layers form concentric wrappings around the blood vessels and duct that the descending gonad drags along behind it. These wrappings, described in more detail in Chapter 10, constitute the coverings of the spermatic cord.

▪ The Thoracic Body Wall

The body wall in the thoracic segments differs from the abdominal body wall in four ways:

1. The thoracic muscle segments are kept separate from each other by ribs and sternum.
2. Unlike the abdominal body wall, the walls of the thorax are enveloped in a superficial cloak or girdle of limb musculature.
3. The rectus series of hypaxial muscles is absent over the front of the sternum.
4. In female human beings, the skin of the thorax encloses a pair of breasts—enlarged skin glands buried in connective tissue and fat.

The three layers of **Intercostal** muscles are the thoracic equivalent of the lateral abdominal muscles. The two outmost layers—the **External** and **Internal Intercostals** (Fig. 5-6)—are serially homologous with the External and Internal Obliques. The **External Intercostal** muscle between each pair of ribs slants *ventrally* downward, as does its serial homolog, the External Oblique. It is poorly developed in *front,* near the sternum, where it is represented only by a sheet of deep fascia (the **external intercostal membrane**). The **Internal Intercostal** muscle is just the reverse. Its fibers slant *dorsally* downward and are repre-

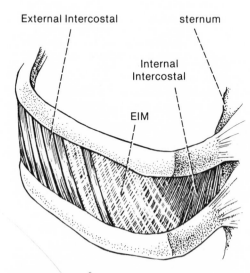

Fig. 5-6 Anterior end of a right intercostal space, showing the two outer layers of Intercostal muscles. At its anterior end, the External Intercostal muscle becomes a collagenous deep fascia, the external intercostal membrane (EIM).

External Intercostal

sternum

Internal Intercostal

EIM

sented only by a sheet of deep fascia (the **internal intercostal membrane**) in *back,* near the vertebral column. The Transversus layer in the thorax is poorly developed and mostly fascial. It is represented by a few small and variable muscles of little functional importance (**Transversus Thoracis** ventrally and the **Innermost Intercostals** laterally).

An incision into the thorax would pierce the same sorts of tissues as would an abdominal incision and in the same order: skin, superficial fascia (including mammary tissue, if any), body-wall muscle (or rib), fascia surrounding the celom, and celomic lining. The thoracic celom is divided into three separate sacs, which are wrapped around the heart and each of the two lungs. These have special names: **pleura** around each lung, and **serous pericardium** around the heart (Fig. 8-1C).

■ The Nerves of the Body Wall

The body-wall muscles are all hypaxial, so they are innervated by ventral rami. The ventral rami of nerves T.1 through T.11 run around the body wall in the spaces between the ribs. They are accordingly called **intercostal nerves.**

A typical intercostal nerve (Fig. 1-12) runs along between the inner two muscle layers of the lateral body wall, just below the rib. It gives off a lateral cutaneous branch halfway along, and its terminal cutaneous branches supply the skin over the belly. Motor fibers pass from each intercostal nerve into the surrounding Intercostal muscles.

The first thoracic ventral ramus is atypical because of its proximity to the nerve plexus of the forelimb; it sends most of its sensory and motor fibers into that plexus. (The first intercostal nerve is present, but diminutive.) The second intercostal nerve (T.2's ventral ramus) may also send a branch directly into the plexus. The last thoracic ventral ramus (T.12) is called the **subcostal** nerve because there is no rib below its segment; it is otherwise like the intercostal nerves.

The abdominal part of the body wall is mostly supplied by intercostal and subcostal nerves—which implies that it is mostly derived from thoracic somites in the embryo. The ventral rami of the lower six thoracic nerves run downward and forward past the end of the rib cage. As each nears the rectus sheath, it gives off a fine **collateral** branch, which runs below the main branch. The collateral branches send motor fibers to the edge of the Rectus Abdominis; the main

Fig. 5-7 The two named branches of the L.1 ventral ramus.

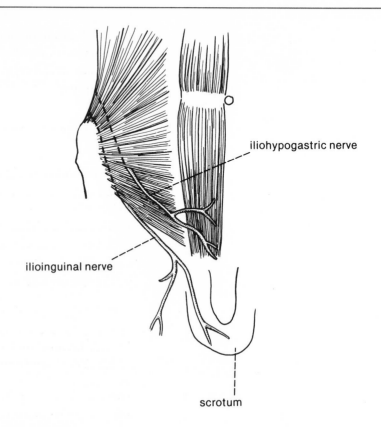

iliohypogastric nerve

ilioinguinal nerve

scrotum

branches continue on behind the Rectus, piercing and supplying that muscle near the midline, and end in a spray of sensory nerves to the skin.

The first lumbar nerve is the last of the typical spinal nerves, and it is close enough to the lower-limb plexus to show a few peculiarities of its own. Its ventral ramus divides into main and collateral branches back near the vertebral column; they are accordingly given separate names (Fig. 5-7). The main branch, the **iliohypogastric** nerve, runs around the lower edge of the abdominal body wall. It resembles the main branch of T.12, but it runs superficial to the Internal Oblique in front, so it does not pierce the rectus sheath or send any motor fibers to Rectus Abdominis. It frequently picks up some motor fibers from nerve T.12 back near the vertebral column. The collateral branch is called the **ilioinguinal** nerve; like any other collateral branch, it runs below (caudad from) the main branch. It is drawn out into the scrotal pouch of the abdominal wall, where it sends sensory fibers to the skin. In females, it innervates the **labia majora**—rounded folds of skin on either side of the vaginal opening, which are the female equivalent of the scrotum.

■ The Blood Vessels of the Body Wall

As each intercostal nerve runs along through the intercostal space, it is accompanied by a small artery. These arteries are branches of larger blood vessels running longitudinally along the inside of the body wall in front and in back.

In back, just ventral to the vertebral bodies, runs the extremely large **descending aorta.** The descending aorta carries blood from the heart down to the thorax, abdomen, and lower limbs. As it passes each intercostal space, it gives off a small **posterior intercostal** artery on either side. In the lumbar segments, the serial homologs of the posterior intercostal arteries are called the **lumbar** arteries. In the embryo, all these branches of the aorta are called **intersegmental** arteries because they travel between body segments (in contrast to spinal nerves, which run within segments and are thus called segmental nerves).

The lumbar and posterior intercostal arteries do not run all the way around to the midline of the belly. The ventral part of the body wall gets its blood via paired longitudinal arteries running along its inner surface, one on each side of the midline. These longitudinal trunks arise from the great arteries that supply the limbs.

From the artery that supplies the lower limb, an **inferior epigastric** artery (Fig. 5-8) runs upward on each side, deep to Rectus Abdominis. It enters the sheath of that muscle and supplies it with blood (Fig. 5-5). A similar small branch from the upper limb's main artery runs down the inside of the thorax beside the sternum. It is called the **internal thoracic** artery. As it descends, it supplies an **anterior intercostal** branch to each intercostal space. These branches end by running into and joining the aorta's *posterior* intercostal branches coming around in the opposite direction. Such a junction of artery with artery, or vein with vein, is called an **anastomosis.** The internal thoracic artery itself ends in much the same way, running down out of the thorax into the rectus sheath and forming anastomoses with the inferior epigastric on the deep surface of Rectus Abdominis. The

Fig. 5-8 Internal thoracic and epigastric arteries form a pair of longitudinal ventral arterial channels inside the body wall. Compare with Fig. 5-5. a., artery.

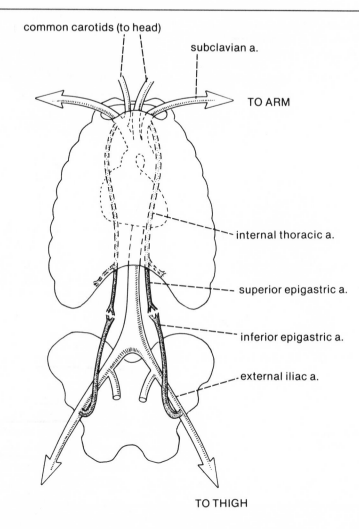

extension of the internal thoracic artery down into the rectus sheath is called the **superior epigastric** artery.

In addition to anastomosing with each other and supplying the Rectus Abdominis, both epigastric arteries send little branches out of the rectus sheath to supply the overlying skin—and to anastomose with the lumbar arteries and other small arteries supplying the abdominal body wall. Cutaneous branches from the internal thoracic arteries similarly supply the skin over the front of the chest.

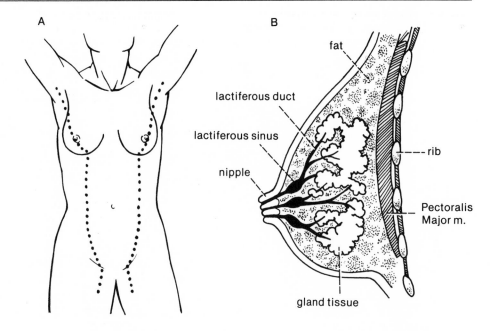

Fig. 5-9 Mammary gland. A. Position of the mammary ridge (*dotted line*). B. Section through breast.

■ The Breasts

In early fetal life, all placental mammals develop a ridge of thickened ectoderm extending along each side of the body from armpit to crotch (Fig. 5-9A). This thickening is called the **mammary ridge,** and it represents a zone of potential mammary-gland development. Different mammals develop mammary glands at different points along the mammary ridge. Some bats have them in the armpit; elephants, sea cows, and monkeys have them on the thorax; sheep, horses, and cattle have them in the groin; and some whales have them alongside the vagina. Among human beings, a single pair of mammary glands normally appears on the thorax. Accessory nipples, however, often appear at other points along the mammary ridge, in both men and women. Accessory nipples figure in American history; the Pilgrim Fathers believed that these anomalies were distinctive of witches.

The mammary gland develops as a branching ingrowth of the mammary ridge on the thorax. This ingrown ectoderm becomes a system of hollow glandular lobes whose ducts converge and open on a raised **nipple.** The spaces between the lobes are filled with fibrous connective tissue and fat. The fatty and glandular tissues proliferate in females at puberty to form prominent **breasts** (Fig. 5-9B). In males, the various parts of the breast are ordinarily rudimentary. The breast is supplied, like any other part of the ventral thoracic skin, by intercostal nerves and by branches of the internal thoracic artery—which used to be called the internal mammary artery for that reason.

■ Other Regions of the Body Wall

The body wall is best-defined in the abdomen and thorax, but it also extends up past the forelimb into the neck and down below the pelvis into the region of the anus and external genitalia. The body-wall elements in these regions are not separated by a celom from the underlying viscera. In the neck (Chapter 22), the body-wall muscles are incomplete and do not form a closed muscular tube around the visceral structures. The postpelvic body wall (Chapter 11) is particularly specialized and complicated. It is represented by several layers of voluntary muscle and fascias that support and surround the openings of the gut, the urinary duct, and the reproductive tracts.

THE THORAX
AND
ITS VISCERA

PART II

The Development of the Mammalian Circulatory Pattern

6

■ Fish Circulation and the Dorsal Aorta

The circulatory pattern in a water-breathing chordate is essentially a simple loop. In *Branchiostoma* (Fig. 6-1), blood flows up through the gill arches on either side of the pharynx and into a **dorsal aorta** on each side. These paired aortae fuse behind the rear end of the pharynx into a single, midline, dorsal aorta, which runs down the middle of the back and gives off lateral branches to the somites and unpaired (midline) branches to the capillary bed of the gut. The blood draining from the gut is collected into a **hepatic portal** vein and led to a specialized outpouching of the gut tube—the equivalent of the vertebrate liver. Here the blood passes through a second capillary bed and is collected once again by a midline **hepatic** vein. This vein joins the paired vessels (**common cardinal** veins) draining the body wall and somites on either side, thereby forming a single great vessel underlying the skin of the belly. This midline vessel, the **ventral aorta,** carries the blood forward and breaks up into multiple vessels that enter the gill arches. Here the cycle begins all over again.

Essentially the same pattern, with variations, is seen in all water-dwelling chordates. Two major structural advances, however, are found in fishes. First, the gill arches bear gills and have replaced the skin as the major site for exchange of respiratory gasses. Second, the posterior part of a fish's ventral aorta is specialized to form a valved and contractile tube of muscle, the **heart,** which forces the blood through the gills and around the circulatory loop under pressure (Fig. 6-2A). Mammals retain a fishlike arrangement in early development; but by the time of birth, the heart and the gill-arch vessels have been greatly remodeled to accommodate yet another evolutionary shift in respiratory apparatus—from gills to lungs.

Fig. 6-1 Circulatory system of *Branchiostoma* (diagrammatic).

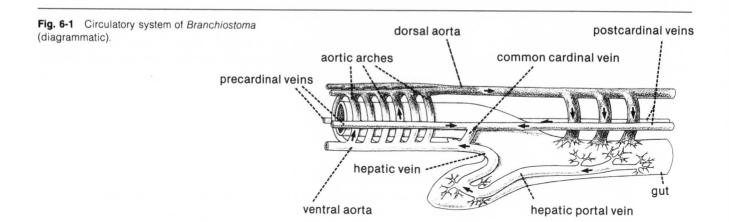

Fig. 6-2 Simplification of the aortic-arch system during vertebrate evolution.
A. Typical fish (left aspect).
B. Aortic arches of lungfish; gills reduced, pulmonary arteries added on to arch VI.
C. Salamander; gills and first two arches lost in the adult.
D. Lizard; ductus arteriosus lost in the adult (persists on left side of embryo).
E. Mammal; carotid duct and right fourth arch lost.

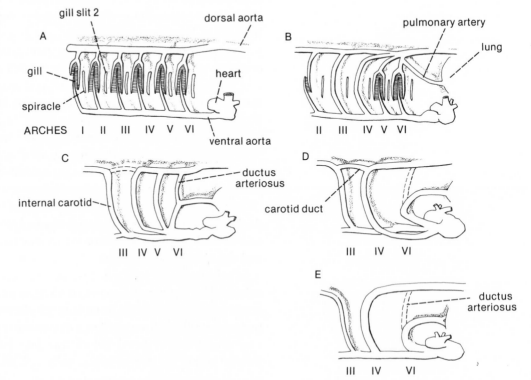

■ Fish Out of Water: Respiration in Terrestrial Vertebrates

The ancestral chordates in the sea absorbed oxygen through those parts of the body surface that came in contact with the water around them: the skin, the lining of the mouth, and the gill slits in the walls of the pharynx. The earliest vertebrates appear to have been freshwater animals, living in streams, ponds, and estuaries and feeding on small invertebrates. This kind of life (something like that of a modern catfish) demands frequent swimming; so it calls for more efficient respiration than a stick-in-the-mud animal like *Branchiostoma* needs. In addition, the oxygen content of fresh water fluctuates seasonally, and freshwater fish may find themselves trapped for weeks in stagnant, deoxygenated ponds. A trapped fish has a better chance of surviving if it has some way of absorbing oxygen from the air.

These demands were met early in vertebrate history by the appearance of two separate but closely related respiratory organs. For more efficient absorption of oxygen from *water,* the ectoderm around the margin of each gill slit became elaborated into **gills**—multiply folded and refolded flaps of highly vascular tissue. The gills replaced the skin as the most important respiratory organ. *Atmospheric* oxygen could be absorbed in time of need by the lining of the mouth. (Even today, many freshwater fishes rise to the surface and gulp air when their water becomes stagnant.) In some early vertebrates, the mouth surface available for absorption of atmospheric oxygen was increased by the development of a double pouch from the ventral lining of the pharynx. These twin outpocketings of the gut, extending back around either side of the heart, were the primitive **lungs**. Lungs are found in several different groups of fishes as well as in land-dwelling vertebrates and were obviously evolved as accessory breathing organs very early in vertebrate history.

Gills are not suited for breathing air; and in terrestrial vertebrates the lungs are usually the principal organs of respiration. The elaboration of the lungs required some big changes in the major blood vessels and the circulatory pattern.

In primitive fishes (Fig. 6-2A), the walls of the pharynx were vascularized by a series of six **aortic arches,** each of which left the ventral aorta, passed upward in front of a gill slit, broke up into a capillary bed in the gill, and returned to a dorsal aorta above the gill slits. The two dorsal aortae fused behind the last gill slit to form a major arterial trunk, the **dorsal aorta,** running back down the body on the ventral surface of the vertebral column.

The lungs were outpocketings from the floor of the pharynx just aft of the gill region. They received their vascular supply from the last (sixth) aortic arch via a side branch that came off before the last arch joined the dorsal aorta. This arrangement is still seen in modern lungfish and salamanders (Fig. 6-2B and C). In amniotes (Fig. 6-2D and E), the sixth arch loses its connection with the dorsal aorta in the adult, and all of the blood that flows into this arch passes through the lungs. (In the amniote *embryo,* the old sixth-arch connection with the dorsal aorta persists on the left side until birth, forming a critical part of the fetal circulatory setup.)

The veins returning from the lungs of primitive land-dwelling vertebrates originally drained directly into the posterior end of the heart, together with the systemic and portal veins. Systemic, portal, and pulmonary (lung) returns were therefore thoroughly mixed in the heart before they were driven through the aortic arches. The blood reaching the lungs was thus already partly oxygenated, and the systemic arterial supply was contaminated with venous blood that had not yet passed through the lungs. This inefficient arrangement is characteristic of all lung-breathing vertebrates, except birds and mammals. (Crocodiles and alligators, the closest living relatives of birds, also have a very birdlike circulatory arrangement.) Because birds and mammals are warm-blooded, they have a high and stable metabolic rate. Their elevated metabolism involves a high rate of oxygen consumption, and calls for a complete separation of arterial blood from deoxygenated venous blood.

■ Circulation in Adult Mammals

Figure 6-3 presents a diagram of the adult circulatory pattern in mammals. As in fishes, one end of the heart receives venous blood from all parts of the body, and the other end sends it forth into the aortic arches. The important difference between fishes and mammals is that all of the stale venous blood returning from a mammal's body is sent through the sixth aortic arch into the lungs, oxygenated, and then returned to the heart before being distributed to the body again. This separation of the pulmonary circuit has been accomplished by developing a median septum that partitions the heart into right and left halves. The blood sent to the sixth (or pulmonary) aortic arch

Unlike fishes, the pulmonary circuit in mammals is separate from the systemic circuit

Fig. 6-3 Circulatory patterns in the adult (A) and fetus (B). Darker vessels carry blood that is proportionately more oxygenated. D, ductus arteriosus; IVC, inferior vena cava; LA, left atrium; N, navel; RA, right atrium; RV, right ventricle; U–G, urogenital.

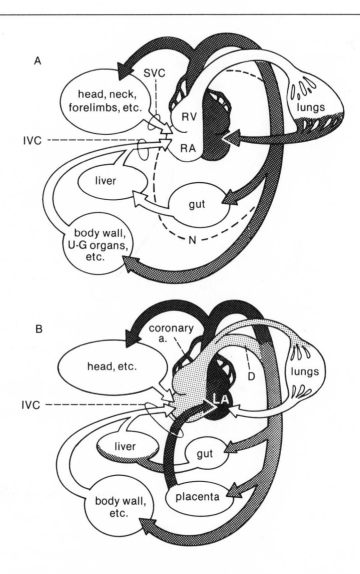

leaves the heart on the right-hand side of this septum; when it comes back from the lungs saturated with oxygen, it reenters the heart on the left side of this septum. From there it is sent out through the remains of the third and fourth aortic arches (Figs. 6-4 and 7-10) to the rest of the body. Venous and arterial blood cannot contaminate each other as they do in typical reptiles.

Fig. 6-4 Simplification of the aortic-arch system in *Homo* during development. A. Ventral view of complete system with all six arches. B. Persisting remnants (*white*) in adult. The complete system never really exists in the embryo because arch I degenerates before arch VI has formed.

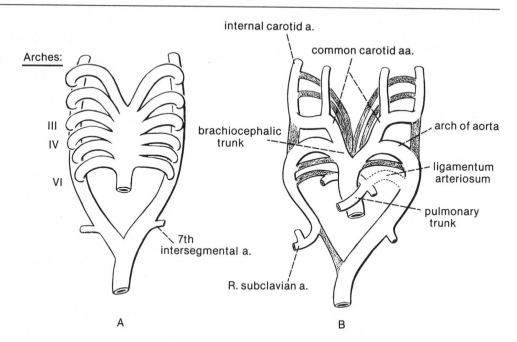

■ The Early Development of the Human Circulatory System

Vascular tissues show up first in the extraembryonic mesoderm of the chorion, where they must develop as soon as possible to begin bringing oxygen and nutrients to the embryo. Shortly after the embryo implants itself in the uterine wall, a network of relatively unorganized small blood vessels forms in the mesoderm of the body stalk and yolk sac. As development progresses, these diffuse plexuses of umbilical capillaries gradually become more organized, and placental blood flow is canalized into larger and larger channels—the umbilical arteries and veins. These remain connected to each other at their distal ends by the placental capillaries, where maternal–fetal exchange takes place.

Blood vessels begin to form inside the embryonic disk before the first somites appear. They coalesce from **angiogenetic** (Gk., "giving birth to vessels") **cell clusters** in the mesoderm around the edges of the yolk sac's mouth (Fig. 6-5). These clusters quickly develop into a network of capillarylike tubules that are lined with endothelium from

Fig. 6-5 Cutaway diagram of the head end of an early human embryo, showing angiogenetic cell clusters (ACC) with overlying celom.

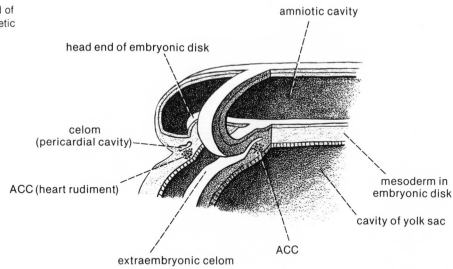

amniotic cavity

head end of embryonic disk

celom
(pericardial cavity)

ACC (heart rudiment)

mesoderm in
embryonic disk

cavity of yolk sac

ACC

extraembryonic celom

which primitive blood cells spring. Vessel formation proceeds by enlargement of some of the channels in this network.

■ The Formation of the Heart and Pericardial Cavity

The angiogenetic cell clusters extend in an arc around the head end of the yolk sac's mouth. Thus the big blood channel that forms from them is at first shaped something like a wishbone, with a short longitudinal trunk in front and two "legs" trailing back around either side of the yolk sac. As development proceeds, the mouth of the yolk sac gets relatively narrower, so the right and left legs (**endocardial tubes**—Fig. 6-6) of this wishbone come together in the midline. They fuse together under the floor of the pharynx to form a single tube—the primordial heart (Fig. 6-7).

The head end of the celomic cavity at first also forms an arc around the head end of the yolk sac's mouth. The developing heart lies between this celomic arc and the yolk sac (Fig. 6-5). As the yolk sac narrows and the ectodermal surface of the embryo grows more rapidly, the expanding head end of the embryo swells out forward and downward over the primoridal heart, and the heart is rolled backward underneath the pharynx (Figs. 6-6 and 6-7). As a result, the cranial end of the celom comes to lie ventral to the heart instead of

Fig. 6-6   Diagrammatic midline (A) and cross (B) sections through the mouth of the yolk sac in a 21-day embryo, showing the wishbone-shaped heart formed from the paired endocardial tubes. The arrow in A indicates the plane of the cross section shown in B.

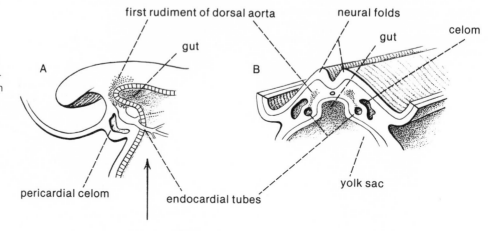

Endocardial tubes, derived from ACC, coalesce to form the tubular heart in the midline.

surrounding its cranial side. The thoracic body wall now grows down from adjacent somites and closes around the heart and the celom. While all this is going on, the endocardial tubes have been coalescing into a tubular heart in the midline. The thoracic part of the celomic cavity expands around the heart, leaving the heart briefly suspended from the ventral surface of the gut by a thin **dorsal mesocardium** (Fig. 6-7) that soon becomes perforated and is resorbed. The heart is then wholly surrounded by the celomic cavity, and is attached to the rest of the body only at its cranial end (where the aortic arches travel forward and dorsally into the celom-wall mesoderm) and its caudal end (where the heart receives the veins returning from gut, placenta, and body wall).

■ The Development of Circulatory Asymmetry

The circulatory system in a four-week human embryo is as tidy and symmetrical as that of a fish (Fig. 6-8). Its pleasing symmetry cannot last. If the pulmonary and systemic circuits are to become separated, the heart must be divided into two differently connected halves: a right half that receives all the deoxygenated blood from the systemic veins and sends it into the lungs, and a left half that drains the oxygenated blood from the lungs and pumps it out into the systemic arteries.

In four-week embryos, the tubular heart hangs below the gut, attached only at its cranial and caudal ends where the major arteries

Fig. 6-7   Heart in a four-week human embryo.
A. Diagrammatic dissection from the side.
B. Cross section through the plane indicated by
arrows in A.

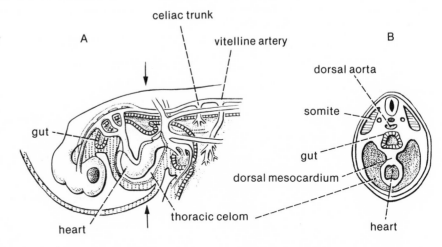

and veins spread into the surrounding mesoderm. The caudal end of the heart tube receives blood from the veins; the cranial end pumps blood around through the aortic arches into the dorsal aorta (Fig. 6-8). A waistlike constriction in the middle of this tube divides it first into two chambers: a caudad **atrium** (L., "courtyard"), into which venous blood is received, and a craniad **ventricle** (L., "little belly"), a more muscular dilation from which blood is expelled into the aortic arches.

The ventricle and atrium are both gradually divided in half by a median septum that grows out of the walls of the heart, producing four chambers: a right and left atrium, and a right and left ventricle. The atrium on each side opens into the ventricle on the same side. The ventral aortic trunk leaving the front end of the heart is also divided by a median septum. Thereafter, the right ventricle empties exclusively into the last (sixth, or pulmonary) aortic arch, and the pulmonary and systemic branches of the aorta are kept separate. Because the septum that forms in the aortic trunk is helical, the definitive aorta and pulmonary trunk twist around each other and the aortic channels leaving the right and left ventricles switch sides as they move away from the heart (Figs. 6-4 and 7-10).

Several venous channels return blood to the tail end of the developing heart. Because the caudal end of the heart is at first jammed up against the mouth of the yolk sac (Fig. 6-6), it is divided into a left and right **venous sinus** (**sinus venosus**); all the tributary veins of the sinuses also come in pairs. There are three sets of these paired venous

Fig. 6-8 Major blood vessels in a human embryo four weeks after conception.

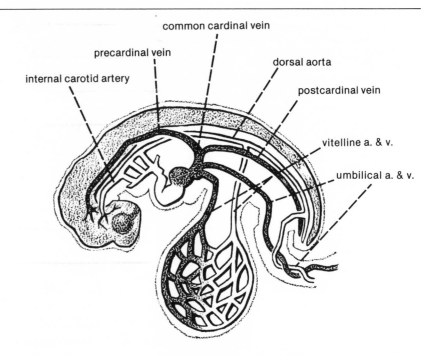

common cardinal vein

precardinal vein

dorsal aorta

internal carotid artery

postcardinal vein

vitelline a. & v.

umbilical a. & v.

channels: (1) The left and right **vitelline** veins (Fig. 6-8) drain the yolk sac. In birds, reptiles, and some mammals, the embryo absorbs its nourishment through these vessels. They are important even in *Homo*, because tributaries of the vitelline veins vascularize the developing liver. (2) The right and left **umbilical** veins pass around either side of the mouth of the yolk sac to drain the allantois—and therefore to drain the placenta. Through these veins, nutrients and oxygen pass from the placenta to the developing human embryo. The right umbilical vein atrophies early; the left persists and shifts over to the midline as the mouth of the yolk sac narrows and eventually disappears. (3) The **common cardinal** veins pass dorsally from the venous end of the heart and divide into **precardinal** and **postcardinal** veins (Fig. 6-8). Tributaries of these veins drain the head and the body wall.

At first, the venous system is bilaterally symmetrical. But if venous and arterial blood are to be kept separate in the air-breathing adult, all the deoxygenated blood coming back to the heart must return to the right side of the heart to be pumped into the lungs. Asymmetry begins to appear in the embryonic venous system about seven weeks after conception. An anastomotic channel develops and runs across to connect the left precardinal vein to its counterpart on the right. Between this anastomosis (the left brachiocephalic vein) and the heart, the left precardinal vein atrophies, and the whole precardinal drainage eventually returns to the right atrium. Similar but more complex anastomoses develop between the postcardinals. Ultimately (Fig. 7-1), only three veins enter the right atrium: (1) a descending **superior vena cava** representing the precardinal drainage; (2) an ascending **inferior vena cava** that forms from bits and pieces of the vitelline, umbilical, and postcardinal systems; and (3) a **coronary sinus,** which is a leftover bit of the sinus venosus that drains blood from the heart's own musculature. The left atrium receives only the four **pulmonary** veins, which form as branches of a single vein that drains the embryonic lungs. In the adult, the pulmonary veins bring oxygenated blood from the lungs back to the left atrium.

Originally a straight tube, the heart soon becomes bent into an S-shape, so that the ventricles lie ventral to the atria (Fig. 7-7). The ventricles get their name from their more *ventral* position. The heart also undergoes a rotation that carries its ventral midline to the left—so, in the adult, little of the original left half of the heart is visible from the ventral aspect.

▪ The Fetal Circulation

In the fetus, the lungs are small and collapsed. They are too small to allow for pushing all the blood from the right atrium through the lung circuit before it can be sent out again through the aorta. There is no point in sending the right atrial blood through the lungs anyway: the lungs are full of amniotic fluid and cannot oxygenate the blood, and the right atrial blood is already the most highly oxygenated blood in the fetus (because it includes the blood returning from the placenta).

Before birth, it would thus be desirable to let most of the right atrial blood pass directly into the systemic circulation, without going through the pulmonary circuit at all. This could be done by leaving a hole in the heart's midline partition or by leaving the sixth (pulmonary) aortic arch connected to the descending aorta, as it is in an adult salamander (Fig. 6-2C).

In fact, both mechanisms are employed in the fetus. Fetal blood flow is diagrammed in Figure 6-3B. You may find it useful to color this diagram with red and blue pencils as you read the following description.

Arterial blood, laden with oxygen and nutrients, returns from the placenta to the fetus through the umbilical vein. Because the umbilical vein empties into the inferior vena cava, the blood returning to the right atrium via the inferior vena cava is purer than that returning via the superior vena cava. Inside the right atrium, the stream of blood from the inferior vena cava manages to avoid mixing thoroughly with the less pure blood (from the superior vena cava), remaining discrete like a warm ocean current in a cold sea. It passes through an aperture, the **foramen ovale,** in the septum that separates right and left atria. From the left atrium, this oxygen-rich blood is sent through the left ventricle, and thus out via the arch of the aorta. Most of it is distributed to the head, neck, and arms; some is distributed to the heart itself through the **coronary** arteries that arise from the base of the ascending aorta (Fig. 6-3). The heart and brain of the fetus thus receive the purest and richest arterial blood during fetal development.

The staler blood returning to the heart through the superior vena cava passes from the right atrium into the right ventricle and thence into the pulmonary trunk. Little of it goes through the lungs, however, because the lateral end of the sixth aortic arch persists on the left side, forming a **ductus arteriosus** that conducts the pulmonary blood supply directly into the dorsal aorta (Figs. 6-2 and 6-4). Because the systemic and placental blood mix together somewhat in the right atrium, the blood passing through the ductus arteriosus is partially oxygenated—though not as much so as the blood that enters the aorta via the foramen ovale and left ventricle.

▪ Circulatory Changes at Birth

If the fetal circulatory pattern were to persist in the newborn, venous blood would continually spill from the pulmonary circuit into the systemic circuit via the foramen ovale and ductus arteriosus. The arterial supply of the entire body would thus be contaminated, resulting in a more or less severe hypoxia (oxygen deficiency). To prevent this, the foramen ovale and ductus arteriosus *must close at the moment of birth.* The mechanisms that accomplish this radical change in circulatory pattern are simple and beautiful:

1. In the fetus, the foramen ovale is covered by a flap valve that allows blood to pass from right atrium to left atrium, but not in the opposite direction.

2. After the child is delivered, the fetal blood vessels in the placenta contract, returning the blood they contain (up to 100 milliliters) to the infant.

3. As the placental circulation shuts down, the child takes its first breath; the lung capillaries fill with blood, and oxygenated blood returning from the lungs floods the left atrium with the next heart-beat.

4. When the lungs inflate, the blood pressure in the right atrium falls below that in the left. This pressure differential holds the inter-atrial flap valve shut, thus closing the foramen ovale.

5. At the moment of the first breath, powerful vasoconstriction in the ductus arteriosus closes it; in a few days, fibrous tissue begins to close the lumen. The ductus soon becomes a vestigial cord, the ligamentum arteriosum (Fig. 6-4B). (The **ductus venosus,** which shunts oxygenated placental blood around the liver into the inferior vena cava (Fig. 6-3B), closes in the same way.) The first breath has converted the fishlike circulatory pattern of the fetus into that of an air-breathing mammal.

The Heart
and the
Great Vessels

7

■ The Anatomy of the Heart

The adult human heart (Fig. 7-1) is about the size and shape of a large artichoke. Its apex points caudally, ventrally, and to the left. As a result of the kinking-up and rotation of the heart tube during fetal life (Figs. 6-8 and 7-7), the right ventricle occupies most of the ventral surface of the heart in the adult and the left atrium is practically invisible from the front. The only part of the left atrium that can be seen in a ventral view is its **auricle** (L., "little ear"), which curls ventrally around the left side of the pulmonary trunk. The right atrium also sports an auricle of its own, wrapped around the base of the ascending aorta. Figure 7-2, an exploded diagram of the four chambers of the heart, shows the spatial relationships of the parts of the heart and the pattern of blood flow between its chambers.

The first rudiment of the heart in the embryo is a wishbone-shaped tube (Fig. 6-6). The legs of the wishbone are venous trunks extending back around the mouth of the yolk sac; the point or apex of the wishbone is the ventral aorta, which carries blood forward toward the aortic arches in the neck region. The early heart tube is made wholly of **endothelium**—flattened mesodermal cells like those in the walls of a capillary, with no power to contract. By the time the first somites form in the embryo, celom-wall mesoderm has condensed around the endothelial heart tube, providing it with a jacket of heart muscle, or **myocardium**. The embryonic heart first begins to beat at this point.

Most of the substance of the adult heart is muscle tissue derived from the embryonic myocardium. The myocardium develops into a thick, spongy layer of muscular strands, surrounded by a denser layer of cortical muscle. The dense cortical layer enlarges and becomes more complicated as development goes on. The primitive spongelike inner layer of myocardium is eventually reduced to a meshwork of

Fig. 7-1 The heart and great vessels. A. Anterior (ventral) aspect. B. Posterior (dorsal) aspect. L., left; R., right.

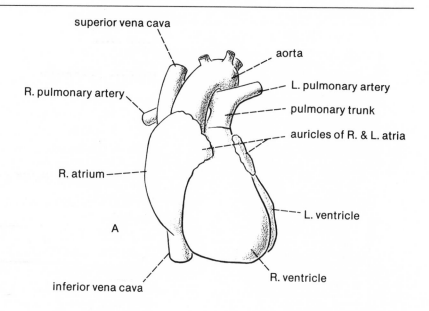

superior vena cava

aorta

R. pulmonary artery

L. pulmonary artery

pulmonary trunk

auricles of R. & L. atria

R. atrium

L. ventricle

A

R. ventricle

inferior vena cava

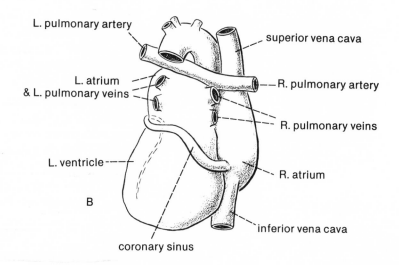

L. pulmonary artery

superior vena cava

L. atrium & L. pulmonary veins

R. pulmonary artery

R. pulmonary veins

L. ventricle

R. atrium

B

inferior vena cava

coronary sinus

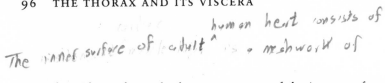
The inner surface of adult human heart consists of a meshwork of

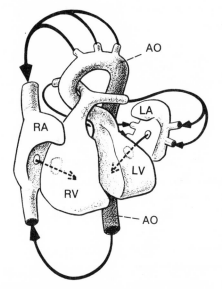

Fig. 7-2 Chambers of the heart. Exploded diagram showing their spatial relations and the pattern of blood flow (*arrows*). AO, aorta; LA, left atrium; LV, left ventricle; RA, right atrium; RV, right ventricle.

irregular ridges of muscle that cover most of the inner surface of the adult human heart (Fig. 7-3). Other parts of the inner surface are smooth. These smooth parts are derived from arteries and veins assimilated into the heart's chambers during fetal growth, and they are thinner and less muscular than the parts derived from the embryonic myocardium.

The atria of the heart have weaker and thinner walls than the ventricles. This is because the ventricles do most of the heart's work, pushing the blood out through the arteries to all parts of the body. All that the atria have to do is receive blood from the veins and shove it forward into the ventricles. The fetal atria therefore do not have to develop thick myocardial walls like those of the ventricles. Instead, they grow chiefly by incorporating the attached veins into their walls. As a result, the inner walls of the atria are mostly smooth. The parts of the atria that develop from embryonic myocardium are covered on the inside with muscular ridges called **pectinate** (L., "comblike") muscles. These ridges cover about half the inner surface of the right atrium; the left atrium retains them only on the inside of the auricle.

The interior of the right atrium is shown in Figure 7-3. The **fossa ovalis** represents the site of the closed-off foramen ovale; it is visible on the wall separating the two atria. The inferior vena cava opens immediately below it. During fetal life, oxygenated blood entering the right atrium from the placenta flows directly through the foramen ovale into the left atrium. This pattern of flow (from inferior vena cava to foramen ovale) is guided by the surrounding ridges: the **limbus** of the fossa ovalis and the **crista terminalis**, which marks the boundary between the right atrium's smooth and pectinate parts. Note that the openings of the three major veins that enter the right atrium—the two venae cavae and the coronary sinus—all lie in the smooth, vein-derived area on the atrium's back wall.

The growing ventricles did not incorporate much of the aorta, and their inner walls therefore retain something of their primitive spongy character. They are covered with muscular ridges, called **trabeculae carneae** (L., "fleshy little timbers") because many of them stretch across the ventricular cavity and are anchored only at their ends. Virtually the whole inner surface of each ventricle is an openwork mesh of these trabeculae (Fig. 7-3).

The right and left atria empty respectively into the right and left ventricles. Each opening from an atrium into a ventricle is guarded by an atrioventricular valve that shuts when the ventricle contracts,

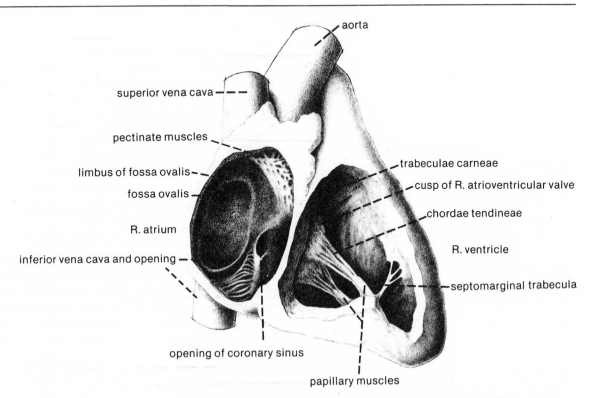

Fig. 7-3 Right atrium and right ventricle, opened to show their interior structures.

thereby preventing regurgitation of ventricular blood back into the atrium. The **left atrioventricular valve** is formed by two flaps, or cusps, drawn out from the margins of the opening. These flaps fly apart like a pair of swinging doors when the left atrium contracts and slam shut when the left ventricle contracts. This bicuspid valve is also called the **mitral valve**, after its resemblance to a bishop's miter. The **right atrioventricular valve** is similar, but it has three cusps. Accordingly, it is sometimes called the tricuspid valve.

When the ventricles contract, these cusps are in danger of being forced back into the atria, like a swinging door swinging open in the wrong direction. This is prevented by two means: (1) The margin of each atrioventricular opening is reinforced by an embedded ring of fibrous connective tissue that acts as a "frame" for the "swinging door." (2) The cusp is prevented from swinging open the wrong way by specialized trabeculae carneae, which attach to its edges and are called the **papillary** muscles (Fig. 7-3). Each arises from a ventricular wall as a thick, muscular projection and inserts into the edges of two adjoining valve cusps via a spray of fine tendinous cords, the **chordae tendineae.** If the chordae simply attached to the inner walls of the ventricles, then the contracting ventricles' shrinkage would cause them to become slack. But the papillary muscles contract when the ventricles do and so maintain the tension in the chordae that is needed to prevent the valves' cusps from being forced into the atria.

Blocked from flowing back into the atria, the blood in the contracting ventricles pours into the great arterial channels leaving the heart: the **ascending aorta** and **pulmonary trunk.** The elastic walls of these arteries stretch greatly when they are distended with blood from the contracting ventricles. So valves are needed here, too—to prevent blood from rushing out of the distended arteries back into the heart when the ventricles relax. The aortic and pulmonary openings are each guarded by a tricuspid valve (Fig. 7-4). The cusps of these valves are small, hammocklike folds of fibrous tissue. When the ventricle contracts, the blood rushing upward through the opening presses the cusps against the side of the vessel; when the ventricle relaxes, the back pressure of the expelled blood makes the collapsed cusps fill and belly out like sails in the wind, pressing against each other and occluding the ventricular opening. Like sails abruptly bellying in the wind, the filling cusps provide a sharp sound, which is audible through a stethoscope. The familiar "lub-dup" sound of the heart is composed of two valve "knocks": the first ("lub") produced by the closing atrioventricular valves at the beginning of ventricular contraction and the second ("dup") by the closure of the aortic and pulmonary valves to bar regurgitation of blood into the relaxing ventricles.

The inner wall of each ventricle is smooth near the ventricular outlet. Like the smooth parts of the atrial walls, these smooth areas are derived from blood vessels that have become incorporated into the chambers of the growing heart. The smooth-walled outlet of the right ventricle is called the **infundibulum** (L., "funnel"); that of the left ventricle, the **aortic vestibule.** Directly around the tricuspid valve that guards each ventricular outlet, the tissue of the ventricular wall is condensed into a dense, fibrous ring like the rings found around the atrioventricular openings. Together, these fibrous rings around the valves provide the heart with a skeleton of sorts, to which the muscle fibers in the cortical myocardium find attachment. Indeed, this skele-

Fig. 7-4 Superior aspect of the heart. The dorsal surface of the heart is toward the bottom of the drawing. The aortic and pulmonary openings are occluded by their tricuspid valves, shown here in the closed position.

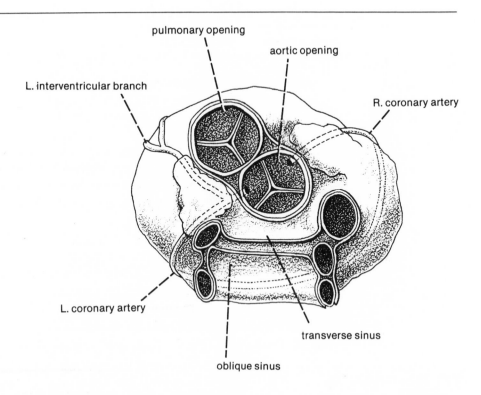

pulmonary opening

aortic opening

L. interventricular branch

R. coronary artery

L. coronary artery

transverse sinus

oblique sinus

ton may sometimes be cartilaginous in man; in certain other large mammals, it is partly ossified.

■ The Coronary Circulation

The heart, like any other living tissue, needs a blood supply. Primitive vertebrate hearts, largely composed of spongy muscular trabeculae with a relatively thin layer of cortical muscle, can get all the nutrients and oxygen they need by absorption from the blood passing through their chambers. (The same thing is true of the early embryonic heart in humans.) In higher vertebrates, one or two **coronary** arteries (Figs. 7-4 and 7-5) grow out from the base of the aorta to provide a more effective blood supply to the thick cortical muscle of the heart. In mammals, including ourselves, there are two coronary arteries. The left coronary artery passes between the pulmonary trunk and left auricle and then runs in a groove between the atrium and ventricle on the left side of the heart; the right coronary artery has a similar course

Fig. 7-5 Pattern of the coronary arteries (A) and cardiac veins (B), viewed from the front. One of the anterior cardiac veins is shown draining into the coronary sinus—a common variation.

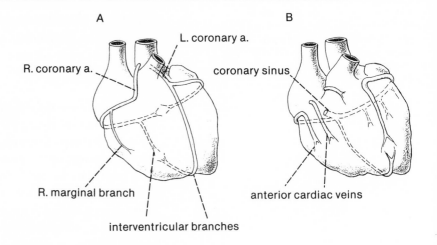

on the right side. **Circumflex** branches of both arteries continue along the atrioventricular groove to the back side of the heart, forming a "waistband" that demarcates the atria from the ventricles. Each coronary artery also gives off an **interventricular** branch that runs downward between the right and left ventricles and supplies their thick, hard-working walls with blood. The right artery usually sends its interventricular branch down the back side of the groove between the ventricles, and the left artery sends its down in front. The definitive coronary arteries therefore constitute a circle and a conjoined half-circle. A **right marginal** branch from the right coronary artery, supplying the right edge of the right ventricle, completes the general picture (Fig. 7-5A).

The venous return from the heart, like any other venous return, must empty into the right atrium. The part of the heart supplied by the proximal end of the right coronary artery is drained by two or three **anterior cardiac** veins, which usually pass directly into the right atrium. The rest of the heart is drained by tributaries of a venous channel called the **coronary sinus**, which runs across the dorsal surface of the heart. Its tributaries accompany the branches of the coronary arteries. The coronary sinus is developmentally part of the heart; it represents that part of the left atrium (or, strictly speaking, its venous sinus) that received the left venous return before the whole systematic venous drainage became channeled to the right side. A few tiny veins (**venae cordis minimae**) drain from the heart wall directly into the atria—a vestige of the primitive arrangement. Those of the left atrium contaminate the oxygenated blood, but apparently not enough to be eliminated by natural selection.

▪ The Pericardial Sac

The heart first appears in the embryo as a longitudinal tube with branching ends. The branches at the head end are the aortic arches; those at the tail end are the great veins. As development proceeds, the venous connections of the heart stay put in the celom wall, but the aortic arches grow and elongate. The cranial end of the heart tube therefore moves down into the thorax, where the hypaxial body wall closes over it. The heart thus becomes increasingly S-shaped and winds up as a twisted bag hanging from a crown of vessels near its cranial end.

The thoracic part of the celom at first is horseshoe-shaped, with the central arc of the horseshoe lying ventral to the heart tube. As the heart descends into the thorax proper, this midline part of the celom expands and wraps dorsally around the heart tube. For a short time, the heart is suspended by a dorsal mesentery, the dorsal mesocardium; but this is soon resorbed, leaving a celomic cavity in the form of a torus—a hollow doughnut shape, with the heart tube thrust through the hole in the middle (Fig. 7-6).

This toroidal cavity communicates on either side with the right and left legs of the original horseshoe, which are themselves continuous with the right and left halves of the celom in the abdomen. In the adult, this single big celomic arc is divided into four separate cavities. The thoracic celom is partitioned off from the abdominal celom by the diaphragm; and the thoracic celom is itself further subdivided into a **pericardial cavity** (around the heart), and two **pleural cavities** (one around each lung). This subdivision of the thoracic cavity takes place while the heart descends into the thorax. As the heart moves caudad past its venous connections, the great veins draining the body wall— the common cardinal veins (Fig. 6-8)—are drawn closer together in the midline. As they move together, they invaginate the celom, and each draws a double fold of celomic lining along with it. These **pleuropericardial folds** (Fig. 8-1) fuse in the midline, thus closing off the pericardial cavity from the pleural cavities.

Like all celomic spaces, the pericardial cavity is lined with a membrane that secretes a thin film of lubricant fluid. This membrane is

Fig. 7-6 Formation of the pericardial sac. Resorption of the dorsal mesocardium (DM in A) converts the original sac into a hollow torus (B).

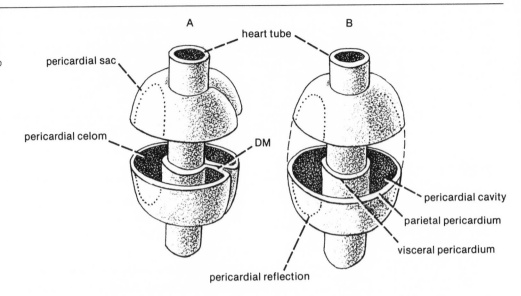

called the **serous pericardium.** It is comparable to (and originally was continuous with) the pleura that surrounds each lung and the peritoneum that surrounds the abdominal viscera. The function of all these bags of celomic lining surrounding mobile viscera is the same: to allow the enclosed viscera to expand and contract without rubbing against or tearing adjacent organs. The part of the pericardial bag that lies directly against the heart is distinguished as *visceral* serous pericardium; the rest of the bag is called *parietal* serous pericardium (Fig. 7-6). Similar terms are applied to other celomic linings, so that we speak of visceral peritoneum, parietal pleura, and so on. The line along which the serous pericardium curves away from the surface of the heart—that is, where visceral and parietal pericardium meet—is called the **reflection** of the serous pericardium. There are two sets of these pericardial reflections, one around the arteries and one around the veins. They correspond to the two ends of the central hole in the original pericardial "doughnut" (Fig. 7-6). Because the atria grow by incorporating veins, many separate veins enter the adult heart, and the margins of the venous reflection wrap around these separate veins and develop hollow fingerlike extensions that project in between them (Fig. 7-8). The largest of these lobules, which sticks up between the two lower pulmonary veins, is dignified by a name of its own— the **oblique pericardial sinus.** As the atria move up behind the ventri-

Fig. 7-7 Bending of the primitive tubular heart (A, B) as it descends into the thorax converts it into a U-shaped structure, with the atria lying dorsal to the ventricles (C). At, atrium; O, oblique sinus of the (serous) pericardium; T, transverse sinus; V, ventricle.

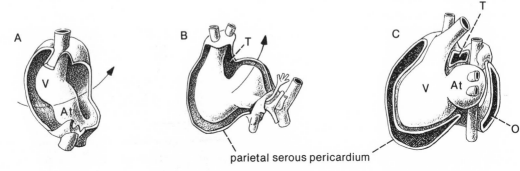

parietal serous pericardium

cles of the developing heart (Fig. 7-7), the original dorsal half of the toroidal pericardial cavity gets constricted into a narrow channel separating the two sets of pericardial reflections. This channel is called the **transverse pericardial sinus** (Figs. 7-4, 7-7, and 7-8).

Mesoderm condenses around the outside of the whole pericardial sac to form a tough external layer, the **fibrous pericardium**. Because this layer is connective tissue, it is continuous with surrounding connective tissues. It has particularly strong attachments to the fascia over the diaphragm below, the fibrous sheaths around the great vessels above, and the periosteum of the sternum in front (via a couple of little **sternopericardial** ligaments).

■ Control of the Heartbeat

The hearts of lower vertebrates will go on beating for hours when removed from the body and placed in an isotonic solution. This experiment demonstrates that the heartbeat is independent of any motor innervation. The motor nerves that supply the human heart do not initiate contraction of the heart's muscles; they only modulate its rate. Like all blood vessels, the heart has a wholly autonomic motor innervation. As you might expect, sympathetic ("fight-or-flight") motor impulses speed it up and parasympathetic impulses slow it down.

The primitive vertebrate heart is a simple muscular tube. In a fish, a wave of contraction begins at the tail end of the heart and rolls forward toward the aortic arches, squeezing the blood from the heart like toothpaste from a tube. But in higher vertebrates, the muscles of the atria are no longer continuous with those of the ventricles. The

Fig. 7-8 Reflections of the serous pericardium. Anterior view of the pericardial sac with the heart removed.

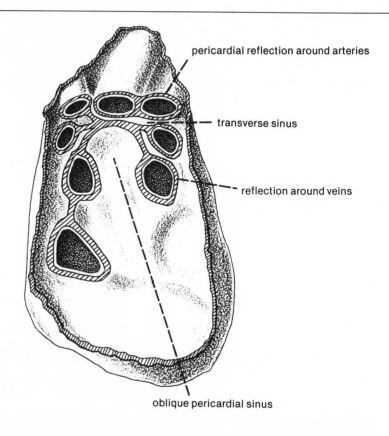

pericardial reflection around arteries

transverse sinus

reflection around veins

oblique pericardial sinus

This prevents waves of contraction starting at the atrial end of the heart from directly spreading into the ventricle.

heart wall has become fibrous between each atrium and its corresponding ventricle, providing a rigid frame for the atrioventricular valve. A wave of contraction starting at the atrial end of the heart is therefore "grounded" when it runs into the fibrous atrioventricular partition. Even if the wave of contraction could cross directly from atrium to ventricles, it would not succeed in squeezing the blood out of the human heart. The folding of the embryonic heart tube has left the inflow and outflow valves of each ventricle sitting close to each other at the top of the chamber and most of the ventricle hanging down below like a bag. If a wave of contraction were to spread directly into the ventricle from the neighborhood of the atrioventricular valve, it would drive the blood down toward the apex of the ventricle (instead of upward and away from it) and would not empty the ventricle effectively.

What is needed, then, is some way of conducting the wave of

contraction from the atria past the fibrous atrioventricular partition and carrying it directly down to the apex of each ventricle. This need has been met by specializing some of the heart's own tissues to form a little imitation nervous system made up of muscle fibers that do not contract but carry a wave of changes in electrical charge comparable to that propagated in a contracting muscle. The **Purkinje fibers** that make up this system are insulated from the surrounding cardiac muscle and stimulate contraction only at their ends, much as an axon does at its synapse. Through this internal conducting system of the heart (Fig. 7-9), a wave of muscle contraction can be transmitted from one point to another without affecting the heart muscle in between.

The "spinal cord" of the heart's imitation nervous system is a band of Purkinje fibers called the **atrioventricular bundle**. This begins in the wall of the right atrium, just above the atrioventricular opening (where its atrial end is enlarged to form an **atrioventricular node**), and runs through the fibrous atrioventricular boundary into the fleshy septum between the two ventricles. There the bundle splits into right and left limbs (**crura**), which run along the inner walls of the corresponding ventricles and branch out over the ventricles' apices. (The

Fig. 7-9 Internal conducting system of the heart. Schematic right anterior view of the right atrium and ventricle.

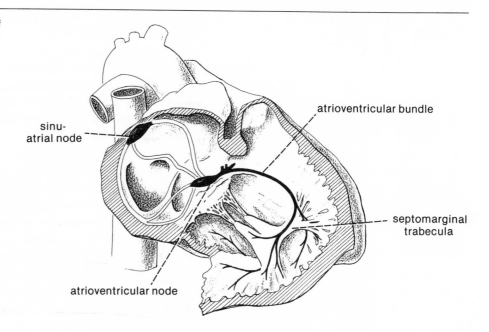

sinu-atrial node

atrioventricular bundle

septomarginal trabecula

atrioventricular node

right limb of the atrioventricular bundle usually runs through a trabecula carnea called the **septomarginal trabecula** [Figs. 7-3 and 7-9] on its way to the right ventricular apex.) Thus, even though a wave of contraction beginning in the right atrium always dies out when it reaches the fibrous atrioventricular septum, it first gets picked up by the atrioventricular node and propagated to the lower ends of the ventricles—and so the ventricular contraction begins in the right place at the right time.

What starts the original wave of contraction in the right atrium? Buried in its wall just below the opening of the superior vena cava lies the pacemaker of the heart, the **sinuatrial node**. This is another nodule of peculiarly modified muscle tissue similar to that of the atrioventricular bundle. It generates periodic impulses that initiate waves of contraction in the right atrium. Vagal parasympathetic fibers reaching the heart synapse on ganglion cells embedded in the walls of both atria. From these atrial ganglia, postganglionic fibers run to the sinuatrial node and atrioventricular node. Impulses traveling along these parasympathetic pathways slow down the heartbeat; sympathetic fibers (which are distributed to ventricles as well as atria) speed it up. But all these autonomic nerves act merely to *modulate* the tempo of the heart's intrinsically coordinated rhythm.

■ The Aorta and Its Branches

The great arterial trunk leaving the heart of a typical vertebrate embryo divides into a series of aortic arches that pass between the gill slits and reunite above the gill region, thereby forming a dorsal aorta on each side. The two dorsal aortae come together in the midline and fuse into a single descending aorta after they get past the last gill arch.

The system of aortic arches develops in the human embryo, but most of it soon disappears. The descent of the heart into the thorax and the specialization of the body-wall branches that supply the upper limb stretch and distort the remaining parts of the system so much that they are not easily recognized. These simplifications and distortions (Fig. 7-10) can be summarized as follows:

1. Aortic arches 1, 2, and 5 disappear.
2. The parts of arch 6 nearest the heart persist and become the pulmonary arteries. The connection of arch 6 to the dorsal aorta persists only on the left side, where it becomes the fetal ductus arteriosus (and the ligamentum arteriosum after birth).

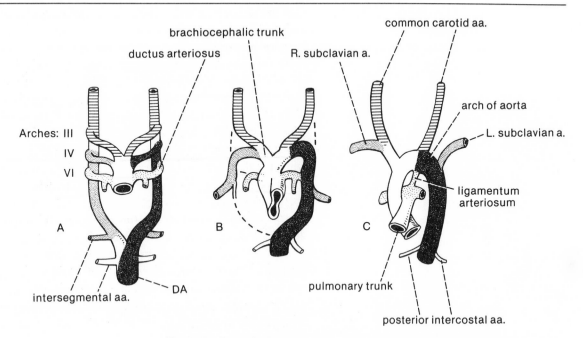

Fig. 7-10 Development of the major arteries in the thorax. Schematic ventral views. A. Arrangement six weeks after conception. B. Arrangement two days later. C. Adult arrangement. Tones on the vessels show the embryonic homologies of the adult's arteries. DA, dorsal aorta.

3. The left and right dorsal aortae disappear between arches 3 and 4, and the right dorsal aorta loses its connection with the midline (descending) aorta.

4. Because the left and right third arches are no longer connected with the descending aorta, all the blood sent into them enters the persisting cranial end of the dorsal aorta and supplies the head; the arch and attached dorsal aorta become the **common** and **internal carotid** arteries. A branch that arises from the middle of each third arch supplies the walls of the pharynx and eventually develops into the **external carotid** artery.

5. Both fourth arches persist and remain attached to their respective dorsal aortae. The left dorsal aorta is complete and carries blood around to the descending aorta. The right dorsal aorta does not. It extends tailward only far enough to reach and supply the enlarged right seventh intersegmental artery, which grows out into the developing right upper limb. That artery and the right fourth arch that feeds it become the right subclavian artery. The left fourth arch—the

only aortic arch that retains all its embryonic connections into adult life—becomes *the* arch of the aorta.

As the heart descends from the cervical region into the thorax, its connections with structures in the neck region become stretched into a cluster of great vessels springing from the top of the arch of the aorta (Fig. 7-10): two common carotid arteries (third arches) and two subclavian arteries (seventh intersegmentals) to the upper limbs. On the right side, the common carotid and subclavian arteries usually wind up sharing a short stem called the **brachiocephalic trunk**.

Apart from the three great vessels springing from the arch of the aorta (and the coronary arteries that grow out from the ascending aorta into the heart musculature), all the aortic branches arise from the *descending* aorta. They all belong to one of three groups (Fig. 10-1A): (1) paired **intersegmental** arteries to the somite derivatives, (2) paired **mesonephric** arteries to the embryonic urogenital system and associated structures, and (3) unpaired midline branches to the gut. The thoracic mesonephric arteries are vestigial and unimportant; the important representatives of this group are confined to the abdomen.

Several of the midline arteries to the gut are retained in the thorax. They are small but functionally important. A few little twigs from the descending aorta supply the esophagus. The lungs, which are out-pocketings of the gut, receive three small **bronchial arteries**—two to the left lung, one to the right—that supply the walls of the air passages. The lung thus receives two streams of blood: one (bronchial) that *supplies* the tissues of the lung and one (pulmonary) that its tissues *process* for the benefit of the whole body. Most of the bronchial blood returns to the heart via the pulmonary veins.

The intersegmental arteries are important in both thorax and abdomen, where they provide the blood supply to the skin and to the muscles derived from somites—that is, the epaxial and hypaxial muscles. Each intersegmental artery leaves the descending aorta and passes laterally into the somitic mesoderm on either side of the vertebral column. In the thorax, the upper part of the descending aorta lies to the left of the midline (because it develops from the left fourth arch), so the right intersegmental arteries have to cross the ventral side of the vertebral column before entering the adjoining muscles.

Each intersegmental artery divides into **dorsal** and **ventral rami**, which follow the corresponding rami of the spinal nerve to somitic muscle and to the skin. The thoracic and lumbar intersegmental arteries are the **posterior intercostal** and **lumbar** arteries, respectively (Chapter 5). The dorsal rami of the arteries enter the epaxial muscles and branch to accompany the nerves. In the embryo, each dorsal ramus also gives off a branch that runs back along the segmental nerve into the vertebral canal, where it enters the subarachnoid space and supplies the spinal cord. Although the dorsal arterial rami form first in the embryo, the ventral rami are much larger in the adult; the adult's dorsal rami seem like mere secondary offshoots from the intercostal and lumbar arteries.

Longitudinal anastomoses link up various branches of the intersegmental arteries, forming collateral channels that run lengthwise along the body. One of these is a ventral channel on each side near the midline of the ventral body wall, which becomes the **internal thoracic** and **epigastric** arteries (Chapter 5). Another set of anastomoses coalesces into tiny arteries running on the ventral surface of the spinal cord. After these longitudinal anastomoses form, some of their segmental tributaries degenerate, and others enlarge to take up the load; for example, most of the intercostal arteries lose their connections to the longitudinal channels accompanying the spinal cord.

The ventral rami of the seventh and the twenty-fourth intersegmental arteries become the arteries to the paired limbs. When the heart moves caudally past the cervical segments into the thorax, it drags the aortic arches down with it. As they move away from the neck region, their intersegmental branches to the cervical somites become tenuous and degenerate one by one until only the seventh one in the series remains. In an adult, this is the subclavian artery. It runs along inside the thorax up into the lower cervical region (where the limb and the heart originally developed side by side). This course brings it out of the upper end of the rib cage, and it passes laterally over the first rib into the limb. The subclavian may be thought of as an enlarged intercostal artery that the heart passed in its descent and whose origin therefore has been pulled to the summit of the remaining aortic arch. Indeed, the subclavian artery of an adult supplies the first two intercostal spaces, via another one of those longitudinal anastomoses— the **costocervical trunk** in the root of the neck (Fig. 21-19). This arrangement reflects the subclavian artery's serial homology with the intercostal arteries; it is an enlarged "intercostal artery" of the lower neck.

■ The Great Veins of the Thorax

For every channel of arterial supply in the body, there is a corresponding channel of venous return. Usually the veins follow the same pathways as the arteries. (For instance, each branch of the major artery to the forelimb is accompanied by a pair of little **venae comitantes** [L., "accompanying veins"] having the same names and covering the same territory as the arterial branches.) Near the heart, however, there are gross differences between venous and arterial pathways. This is to be expected, because the systemic veins return to the right side of the heart and the systemic arteries arise from the left side.

Blood from the lower limbs, pelvis, and abdomen returns to the heart through the *inferior* vena cava. This vessel has a very short course in the thorax because it enters the right atrium immediately after piercing the diaphragm. It need not concern us now.

The *superior* vena cava returns deoxygenated blood from the forelimbs, head, neck, and most of the abdominal and thoracic body wall. It develops from the right common cardinal and precardinal veins that drain the body wall of the embryo (Fig. 6-8). The superior vena cava has only three tributaries (Fig. 7-11): the **azygos** vein and the two **brachiocephalic** veins.

The azygos (Gk., "unpaired") vein develops from the right postcardinal vein. Like that postcardinal vessel, it drains the thoracic segments of the body wall on the right side. Running upward along the right side of the vertebral bodies, the azygos vein receives a subcostal vein and a vein from each intercostal space (except the first). It then arches forward over the root of the right lung to enter the superior vena cava. The azygos vein is paralleled on the left by remnants of the left postcardinal system, which drain the body wall and enter into the azygos vein by a variable number of anastomotic channels (**hemiazygos** veins) crossing behind the aorta.

The brachiocephalic veins carry the blood returning from the head, neck, and upper limbs. The brain and parts of the face are drained on each side by the **internal jugular** vein, descendant of the embryonic precardinal vein. The upper limb is drained by the **subclavian** vein, which receives as a tributary the **external jugular** vein bearing venous blood from the superficial layers of face and neck. Subclavian and internal jugular veins fuse on each side to form a brachiocephalic vein. On the right, this is a short vessel that soon enters the superior vena cava. The left brachiocephalic vein is longer (Fig. 8-5). It has to

Fig. 7-11 Azygos and hemiazygos veins and their connections. Anterior view with the heart and inferior vena cava removed. AHV, accessory hemiazygos vein.

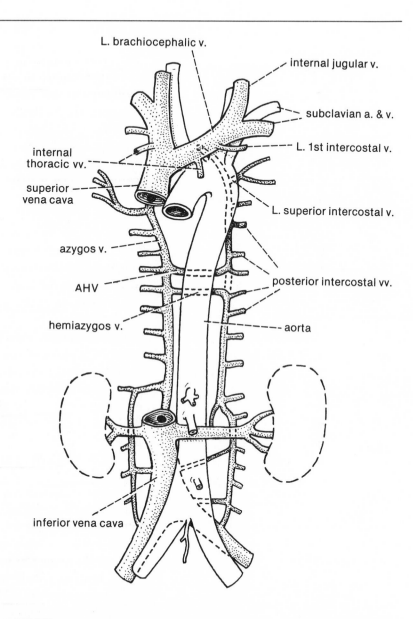

cross the great arterial vessels to get to the superior vena cava on the right side of the body. It crosses ventral to them. Contrast this with the left-side veins draining the intercostal spaces, which cross to the right behind (dorsal to) the aorta. (This reflects the fact that the left brachiocephalic vein develops as a secondary anastomosis between the common cardinal veins, replacing the atrophying left common cardinal; hence it lies in the plane of the common cardinal veins, ventral to the descending aorta [Fig. 6-8].)

Each brachiocephalic vein receives the venous drainage of the vein accompanying the internal thoracic artery and also that from the first intercostal space. The left brachiocephalic additionally is joined by a vein (the **left superior intercostal** vein) that drains the second and third intercostal spaces. The stem of this vessel is a remnant of the left common cardinal vein. In some mammals, and occasionally in man, it has a connection with the coronary sinus on the back of the heart, forming a vestigial superior vena cava on the left side.

■ The Lymphatic System

Not all the fluid distributed via the arteries returns through the veins. Some of it returns through an alternative network of vessels called the **lymphatic system**. The lymph vessels carry, not blood, but tissue fluids trickling back to the bloodstream from the interstitial spaces between cells.

Lymphatic drainage begins in the **lymph capillaries**. They are blind pouches of endothelium, a single layer of cells in thickness, and have no connection with the blood capillaries. Lymph capillaries will accept larger particles than blood vessels will, including such things as carbon particles (from the inner surface of the lungs), emulsified fat droplets (from the intestinal contents), and bacteria and other parasitic organisms.

Lymph capillaries coalesce to form larger collecting vessels, called **lymphatics**. Like many veins, lymphatics contain valves that force the fluid they collect to move in one direction only. The collected fluid (called **lymph**) is pushed along principally by pressure from adjoining muscles, viscera, and arteries, with some help from smooth muscle in the walls of the lymphatics themselves. The collected fluid soon arrives at one of the dozens of **lymph nodes** found throughout the body. Here the lymph is forced through a maze of microscopic sinuses containing white blood cells (mainly B and T lymphocytes) that engulf and destroy bacteria or other intruders.

Why should anyone bother to learn the anatomy of such an inconstant and amorphous system? Clinicians need to learn it because the lymph channels are highways for the spread of infections or cancer, and the spread of such diseases can be monitored and assessed by palpation or biopsy of the lymph nodes. A lymph node containing invading organisms becomes enlarged as lymphocytes proliferate inside it to combat the infection, so the condition of the lymph nodes reflects the extent and spread of localized infections. Because lymph nodes trap and harbor abnormal cells, they are secondary centers in the metastasis of many forms of cancer. When a malignant tumor is excised, neighboring lymph nodes often need to be dissected out and removed as well.

All the lymph in the body returns to the brachiocephalic veins. Most of it is collected and emptied into the left brachiocephalic vein by a single big lymphatic, the **thoracic duct**, which drains lymph from the entire body below the diaphragm and also from the thoracic body wall (Fig. 7-12). The thoracic duct begins on the front of vertebral body T.12 or L.1 and runs up through the thorax along the front of the vertebral column. At first it lies to the right of the midline, but it moves over to the left side when it reaches vertebra T.5 or thereabouts. (Its two ends differ in this way because it developed from originally paired lymph trunks; its lower part is derived from the right member of the pair, and its upper, terminal end derives from the left member.) As the thoracic duct enters the neck, it hooks around behind the common carotid artery and ends by emptying into the left brachiocephalic vein—or into one of that vein's two major tributaries, the left subclavian and internal jugular veins.

The other lymphatic trunks also empty into the beginning of the brachiocephalic vein (or its two tributaries). On the right side, there are usually three terminal lymph trunks: the **jugular** trunk from the head and neck, the **subclavian** trunk from the upper limb (and the adjoining side of the rib cage), and the **bronchomediastinal** trunk from the heart and lung. They sometimes hook up with each other in various ways before ending in the brachiocephalic vein. All three may unite to form a short **right lymphatic duct** (Fig. 7-12). The corresponding lymph trunks on the left side usually empty into the thoracic duct, but they too may have separate venous connections. The openings of all these lymphatics into the veins are guarded by bicuspid valves that prevent blood from backing up into the lymph vessels.

If lymphatics—even the thoracic duct—are blocked or tied off, usually nothing significant happens. Because the lymphatic vessels are so anastomotic, injuries or obstructions seldom interfere with lymph drainage. Lymph that cannot get back to the bloodstream through one lymphatic will take a circuitous path and return via another lymph trunk. But a general blockage of lymph channels from any area of the body—for example, in the disease called elephantiasis, in which the lymph nodes become crammed and congested with the eggs

Fig. 7-12 Lymphatic system in the thorax (schematic).

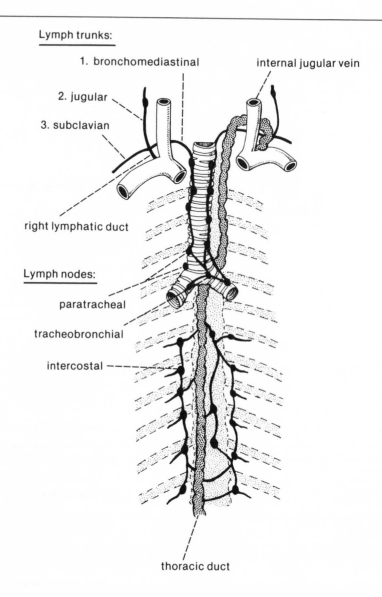

Lymph trunks:

1. bronchomediastinal

internal jugular vein

2. jugular

3. subclavian

right lymphatic duct

Lymph nodes:

paratracheal

tracheobronchial

intercostal

thoracic duct

of parasitic worms—will cause tissue fluids to accumulate, thereby producing swellings that may reach grotesque proportions. This phenomenon shows why the lymphatic system is needed: it provides a route through which fluids and dissolved substances (especially macromolecules and particulates) can drain away from the body's tissues without having to force their way "uphill" against osmotic gradients into the blood capillaries.

The Thorax

8

The **trachea,** or windpipe, is a tubular outgrowth of the gut. It begins as a bud from the floor of the pharynx and grows tailward into the rib cage. Here it forks, and each fork (called a **primary bronchus**) keeps on growing and dividing like a branching tree, resulting in the formation of two **lungs** inside the rib cage. As the embryonic lungs grow out from the tail end of the trachea, the celom wraps around them. Covered with a film of celomic lining, the lungs expand around either side of the heart and press against the upper abdominal viscera.

The abdominal and thoracic parts of the celom are broadly confluent with each other in embryonic life (Fig. 8-1). In amphibians and most reptiles, they remain confluent in the adult, which thus has only two celomic cavities—the pericardial cavity and a single, big celomic space that envelops the abdominal viscera (and sends left and right extensions up on either side of the heart to wrap around each lung). In mammals, however, the thorax and abdomen are separated in the adult by a muscular partition called the **diaphragm.** An adult mammal thus has at least four celomic cavities—one around the heart, one around each lung, and one more in the abdomen. (Human males also have two more in the scrotum, surrounding the testes.)

Like most mammalian peculiarities, the diaphragm is associated with a high metabolic rate. It permits a more rapid and efficient turnover of respiratory gasses. Primitive air-breathing fish, like modern lungfish or frogs, had to rely on swallowing movements to gulp air into their lungs. Early reptiles evolved an improved method of breathing by suction, known as **thoracic respiration.** The breakthrough that made thoracic respiration possible was the appearance of a true rib cage, produced by stretching some of the thoracic ribs down to touch the sternum. The ribs that extended to the sternum had a joint at each end, and they could rotate around the axis defined by the two joints. When a typical reptile inhales, its ribs swing toward its head, with each rib rotating around its vertebral and sternal ends.

Fig. 8-1 Subdivision of the embryonic celom. A. Schematic cross section through the heart of a five-week embryo. The pleural and pericardial cavities are broadly open into each other and the abdominal celom. B. Similar section at seven weeks: the pleuropericardial folds have fused dorsal to the heart, separating pericardial and pleural cavities. A small opening into the abdominal celom persists on the right; this would normally close during the sixth week. C. Diagram of the six celomic spaces in a male adult. H, heart; L, lung; T, testis.

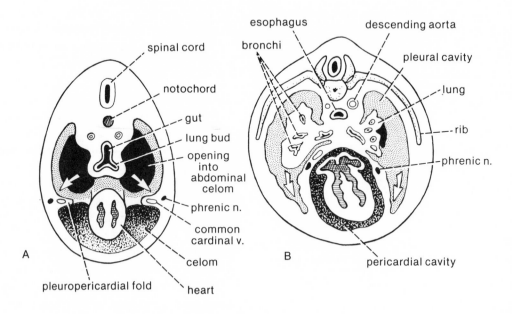

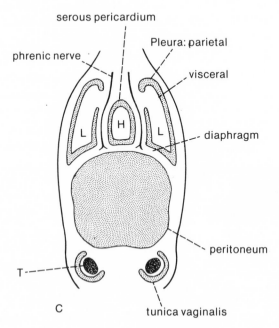

This movement, which is usually compared to lifting the handle on a bucket (Fig. 8-2), increases the side-to-side diameter of the thorax and thus increases thoracic volume. Air rushes into the lungs to fill this added volume. The inhaled air is pushed out again by dropping the costal "bucket handles" back toward the vertebral column again. Hug your rib cage, inhale deeply, and observe where and how your thorax expands to draw air in.

The pumplike action of thoracic respiration was an improvement over gulping air like a fish. But it was not very efficient by itself, because part of the thoracic volume was filled on inhalation by the stomach, liver, and other abdominal viscera slithering up into the thorax. You can get some idea of how this affects respiratory volume by contracting your abdominal muscles sharply ("sucking in your gut") when you inhale, thus shoving your stomach and liver up into your rib cage. Some device was needed to make these viscera stay put so that the volume added by lifting the ribs would be wholly filled by inrushing air.

In most modern reptiles, this problem has been handled by introducing a sheet of elastic connective tissue stretched across the abdominal end of the rib cage. When the ribs swing outward in inhalation, this partition becomes taut, preventing the abdominal viscera from moving up into the thorax. Thus, all the volume added to the thorax by the outward swing of the ribs contributes to the expansion of the lungs instead of being partly wasted in sliding the stomach and liver back and forth.

Fig. 8-2 Rib movements in breathing. When we inhale, our ribs swing out and sideways (B) like the handle on a bucket (A). They also rotate around an axis determined by each rib's two joints with the vertebrae (C), which causes the thorax to expand ventrally as well (*dotted lines*).

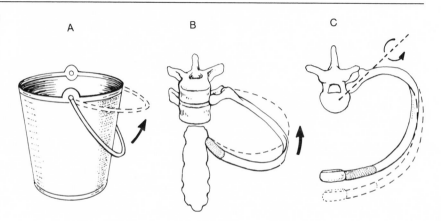

In mammals, this arrangement is still further improved by making the partition out of voluntary muscle. This muscular dome, the diaphragm, forms the floor of the human thorax (Fig. 8-3). When it contracts, it flattens out, increasing the volume of the thorax and shoving the abdominal viscera directly below it down toward the pelvis. Mammals can therefore breathe without moving their ribs, merely by contracting and relaxing the diaphragm. This kind of breathing is called **abdominal respiration.** The acquisition of a diaphragm in mammals probably explains why mammals lack ribs in their abdominal body wall; the abdomen must be able to bulge out freely to accommodate the viscera that are shoved tailward when the diaphragm contracts.

Abdominal breathing is characteristic of human babies. Babies' ribs are mostly cartilaginous; and they lie in a more horizontal plane, so the "bucket handles" are already fixed in the lifted position and cannot be lifted much to expand the thorax. In adults, the ribs have the bony rigidity and the orientation needed to transmit and with-

Fig. 8-3 Midline section of diaphragm (*black*) seen from the left side, showing the vertebral levels at which it is pierced by the inferior vena cava (IVC), esophagus (ES), and aorta (AO). The heart (H) is shown as a dotted outline.

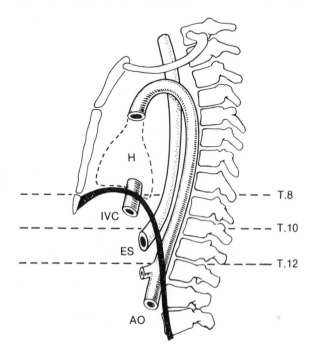

stand the stresses of thoracic breathing, so both abdominal and thoracic breathing are normally combined in each inhalation.

■ Anatomy of the Human Diaphragm

The diaphragm is a sheet of hypaxial muscle, derived mostly from cervical body segments. Its muscle fibers can be thought of as the missing parts of the incomplete layer of body-wall muscles in the neck, torn away and carried tailward by the expanding lungs as they grew down from the pharynx. In the adult, these originally cervical fibers are attached all around the caudal margin of the rib cage (including the lower end of the sternum) and to the top three lumbar vertebrae. From this ring-shaped origin, the diaphragm's muscle fibers converge on a tendinous patch lying just below (caudal to) the heart. The diaphragm is therefore dome-shaped, with the heart sitting atop the apex of the dome (Fig. 8-3). The dome's tendinous apex is called the **central tendon** of the diaphragm. It is roughly V-shaped, with the legs of the V extending dorsally around either side of the vertebral column. This tendinous part of the diaphragm is derived from the **septum transversum** (Fig. 9-4), a mass of unsegmented mesoderm that started out as a partition between the amniotic cavity and the yolk sac back when the heart was sitting out in front of the embryonic head. The heart remains attached to the central tendon indirectly via ligaments binding the fibrous pericardium to the apex of the V, so the heart rides up and down on the diaphragm as we breathe.

When the diaphragm is at rest, the apex of the central tendon lies in front of vertebra T.8 or T.9; in deep inhalation, it may fall as low as T.11, carrying the heart with it. Because the diaphragm's ventral attachments are at sternal level (about T.9) and its dorsal attachments are to the lowest ribs and upper lumbar vertebrae, the dorsal surface of the diaphragm slopes steeply tailward (Fig. 8-3).

The aorta, inferior vena cava, and gut run longitudinally between thorax and abdomen, so they must pass through holes in the diaphragm. The descending aorta, lying just ventral to the vertebral column, squeezes through between the vertebral bodies and the edge of the diaphragm. The diaphragm's edge is formed here by a tendinous arch over the aorta, the **median arcuate** ligament, from which some muscle fibers of the diaphragm take origin (Fig. 8-4). To either side of this median ligament, the diaphragm is thickened to form a

Fig. 8-4 Lower surface of diaphragm and its attachments. IVC, inferior vena cava.

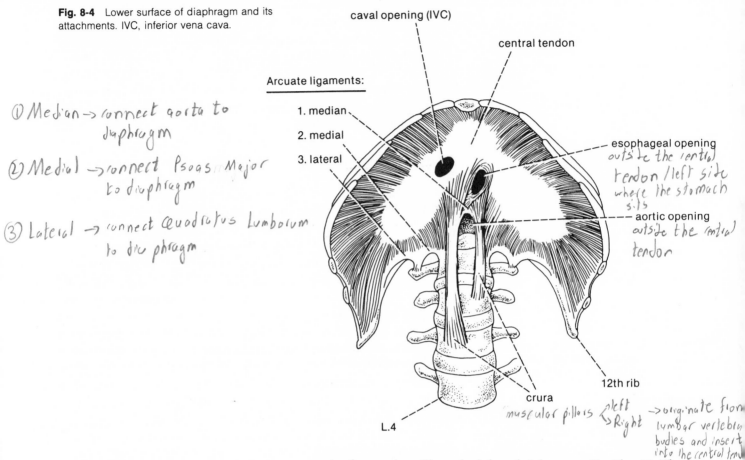

(handwritten annotations)

① Median → connect aorta to diaphragm

② Medial → connect Psoas Major to diaphragm

③ Lateral → connect Quadratus Lumborum to diaphragm

caval opening (IVC)

central tendon

Arcuate ligaments:

1. median

2. medial

3. lateral

esophageal opening *outside the central tendon / left side where the stomach sits*

aortic opening *outside the central tendon*

12th rib

crura
muscular pillars { left, Right } → *originate from lumbar vertebra bodies and insert into the central tendon*

L.4

pair of muscular pillars, the left and right **crura** (L., "legs"). The crura originate from the lumbar vertebral bodies and fan out craniad to insert into the central tendon. Because the heart rides on the central tendon and the inferior vena cava passes directly into the right atrium of the heart, the **caval opening** for that vein lies in the tendon, just to the right of the midline. The third big opening in the diaphragm lies just outside the central tendon, cradled in the notch of the V. Through it passes the **esophagus,** the thoracic part of the gut that connects the pharynx with the stomach. The esophageal opening lies on the left side, where the stomach sits. The muscle fibers of the diaphragm's *right* crus, oddly enough, divide and swing over to the left to form a loop around the esophagus. This loop may have some limited sphincteral action on the esophagus. Two longitudinal hypaxial muscles lying alongside the vertebral column pass between the body wall and the edge of the diaphragm and are therefore (like the aorta) bridged by tendinous arches from which diaphragmatic fibers arise (Fig. 8-4): the **medial** (not median) **arcuate** ligament bridging the hind-limb muscle Psoas Major and the **lateral arcuate** ligament bridging Quadratus Lumborum. All these dorsal tendinous arches along the back edge of the diaphragm are tacked down to the bodies and transverse processes of the upper lumbar vertebrae.

▪ The Lungs and Pleura

The trachea lies in the midline of the thorax, ventral to the esophagus and dorsal to the ascending aorta and the three great branches from the peak of the aortic arch. The trachea ends by dividing into the two **primary bronchi,** each of which subdivides further into **secondary** and **tertiary** bronchial branches inside each lung. The resulting "bush" is known as the **respiratory tree.** Its surface area is huge, providing roughly 100 square meters of respiratory epithelium for gas exchange. The lung is composed of the respiratory tree and the highly vascular mesodermal tissues that surround it. As the fetal lungs form around the proliferating bronchi, branches of the great pulmonary vessels grow into each lung and branch along with the branches of the respiratory tree, getting ready to flood the lung's tissues with right ventricular blood and drain oxygenated blood back to the left atrium in postnatal life. The arterial branches generally run in front of (ventral to) the branches of the bronchial tree. The upper (superior) pulmonary vein on each side enters the lung *in front of* the primary bronchus and drains the ventral parts of the lung; the lower (inferior) vein runs *behind* the bronchus and drains the more dorsal parts. As usual, the veins are more likely than the arteries to deviate from the standard setup; there may be one or three veins on either side. The point where the bronchus and vessels disappear into the substance of the lung is called the **root** of the lung.

Because the heart lies mostly to the left of the midline, the left lung has less room on its side and is smaller than the right lung. This difference between the two lungs shows up in the respiratory tree. The right primary bronchus divides into three secondary bronchi, but its counterpart on the left has only two secondary branches.

The celomic space surrounding each lung is called a **pleural cavity.** The two pleural cavities are separated by the mass of structures in the midline of the thorax—the heart and its great vessels, the gut derivatives (trachea and esophagus), and the thymus gland or its remnants in front. The massive partition formed by these organs, interposed between the two lungs (and their pleurae), is called the **mediastinum** (Figs. 8-5 and 8-6). Each pleural sac is a bag of a synoviumlike connective tissue, wrapped around a lung all the way back to its root—somewhat like a closed plastic bag folded around the cap of a mushroom (Fig. 8-1C). The space inside the bag is the pleural cavity. Normally, this space is negligibly thin, containing only a film of a watery lubricant fluid. The connective tissue that forms the bag is called **pleura.** It is conventionally divided into **visceral pleura,** in contact with the lung's surface, and **parietal pleura,** adhering to the inner walls of the thorax. The pleura is elastic. If it were not, the lungs and the surrounding structures would not be able to expand during inhalation.

Each secondary bronchus collects a more or less separate mass of

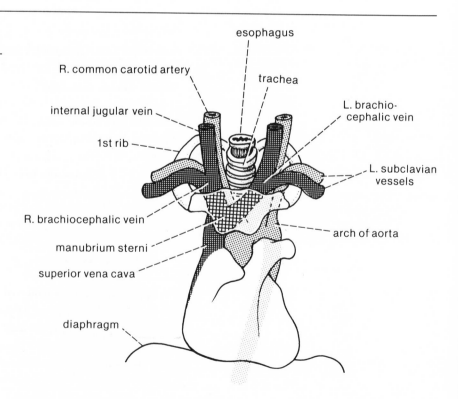

Fig. 8-5 Principal mediastinal organs, seen from in front with thorax removed. The first rib forms a collar around the great vessels emerging from the mediastinum.

esophagus

R. common carotid artery

trachea

internal jugular vein

L. brachio-cephalic vein

1st rib

L. subclavian vessels

R. brachiocephalic vein

arch of aorta

manubrium sterni

superior vena cava

diaphragm

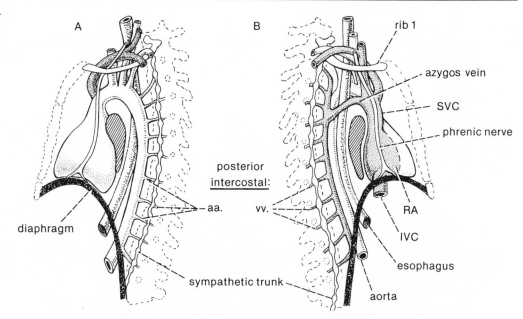

Fig. 8-6 Contents of the mediastinum, viewed from the left (A) and right (B) sides. Uniform stipple indicates right atrium (RA) and veins; the roots of the lungs are diagonally hatched. aa., arteries; vv., veins; IVC, inferior vena cava; SVC, superior vena cava.

lung substance around its branches, forming little sub-lungs called **lobes.** The divisions between them are visible grossly because the visceral pleura dips in between them. There are, of course, three lobes in the right lung and two in the left, corresponding to the number of secondary bronchi in each. Although each tertiary bronchus also supplies its own separate subdivision of a lobe, these smaller units or **bronchopulmonary segments** are not separated by folds of visceral pleura the way the lobes are. They therefore cannot be seen in dissection. The usual arrangement of tertiary bronchi is shown in Figure 8-7. It is of considerable clinical importance, because infections or obstructions may affect only a single tertiary bronchus and hence may be confined to a single bronchopulmonary segment.

The various parts of the parietal pleura are named for the part of the thoracic walls to which they adhere—**diaphragmatic** pleura over the upper (thoracic) surface of the diaphragm, **costal** pleura over the inside of the rib cage, and **mediastinal** pleura lying against the mediastinum. The parietal pleura also bulges out a little through the superior thoracic outlet, forming a dome known as the **cupola** of the pleura. This bulging dome is protected by the clavicle in front and by the head of the first rib in back and is supported by the apex of the lung

Fig. 8-7 Lungs, lobes, and segments. U, upper lobe; M, middle lobe; L, lower lobe. Bronchopulmonary segments: 1, apical; 2, apicoposterior; 3, anterior; 4, lateral; 5, medial; 6, posterior; 7, superior; 8, anterior basal; 9, lateral basal; 10, medial basal; 11, posterior basal; 12, inferior lingular; 13, superior lingular.

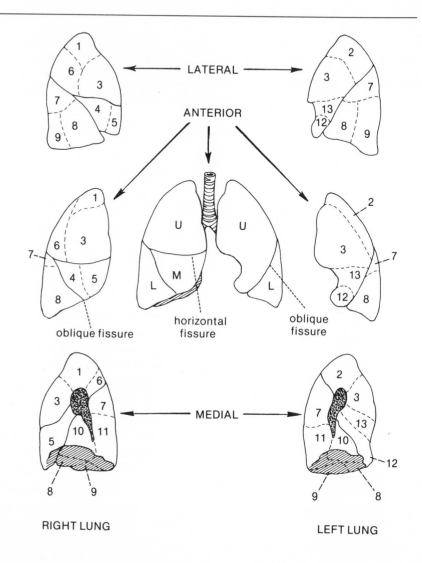

RIGHT LUNG   LEFT LUNG

pressing against it from underneath. Because the lung cannot expand upward past this pleural cupola during inhalation, it must expand downward. It does this by sliding into and filling the potential space between the costal and diaphragmatic pleura when the diaphragm descends. This potential space between the lower ribs and the sloping dorsal face of the diaphragm is called the **pleural recess.** The function of the pleura is to lubricate the movements of the lungs as they slide up and down inside the rigid rib cage with each cycle of breathing. When infection or scarring leaves the inside of the pleural sac less slippery, there may be chafing between visceral and parietal pleura, whereupon breathing becomes painful. This condition (or any other inflammation of the pleura) is known as **pleurisy**.

■ Mechanics of Breathing

During quiet breathing, the diaphragm is the most important respiratory muscle in adult human beings. The role of the Intercostals is debated. Electromyographic studies suggest that the **Scaleni** may be more important than the Intercostals in lifting the ribs during inspiration, especially during deep inspiration. The Scaleni, which represent the remnants of the lateral body-wall layers in the neck, extend from the cervical transverse processes down to the first two ribs. The first costal cartilage has no synovial joint with the sternum but is joined directly to the manubrium by a synchondrosis. Therefore, when the Scaleni contract, the first ribs and the sternum swing forward and upward as a single unit. *Anteroposterior* diameter of the rib cage is increased directly by this means and by rotation of each rib on its two vertebral facets (Fig. 8-2). The indirect pull exerted by the Scaleni on the other ribs (via the intercostal muscles) raises the costal "bucket handles" and thus increases the *transverse* diameter of the thorax. The Intercostals help to lift the ribs but do not draw them closer together. If you press your left fingertips to the right side of your neck in front, just above the first rib, you may be able to feel the Scaleni contract when you inhale deeply.

In forced breathing, all the muscles attaching to or wrapping around the rib cage can come into play. You can easily feel the lateral muscles of your own abdominal wall contracting when you cough; this helps push the diaphragm upward and anchors the lower ribs so that the Internal Intercostals can draw the ribs downward. A vigorous cough produces a sudden increase in intraabdominal pressure and so may precipitate a rupture of a loop of intestine through one of the weaker spots in the abdominal wall. Some of the limb muscles that originate from the rib cage also aid in forced exhalation, as you can observe by coughing with your hand thrust into your armpit and feeling the surrounding shoulder muscles contract.

■ Somatic Innervation of the Respiratory Apparatus

The diaphragm and intercostal muscles are under voluntary control. They are striated, body-wall muscles and receive no autonomic innervation. This comes as a surprise to many people, for breathing is not usually a voluntary activity and continues even during sleep or unconsciousness.

Breathing is an excellent example of an involuntary behavior powered by voluntary musculature. Another familiar example is the involuntary retraction of one's hand from an unexpected pain such as a paper cut or a bee sting. In such cases, the "decision" to contract striated muscles is made by the spinal cord or the brain stem without consulting the higher brain centers that are involved in conscious volition. You can breathe voluntarily (otherwise speech would be impossible), but if you neglect to do so, the respiratory centers in the brain stem will undertake the job on their own without waiting for "permission" from the cerebral cortex. This allows breathing to go on when you are asleep, or anesthetized, or knocked unconscious.

Most of the musculature of the diaphragm is derived from cervical hypaxial musculature that descended into the thorax ahead of the growing respiratory tree. When it descended, it dragged along its motor nerve from the **cervical plexus** of ventral rami. This nerve, the **phrenic** nerve, comprises fibers from spinal nerves C.3, C.4, and C.5. Because the diaphragm gets its motor innervation from all the way up in the midcervical region, spinal-cord injury at the level of vertebra C.5 that produces virtually complete paralysis below the neck will not affect the diaphragm—and may have little effect on breathing.

Early in embryonic life, the phrenic nerves lie on the inner surface of the body wall (Fig. 8-1A). As the common cardinal veins are drawn toward the midline, pulling across the folds of celomic lining that wall off the pleural cavities from the pericardial cavity, the phrenic nerves are drawn with them (Fig. 8-1B). In the adult, the phrenic nerves therefore run down out of the neck, lateral to the major vessels above the heart, and pass between the lung and the heart—that is, between the fibrous pericardium medially and the parietal pleura laterally—to reach the diaphragm on either side of the pericardial sac (Fig. 8-1C). There they pierce the diaphragm near its apex and send branches across its abdominal surface. In dissection, the phrenic nerves can be seen through the mediastinal pleura on each side, running across the lateral aspect of the fibrous pericardium just in front of the root of the lung (Fig. 8-6).

■ The Autonomic Nerves of the Thorax

The vagus nerves carry the **parasympathetic** outflow from the brain to the gut and its muscles. In the thorax, the vagus on each side lies in direct contact with the esophagus, the thoracic part of the gut. The only structures that pass in between vagus and gut are the aortic arches. In early embryonic life, the aortic arches lie against the gut in the neck and the vagus passes caudally around them to reach the last gill arch. As development continues, the heart descends into the thorax, taking the remnants of the aortic-arch system with it. The descending aortic arches pull the vagal fibers to the gill-arch muscles out into a loop. This loop is called the **recurrent laryngeal** nerve (Fig. 8-8).

The left and right recurrent laryngeal nerves differ, because of asymmetrical development of the aortic-arch system. On the right, the lateral end of the sixth arch disappears, and the vagus reaches the gut after it passes the fourth aortic arch (subclavian artery). On the left, the sixth arch persists as the ductus arteriosus in the fetus and the ligamentum arteriosum in the adult, and the vagus must pass these structures before it can reach the gut. The adult's *right* recurrent laryngeal nerve therefore hooks around the subclavian artery, but the *left* one comes off the vagus further down in the thorax and hooks around the ligamentum arteriosum (Fig. 8-8).

Because the lungs are derivatives of the gut, the smooth muscles lining the trachea and bronchi are innervated like other gut muscles, by vagal parasympathetic fibers. Spastic constriction of these muscles narrows the airways and can produce bronchial asthma. This condition can be relieved by administering epinephrine or other drugs with effects mimicking those of sympathetic innervation.

Sympathetic impulses to the thoracic viscera begin in the thoracic segments of the spinal cord, enter the sympathetic trunk via a white ramus communicans from a thoracic ventral ramus—and then run up into the neck, synapse in the cervical part of the trunk, and run down into the thorax again. This seemingly illogical pathway is the logical consequence of two facts discussed earlier: (1) the thoracic viscera develop in the cervical region, and (2) sympathetic outflow from the spinal cord is restricted to segmental nerves T.1 to L.2. Because there are no sympathetic fibers in the cervical nerves' ventral roots, the body's cervical segments must get their sympathetic innervation from thoracic fibers that run up into the cervical extension of the sympathetic trunk and synapse. From there, postsynaptic fibers leave the

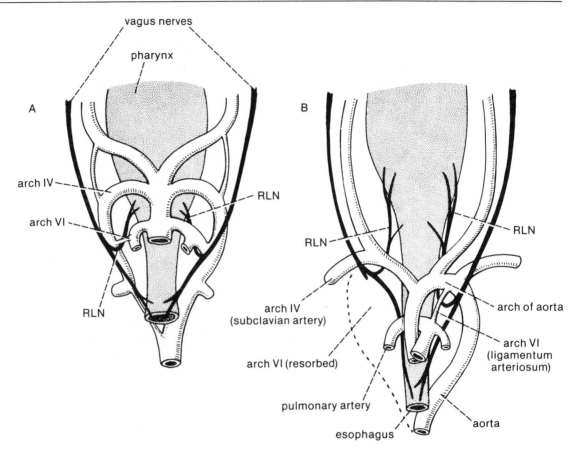

Fig. 8-8 The recurrent laryngeal nerves (RLN) are at first bilaterally symmetrical (A). They become asymmetrical because the lateral end of the right sixth arch is resorbed as the heart and aortic arches descend into the thorax (B).

cervical ganglia of the trunk and run to the cervical structures. The heart and lungs get innervated in this way early in ontogeny and then later descend into the thorax. As they descend, they drag their post-synaptic sympathetic nerves with them, forming **cardiac** nerves (Fig. 9-16) that extend down from the cervical (and upper thoracic) para-vertebral ganglia to the thoracic viscera.

The cardiac nerves are joined by parasympathetic fibers from the vagus on each side, forming skeins of autonomic motor fibers that wrap ventrally around the esophagus and over the roots of the lungs,

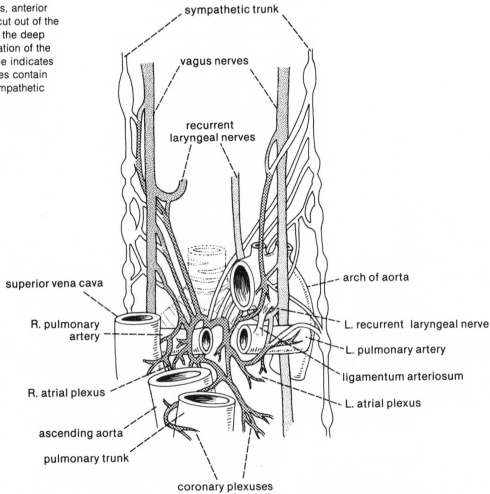

Fig. 8-9 Thoracic autonomic nerves, anterior (ventral) view. Sections have been cut out of the aorta and pulmonary trunk to reveal the deep cardiac plexus in front of the bifurcation of the trachea (*dotted outline*). Light stipple indicates vagal fibers: coarsely stippled nerves contain both sympathetic and vagal parasympathetic fibers.

sympathetic trunk

vagus nerves

recurrent laryngeal nerves

superior vena cava

R. pulmonary artery

R. atrial plexus

ascending aorta

pulmonary trunk

arch of aorta

L. recurrent laryngeal nerve

L. pulmonary artery

ligamentum arteriosum

L. atrial plexus

coronary plexuses

ending up in a plexus behind the heart (Fig. 8-9). This **deep cardiac plexus,** lying in front of the bifurcation of the trachea, surrounds the roots of the pulmonary arteries. From this plexus, some fibers follow the pulmonary arteries into the lungs, forming a **pulmonary plexus** around these arteries; others pass into the heart. The ones that enter the heart can be grouped into two **atrial plexuses** on the back of the heart and two **coronary plexuses** that innervate the ventricles and coronary arteries. The fibers in each atrial plexus arise from the sympathetic trunk and vagus more caudally than do the fibers in the coronary plexuses. This arrangement reflects the fact that the venous (atrial) end of the heart was originally caudal (Fig. 6-8). Most of the vagal fibers reaching the heart pass into the atrial plexuses to convey pulse-slowing impulses to the heart's intrinsic "pacemaker" system; the few vagal fibers that reach the coronary plexuses may have a vasoconstrictive effect on the coronary arteries, but this is not certain.

■ The Lymphatics of the Thorax

Because cancers of the breast and lung are common, the lymphatic vessels and lymph nodes of the thorax are clinically important. Lymph draining from the thorax and its contents follows one of three routes:

1. Lymph from the superficial tissues—the skin, the breast, and the limb muscles attached to the outside of the rib cage—drains toward the **axillary** nodes in the armpit. It returns from those nodes to the bloodstream via the subclavian trunk.

2. Lymph from the lungs and heart drains toward the important cluster of **tracheobronchial** nodes grouped around the bifurcation of the trachea. Lymphatics emerging from those nodes join others draining from **diaphragmatic** nodes on the upper surface of the diaphragm, from **brachiocephalic** nodes lying in the upper mediastinum, and from **parasternal** nodes alongside the sternum that receive lymph from the anterior intercostal spaces (corresponding to anterior intercostal branches of the internal thoracic blood vessels). The composite lymph vessels thus formed are the bronchomediastinal lymph trunks, which carry the lymph back to the bloodstream as described earlier (Fig. 7-12). Note that lymph draining from a cancerous breast may carry tumor cells into the thorax, via the anterior intercostal drainage.

3. Lymph from the posterior ends of the intercostal spaces passes through **intercostal** nodes and thence into the thoracic duct. The upper right intercostal spaces drain into the right lymphatic duct or into some tributary of that vestigial and variable right-side equivalent of the thoracic duct. The lower intercostal nodes may be connected with each other and with the abdominal lymphatics by longitudinal trunks (Fig. 7-12), which dissectors sometimes mistake for the sympathetic trunk.

THE ABDOMEN
AND
THE PELVIS

PART III

9

The
Abdominal
Viscera

■ The Abdominal Gut

The vertebrate digestive tract is a tube with two openings—the mouth and the anus. Although it is a simple, straight tube early in prenatal life, it is neither simple nor straight in the adult. It is not straight because it is about nine meters long and has to be thrown into complicated convolutions to fit inside a human body. It is not simple because it has developed various outpocketings or diverticula, thereby forming accessory viscera such as the lungs and the liver.

The *thoracic* part of the gut (the esophagus) elongates during ontogeny at about the same rate as the thoracic walls; so it remains simple and straight. In contrast, the *abdominal* part of the gut becomes long and convoluted, filling most of the abdomen. Most of the abdominal volume that is not filled by the gut is occupied by two gut diverticula, the liver and the pancreas. The abdominal gut proper is divided into three major sections: the stomach, the small intestine, and the large intestine or colon.

The **stomach** is an elastic bag lying just below the diaphragm. It receives chewed food from the esophagus at the top and churns it into a sour slurry for discharge into the small intestine. Anyone who has ever vomited is unpleasantly familiar with the appearance, consistency, and taste of stomach contents. Vomiting is one of the reasons for the stomach's existence. If the esophagus continued straight on into the small intestine, unwholesome or poisonous food could not be easily rejected once it has been gulped down. The stomach serves as an easily emptied testing chamber. Swallowed food is held in the stomach for some time by contraction of a muscular ring surrounding the stomach's lower outlet. This **pyloric sphincter** not only retains food in the stomach until it has been found suitable for digestion; it also regulates the rate at which stomach contents are allowed to move on after they have proved acceptable. Enough food to keep the small intestine occupied for hours can be packed away in the expansible stomach in a few minutes and held there by the pyloric sphincter until the intestines are ready to receive it.

The stomach's upper (esophageal) opening lies on the left side of the body, and its pyloric outlet lies on the right side of the body. The stomach therefore crosses the midline. It does this by curling downward across the front of the aorta and inferior vena cava. Its whole left side is ballooned outward to form a large sack (Fig. 9-1). The upper end of this leftward bulge is especially large and bulbous. It is called the **fundus,** and it presses up against the underside of the diaphragm. The concave right edge of the stomach is called the **lesser curvature** and the convex left edge is the **greater curvature.** The distal end of the stomach, where it empties into the small intestine, is known as the **pylorus** (Gk., "gatekeeper"). The lining of the stomach is thrown into folds, wrinkles, and pits, giving it a large surface area. Many glands of different sorts are embedded in the stomach's wall and discharge their secretions into its interior. These secretions include digestive enzymes, mucus, and a watery fluid containing hydrochloric acid.

The **small intestine** is conventionally divided into three sections: the **duodenum** at the stomach end, the **ileum** at the other end, and the **jejunum** in between. Although there are no sharp boundaries between the three parts of the small intestine, there are characteristic differences between them, which reflect their differences in function. After the stomach contents pass into the small intestine, they are mixed with digestive juices that the liver and pancreas dump into the middle stretch of the duodenum. Most of the work of extracting nourishment from the intestinal contents is done in the lower duodenum and the jejunum, downstream from the point where the liver and pancreas add their secretions. These parts of the small intestine have a very rich blood supply (and thus look reddish in a living person), and their walls are thick because they are thrown into a series of **circular folds** (plicae circulares) that increase their surface area (Fig. 9-2). Compared with the jejunum, the ileum is thinner walled, less reddish and vascular, and distinguished by big interior patches of aggregated lymphatic tissue (Peyer's patches).

The **large intestine,** as its name implies, has a larger lumen than the small intestine has, and its contents move along more slowly. This encourages the growth of bacteria. The swift movement and high

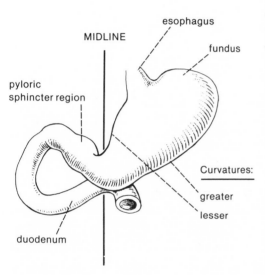

Fig. 9-1 Stomach and duodenum. Ventral view.

Fig. 9-2 Section of the jejunum, opened to show circular folds. The anastomotic arteries lying in its mesentery supply it via numerous **vasa recta** (L., "straight vessels").

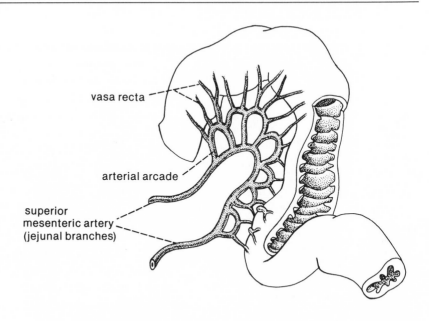

vasa recta

arterial arcade

superior mesenteric artery (jejunal branches)

acidity of the contents of the stomach and upper part of the small intestine tend to keep that part of the gut fairly free of microorganisms; but bacteria find a more congenial environment in the colon, where they multiply until they form about 10% of the dry weight of the intestinal contents. Normal intestinal bacteria aid in digestion by breaking down constituents of our food that we cannot digest without their help—for example, cellulose and pectin. They metabolize these compounds and synthesize vitamins and other trace nutrients that the walls of the colon absorb. In rabbits, horses, and many other animals that have a high-cellulose diet, the colon is long and expansive, with a long, blind pouch called the **cecum** (L., "blind") sticking out from it where the small intestine ends and the colon begins. In these animals, this bag provides a sort of compost heap for fermentation and breakdown of grass and leaves. Human beings have a short cecum, a bit broader than it is long, hanging down from the ileocolic junction (Fig. 9-3). The dorsal side of its tip bears a slender worm-shaped extension, the **vermiform** (L., "worm-shaped") **appendix.** The human appendix has masses of lymphatic tissue in its walls and seems to provide a local defense against infection from microorganisms in the colon. It is large and specialized compared with the equivalent

cecum = first part of the colon. It bears the

Fig. 9-3 Schematic of the abdominal gut.

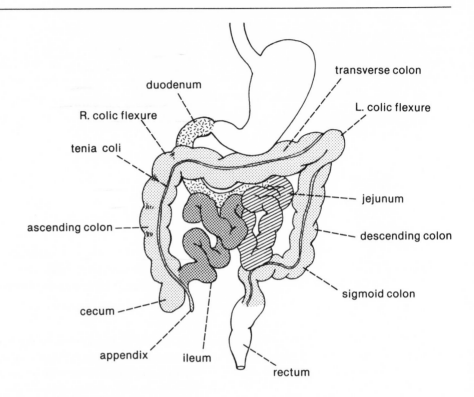

structures in monkeys. People sometimes speak of it as a vestigial organ, as though it were a useless remnant of a long cecum like that of a rabbit. It is not. Like any other mass of lymph tissue, the appendix is prone to infection. An acute infection may cause it to rupture when the walls of the cecum contract, thus spilling intestinal contents and bacteria into the abdominal celom. Before antibiotics, rupture of the appendix ordinarily resulted in a fatal celomic infection (peritonitis) and rapid death.

The colon begins in the lower right part of the abdomen. From there, it runs up to touch the lower edge of the liver, where it bends abruptly to cross the abdomen from right to left, forming a graceful drape below the stomach's greater curvature (Fig. 9-3). When it reaches a point near the left edge of the stomach, it kinks again and runs down the left side of the abdomen to end in the rectum and anus. The two kinks in the colon are called the right and left **colic flexures,** and they divide the colon into three sections—ascending, transverse, and descending. The lower end of the descending colon forms a sinuous loop called the **sigmoid** (Gk.,"S-shaped") **colon.** Three longitudinal bands of muscle called **teniae coli** (L., "ribbons of the colon") begin at the appendix and run along the entire length of the colon's outer surface. They are taut, and their tension throws the underlying colic wall into a series of bulges and intervening "tucks" or puckerings. The bulges are called **haustra.**

■ The Abdominal Celom and Mesenteries

The abdominal part of the celom is the **peritoneal cavity,** and the serous tissue enclosing it is called the **peritoneum.** In the typical body segment, the celom is an empty cavity wrapped around the ventral side of the gut. The gut is not entirely surrounded by the celomic cavity but remains connected to the dorsal wall of the celom by a mesenteric sheet (Fig. 1-12) containing vessels and nerves. The part of the abdominal celom that surrounds the ileum and jejunum fits this typical description. However, the ileum and jejunum are so much longer than the abdomen that they have to loop back and forth, filling the abdomen with sinuous coils of gut and converting their dorsal mesentery into a fan-shaped structure that looks something like a pleated curtain gathered together at one end.

The celomic relationships of the rest of the abdominal gut are more complicated. Although the embryo starts out with a tidy, bilaterally symmetrical arrangement like that seen in the typical body segment, this symmetry is rapidly lost as the gut elongates and twists around and various mesenteries adhere to each other or to parietal peritoneum. These ontogenetic processes greatly distort the original setup.

The chordate celom forms as a cavity in mesoderm. In amniotes, this cavitation begins in extraembryonic mesoderm; so the celom initially forms as the chorionic cavity—outside the embryo—and only later spreads into the embryonic disk. The celom spreads into the embryo around the mouth of the yolk sac, where it burrows into the mesoderm and wraps itself up dorsally around the sides of the gut tube. From the region of the yolk sac, the growing intraembryonic celom sends extensions forward and backward along the left and right sides of the gut. These right and left celomic extensions fuse with each other around the ventral side of most of the abdominal gut, thus forming a single cavity with a U-shaped cross section. The right and left celomic extensions also merge together in the thorax, thus forming a celomic arc across the ventral surface of the heart. In between the thorax and the lower abdomen, however, in the region of the stomach and duodenum, these left and right celomic cavities stay separate—or, to put it another way, this part of the gut has not only the usual dorsal mesentery but also a **ventral mesentery,** a double fold of celom lining running from the gut to the inside of the ventral body wall. This **ventral mesogastrium** (Fig. 9-4) extends all the way from the navel up to the lower surface of the diaphragm.

The ventral mesentery persists here because of the liver and its vascular connections. The liver, the largest gland in the body, develops as a branching glandular outgrowth of the duodenum, to which it remains connected by its "stem", the **common bile duct.** Through this duct, the liver expels excretory products and emulsifying agents (to promote fat absorption) into the gut. A saclike outgrowth of the bile duct, the **gallbladder,** stores the trickling liver secretions when they are not needed and contracts to squirt them out through the common bile duct into the duodenum when the need arises.

Although the liver's digestive functions are important, its major function is as a metabolic buffer between the gut and the rest of the body. The gut lining is not very selective about what it absorbs; it is equally happy moving nourishing sugar or poisonous alcohol into the bloodstream. To prevent undesirable substances from being picked

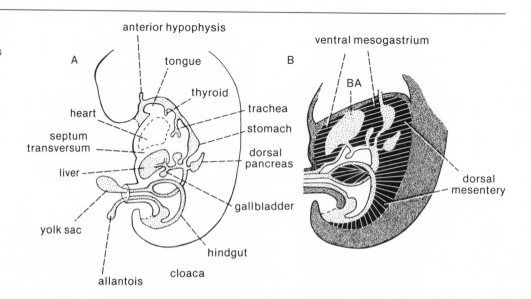

Fig. 9-4 Abdominal viscera in a 9-mm human embryo. A. The gut and its outpocketings. B. Its mesenteries. BA, bare area of liver.

up by the gut and dumped directly into the systemic circulation, all the blood draining from the abdominal parts of the gut is brought together into a single **portal** vein that enters the liver and breaks up into capillarylike vessels called **sinusoids.** The liver cells surrounding the sinusoids remove poisons and excess nutrients from the blood and metabolize or store them. Thus purified and filtered, the blood from the sinusoids is gathered together again into a variable number (from eight to twenty-three) of short **hepatic** veins that carry blood away from the liver. They empty into the inferior vena cava where it lies in contact with the liver, just below the caval opening in the diaphragm.

All these venous channels in the adult, from the portal vein's main tributaries up through the liver sinusoids to the upper end of the inferior vena cava, are derivatives of the **vitelline** veins that drained the blood from the embryo's yolk sac (Fig. 9-5). The liver grows out of the gut into the septum transversum (Fig. 9-4) underneath the heart. As it expands, it gradually surrounds the vitelline veins. The parts of those veins that the liver surrounds branch and break up to

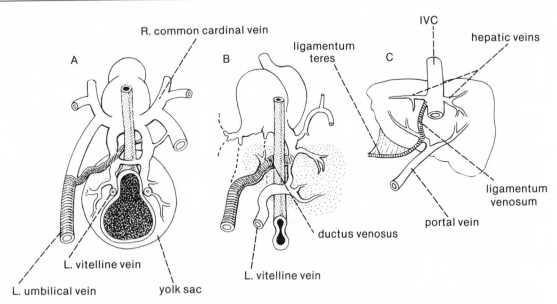

Fig. 9-5 Successive stages (A, B, C) in the development of the hepatic portal system, seen from the dorsal aspect. In postnatal life (C), the vessels that brought in placental blood (*hachure*) degenerate into fibrous cords (ligamentum teres, ligamentum venosum). Stippled area in B indicates the location of the developing liver.

form the liver sinusoids; the parts near the heart form the hepatic veins (and the upper end of the inferior vena cava); and the parts down near the mouth of the yolk sac form the portal vein and its main tributaries (the **splenic** and **superior mesenteric** veins that drain the abdominal gut).

The umbilical veins (originally the veins of the allantois) that return oxygenated blood from the placenta to the body also come to feed into the vitelline veins (Fig. 9-5). Thus, even after the yolk sac and its vasculature degenerate and disappear, the fetal liver remains connected to the navel by the umbilical veins, so the ventral mesentery enclosing the liver and these veins persists from navel to stomach. The liver lies in the middle of this mesenteric sheet, dividing it into two parts: the **lesser omentum** between liver and stomach, and the **falciform** (L., "sickle-shaped") ligament between liver and navel (Fig. 9-9).

▪ The Abdominal Circulation and Its Development

The abdominal gut is supplied with blood by midline arteries coming off the aorta. There are three of these arteries in the adult human abdomen (Fig. 9-10): the **celiac trunk** that supplies the stomach and upper duodenum (and the attached liver), the **inferior mesenteric artery** to the descending and sigmoid colon, and the **superior mesenteric** artery to the parts of the gut in between (lower duodenum, jejunum, ileum, cecum and appendix, ascending colon, and transverse colon). The superior mesenteric artery of the embryo also sends blood to the yolk sac; so it is known as the vitelline artery in early prenatal life (Fig. 9-6).

The aorta extends into the tail in a fish, giving off midline branches to the gut all the way down to the anus. It also gives off intersegmental arteries supplying the body wall and its muscles, including the hind fins that project from the body wall near the anus. In human beings, the hind "fins" are enormous and the tail is vestigial. As a result, the intersegmental arteries to our lower limbs are greatly enlarged, and the tail end of the aorta degenerates into a tiny threadlike vessel. It is so tiny and threadlike that classical anatomists did not recognize it as a continuation of the descending aorta; so they gave it a different name (the median sacral artery). The human aorta seems to end in front of vertebra L.4 by splitting into two big vessels—the **common iliac** arteries (Fig. 9-7). These are the bloated derivatives of

Fig. 9-6 Major arteries (white) and veins (stippled) of a human embryo of four weeks, as seen from the left side.

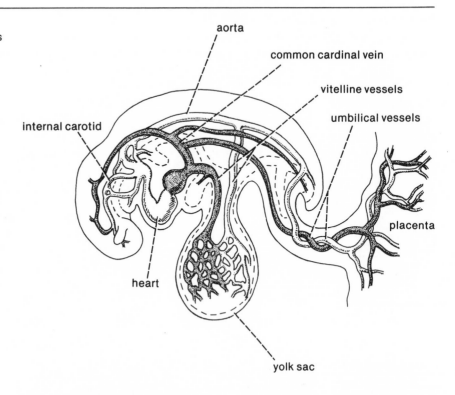

the little intersegmental arteries that grow out into the budding hind limbs of the human embryo. These arteries have taken over the job of supplying the pelvic gut and its derivatives. They run down to the upper edge of the sacrum, where each divides into an **external iliac** branch (to the lower limb) and an **internal iliac** branch that enters the pelvis to supply blood to the pelvic gut and other viscera.

The allantois forms in the human embryo as a diverticulum from the pelvic part of the gut; so it is also supplied with blood via the internal iliac artery during fetal life. The arteries of the allantois are extremely important in higher mammals because they vascularize the fetal tissues in the placenta. They are accordingly renamed the **umbilical** arteries in the human fetus (Fig. 9-6). There are two umbilical arteries (one from each internal iliac artery). They run up out of the fetal pelvis along the inner surface of Rectus Abdominis to enter the umbilical cord. Blood from these arteries courses through the capillary bed of the placenta, giving off waste products and picking up oxygen—the ancient functions of the reptilian allantois. The blood

Fig. 9-7 Lower end of the aorta and its branches in the adult. Ventral view.

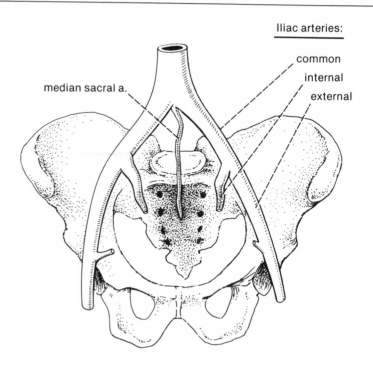

Iliac arteries:

median sacral a.

common

internal

external

vessels of our allantois, unlike those of a reptile or bird, also pick up *nutrients* from the mother's blood, thus usurping the ancient function of the yolk sac. In a human adult, vestiges of the allantois and its arteries persist on the inner face of the belly muscles as three fibrous cords climbing out of the pelvis to converge on the navel—the degenerated allantois (the **urachus**) in the midline, with an obliterated umbilical artery to either side of it.

Blood returning from the placenta is laden with oxygen and nutrients. At first, this blood has its own direct pathway back to the heart via paired allantoic vessels called **umbilical** veins (Figs. 9-5 and 9-6). But as the multiple venous returns from the abdomen merge and coalesce to form a single channel (the inferior vena cava) draining into the right atrium, the umbilical veins lose their direct connection with the heart. They wind up emptying into the hepatic portal vein along with the rest of the blood from the abdominal gut. (The allantois is, after all, a specialized part of the gut.) The right umbilical vein soon degenerates, thus leaving only one functioning channel through which food and oxygen can reach the developing fetus. It is desirable to avoid putting the placental blood return through the capillary bed in the liver, where it would become contaminated with deoxygenated blood. Accordingly, a new, more direct pathway from the placenta to the heart is formed during the second month of prenatal life. This shunt, the **ductus venosus,** runs from the portal vein straight to the inferior vena cava just below the heart and carries the fresh placental blood around the liver (Fig. 9-5) with little contamination from the staler portal drainage. At birth, when blood stops flowing into the body through the navel, the umbilical vein and ductus venosus close off. They too degenerate into fibrous cords. The umbilical vein becomes the **round** ligament (ligamentum teres) **of the liver,** and the ductus venosus becomes the **ligamentum venosum.** Together, these two cords tie the adult's portal vein to the navel in front and the inferior vena cava in back.

The anatomy of the adult liver is partly determined by all the functional and vestigial blood vessels that are attached to it and divide it into lobes (Fig. 9-8). For reasons discussed below, the adult liver lies mostly in the upper right quadrant of the abdomen, pressed up against the abdominal face of the diaphragm. The diaphragm gives it its general shape; it is a sort of fleshy cast of the diaphragm's dome-shaped underside. Most of the surface of the liver is surrounded by the flattened peritoneal sac, and is therefore clothed in visceral peritoneum. But the back of the liver's right lobe lies against and partly surrounds the inferior vena cava; and the two are connected there by the hepatic veins through which the blood in the liver returns to the heart. Because the peritoneal cavity does not intrude between the liver and the inferior vena cava, the adjacent parts of the liver thus lie in direct contact with the diaphragm. This area of direct contact is the **bare area** of the liver (Fig. 9-8B).

■ The Loss of Bilateral Symmetry

Because the ventral mesentery persists in the region of the liver, the fetal stomach and liver are enclosed in a single midline septum of mesentery, which runs from the aorta in back to the navel in front (Fig. 9-9). This septum divides the head end of the peritoneal cavity into left and right halves. It is called the **mesogastrium** (that is, mesentery of the stomach).

As the liver becomes intimately connected to the veins on the right side that are coalescing to form the inferior vena cava, the liver shifts

Fig. 9-8 Ventral (A) and dorsal (B) views of the adult human liver. C, caudate lobe; Q, quadrate lobe. The ligamentum venosum, represented in (B) by a dashed line (from ligamentum teres to a hepatic vein), separates the caudate lobe from the left lobe.

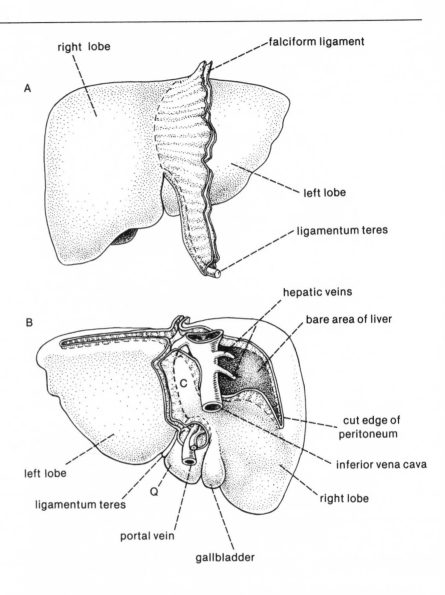

The liver starts at the midline and then moves toward the right

out of the midline toward the right. The stomach correspondingly rotates to the left. As the liver and stomach rotate around each other, the mesogastrium becomes S-shaped in cross section (Fig. 9-9B). The umbilical vein and the falciform ligament enclosing it pass to the right from the navel to reach the liver. The liver's original dorsal connections—nerves, arteries, portal vein, and common bile duct—come to

Fig. 9-9 The abdominal gut and its outgrowths, seen from the left side (diagrammatic). A. Bilaterally symmetrical condition. B. Arrangement after gut rotation.

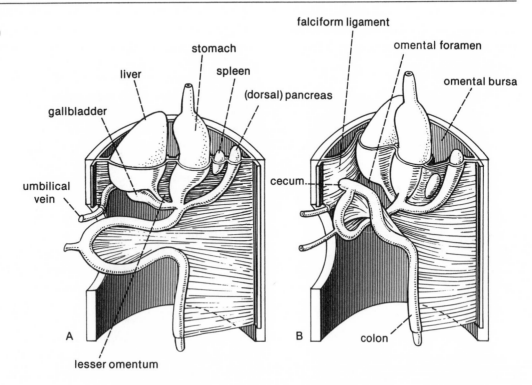

run transversely in the lesser omentum, which is the part of the mesogastrium that stretches between the stomach and liver.

Because of this rotation of the stomach and liver, the part of the celom that originally lay to the right of the lesser omentum comes to lie mostly behind it—that is, dorsal to it. Like its counterpart on the left, this right-sided celomic extension becomes separated from the thoracic celom by the diaphragm. It winds up forming a blind pouch lying dorsal to the stomach and lesser omentum. This pouch is called the lesser peritoneal sac, or (more properly) the **omental bursa.** It communicates with the rest of the abdominal celom (the so-called greater sac) through a narrowed aperture behind the caudal edge of the lesser omentum. This aperture, the **omental** or **epiploic foramen** (Gk. *epiploon* = L. *omentum*), is clinically important because a loop of small intestine can be forced through it into the omental bursa, thereby resulting in a sort of internal hernia with consequent intestinal strangulation.

While the embryonic stomach and liver are rotating around each other, the abdominal part of the gut has been growing longer. At this stage of development, the abdomen is short and most of the space inside it is filled by the liver; so the elongating gut protrudes outside the abdominal wall into the umbilical cord (Fig. 9-9) and forms the **primary intestinal loop** with the degenerating yolk sac at its apex. The whole protruding loop is supplied with blood by the vitelline artery that originally supplied the yolk sac.

At first, the primary intestinal loop lies in the midline plane. As the gut grows longer, the loop starts to twist and fold up. It twists counterclockwise around the vitelline artery (Fig. 9-9). The yolk sac soon atrophies, but the part of its artery that supplies the loop of gut persists. In adult life, it is called the **superior mesenteric** artery.

With further development, the trunk grows longer, making more room in the abdomen available for the intestines. The primary intestinal loop then slides back into the abdominal cavity, twisting further counterclockwise to a total of about 270°; and the large intestine winds up arranged in a loop that carries it ventrally across the upper (cranial) end of the small intestine and back down towards the pelvis again. All the parts of this loop (Fig. 9-10) are still attached to the dorsal celom wall by a twisted web of mesentery containing a fan of anastomosing branches from the superior mesenteric artery. These arterial branches supply the derivatives of the primary intestinal loop; the jejunum, ileum, cecum, and ascending and transverse colon. The rest of the colon, from the left colic flexure down to the rectum, is supplied via another midline mesenteric branch of the aorta—the **inferior mesenteric** artery (Fig. 9-10). The two mesenteric arteries meet and anastomose with each other at the left colic flexure.

■ The Celiac Trunk and the Dorsal Mesogastrium

The stomach and duodenum are not derivatives of the primary intestinal loop. Their dorsal mesentery (the dorsal part of the mesogastrium) contains a different artery, the **celiac trunk** (Figs. 9-10 and 9-13). This supplies the stomach and duodenum, as well as four other viscera that develop within the mesogastrium.

Three of these other mesogastrial viscera develop as outgrowths from the duodenum. The most cranial of these three outgrowths becomes the liver (and gallbladder). The other two fuse to form the pancreas. Originally, there is a *dorsal* pancreas that grows out of the duodenum into the *dorsal* mesogastrium, and a smaller *ventral* pan-

Fig. 9-10 Schematic ventral view of the two mesenteric arteries. The superior mesenteric artery forms large anastomotic loops within the mesentery of the small intestine and the (fused) mesentery of the ascending colon. It anastomoses with the inferior mesenteric artery at the left colic flexure.

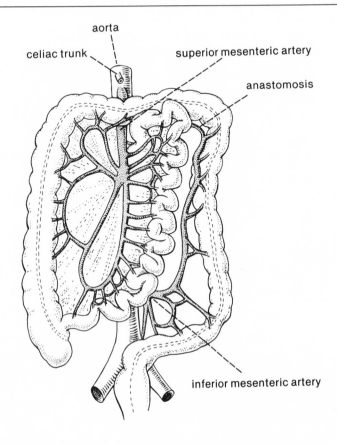

creas that grows out (from the lower end of the common bile duct) into the *ventral* mesogastrium. As the liver swings to the right, the common bile duct rotates around behind the duodenum, carrying the ventral pancreas with it; and the two pancreases touch and fuse into a single gland (Fig. 9-11). The ventral pancreas becomes the **head** of the pancreas, with the duodenum winding along its right margin. The dorsal pancreas becomes the long **body** of the pancreas. When the ventral pancreas swings around behind the duodenum, it moves to the left behind the superior mesenteric artery and its vein; so the definitive pancreas winds up hook-shaped, with the superior mesenteric vessels running ventrally downward through the hook (Fig. 9-12).

The dorsal pancreas usually loses its separate duct; it expels its digestive juices through a secondary connection that opens up be-

Fig. 9-11 Development of the pancreas. The ventral (v) and dorsal (d) pancreatic rudiments develop separately (A), but come into contact as the stomach (S) and liver rotate around each other (B and C). Usually, the dorsal pancreas will lose its own duodenal opening and come to empty directly into the common bile duct (D). The duodenum is cut open in (D) to show the major duodenal papilla.

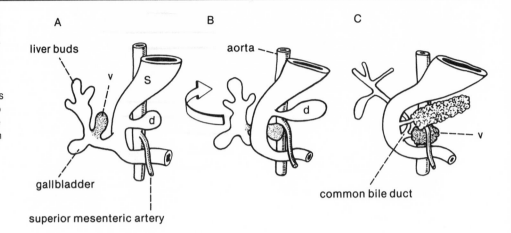

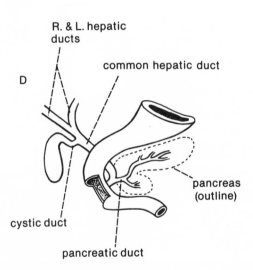

tween its ducts and those of the ventral pancreas (Fig. 9-11C and D). The dorsal pancreas may, however, retain its original duct, and the ventral pancreas may empty directly into the common bile duct or develop a separate opening into the duodenum. Thus, there may be one, two, or three openings here for digestive glands. Usually there is only one, which is guarded by a little sphincter of smooth intestinal muscle. It is marked by a small bump on the inside of the duodenum, the **major duodenal papilla,** which bears the common bile duct's opening on its apex.

In addition to the stomach, duodenum, and the three duodenal outgrowths, the mesogastrium also contains the **spleen**, which is not derived from the gut tube. This soft, blood-filled viscus starts to develop in the dorsal mesogastrium before the stomach and liver have finished their rotation around each other. The spleen is a vascular organ that has no equivalent in the typical body segment. It manufactures various sorts of blood cells, scavenges damaged red cells and other debris from the blood, and produces antibodies. All these functions can be taken over by other tissues, so the spleen can be removed surgically without causing any serious harm.

The celiac trunk arises from the aorta just below the diaphragm (Fig. 9-12) and divides at once into two large branches and a third, smaller branch (Fig. 9-13). The two large branches are the **common hepatic** artery (Gk. *hepat-*, "liver") and the **splenic** artery (Gk. *splen*, "spleen"). Their distributions reflect the embryological picture sketched above. The common hepatic artery is the artery of the ven-

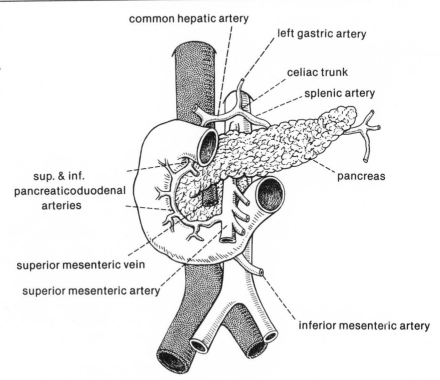

Fig. 9-12 The superior mesenteric vessels run ventrally downward through the hook formed by the adult pancreas. Their inferior pancreaticoduodenal branches help to supply the duodenum and head of the pancreas. The body of the pancreas is supplied by the splenic artery, which is partly embedded in the back of the gland.

common hepatic artery

left gastric artery

celiac trunk

splenic artery

pancreas

sup. & inf. pancreaticoduodenal arteries

superior mesenteric vein

superior mesenteric artery

inferior mesenteric artery

tral mesogastrium. It supplies, not only the liver, but also the other structures that develop in the ventral mesogastrium—the gallbladder and the head of the pancreas. Similarly, the splenic artery supplies the viscera that form in the dorsal mesogastrium—the spleen and the body of the pancreas. Both arteries also help supply the mesogastrial parts of the gut tube proper—the stomach and duodenum. The third branch of the celiac trunk, the **left gastric** artery, furnishes an additional route along which blood can reach the stomach.

The splenic artery meanders left behind the stomach to reach the spleen (Fig. 9-13). Along this route, it is embedded in the body of the pancreas, which it supplies. The common hepatic artery runs in the opposite direction, through the ventral mesogastrium (lesser omentum), to reach the liver. The common hepatic artery sends off a large **gastroduodenal** branch to the head of the pancreas, the duodenum, and the greater curvature of the stomach—and the splenic artery sends off branches to the greater curvature as well. The whole greater curvature is thus outlined by anastomotic arterial branches. Another branch from the common hepatic artery anastomoses with the left

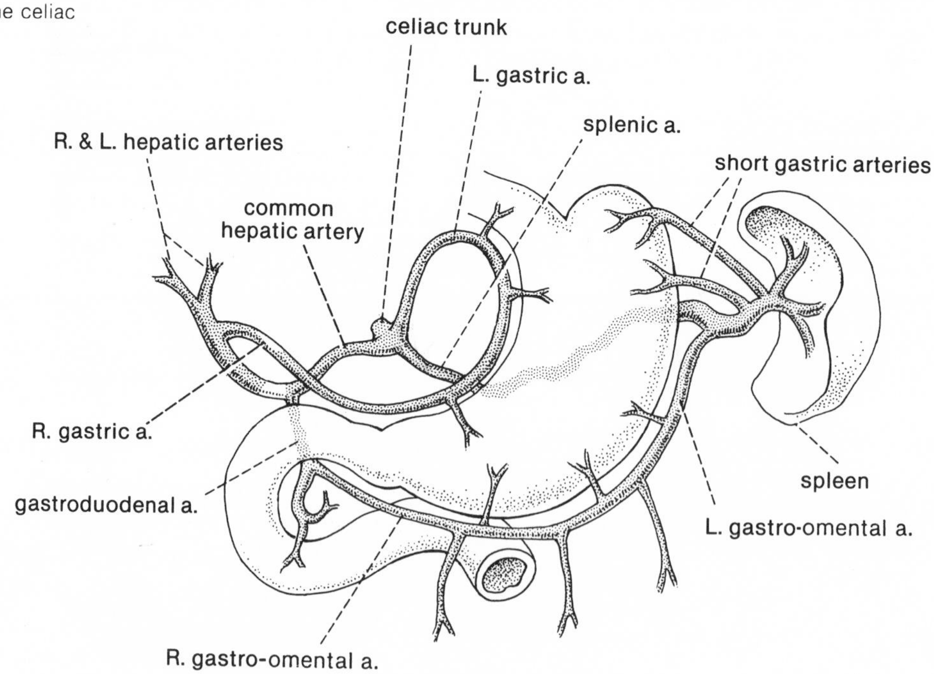

Fig. 9-13 Schematic ventral view of the celiac trunk and its main branches.

gastric to form a parallel arterial loop along the stomach's *lesser* curvature. Still another anastomosis is found on the duodenum, where pancreaticoduodenal branches of the common hepatic's gastroduodenal branch meet similarly named branches running upwards from the superior mesenteric artery (Fig. 9-12). The richly anastomotic arterial arrangement here is typical of the abdominal gut. The branches of the superior mesenteric artery that fan out through the mesentery of the jejunum, ileum, and colon also anastomose with one another, forming looping arterial **arcades** (Fig. 9-10) along the gut's mesenteric border.

■ Mesenteric Expansions and Adhesions

Late in fetal life, much of the dorsal mesentery of the abdominal gut becomes fused to the parietal peritoneum on the dorsal wall of the celom. These mesenteric adhesions leave the ascending and descending colon and most of the duodenum immobilized, unable to twist and swing around the way the jejunum and ileum can. Most of the dorsal mesogastrium also fuses to the parietal peritoneum, thus fixing the body of the pancreas firmly in place. Fusion of the duodenal mesentery similarly immobilizes the head of the pancreas. These fixed viscera—pancreas, duodenum, ascending and descending colon—are sometimes described by surgeons as "retroperitoneal," as opposed to mobile, "intraperitoneal" viscera such as the stomach and sigmoid colon. Of course, no viscera are really intraperitoneal in the sense of being inside the peritoneal cavity; the "intraperitoneal" viscera just retain mesenteric "leashes" that allow them more mobility.

Mesenteric fusion sometimes fails to occur. In such cases, the entire colon remains mobile, and there is often an associated deficiency in the rotation of the primary intestinal loop. People with this relatively common malformation usually experience no problems, but they run a risk of the colon's getting twisted and tangled around the duodenum or herniating out through weak points in the lower abdominal wall, where intraabdominal pressure is highest. Such twisting or herniation can result in a dangerous and potentially fatal interruption of blood flow to that part of the gut. Typical four-footed mammals such as dogs retain unfixed viscera but do not seem to have these problems. This suggests that our pattern of mesenteric fusions became necessary when our ancestors developed a more erect posture, which produced a 90° shift in the direction of the gravitational pull on the intestines. The more upright apes and monkeys, which swing through the trees by their arms, have more or less humanlike mesenteries, whereas quadrupedal monkeys that run atop branches on all fours have a more doglike mesenteric arrangement.

Not all the dorsal mesogastrium becomes fused in the human fetus. The part between stomach and (dorsal) pancreas remains intact, leaving the enclosed spleen with a short mesentery of its own and considerable mobility. The free dorsal mesogastrium along the stomach's greater curvature becomes expanded into a large pouch of peritoneum, the **greater omentum,** which hangs down from the greater curvature like an apron over the front of the other abdominal viscera (Fig. 9-14). This pouch covers the ventral side of the transverse colon and fuses secondarily with the colon's mesentery. In the adult, the transverse colon is therefore attached to the posterior surface of the greater omentum, which supports it against the downward pull of gravity and limits its movement. The greater omentum is laden with tags and sheets of extraperitoneal fat, and serves as a major site of fat deposition. However, its main function is to act as a second line of defense against intraperitoneal infection. It walls off such infections by adhering to any inflamed spots on the parietal peritoneum in front of it. (Most dissecting-room cadavers have a few such adhesions.) The greater omentum is richly vascularized by arteries emanating from the anastomotic loop along the stomach's greater curvature (Fig. 9-13). The arteries forming that loop are called **gastroomental** or **gastroepiploic** (Gk., "stomacho-omental") arteries for that reason.

■ The Veins and Lymphatics of the Abdominal Gut

The smaller veins of the gastrointestinal tract correspond closely to the arteries, but the larger channels into which they flow are differently arranged because they are all tributaries of the portal vein. Because there is no point in draining blood from the liver back into the liver, there is no portal-vein tributary corresponding to the hepatic artery, and the venous pattern accordingly has to differ somewhat from the arterial arrangement.

The portal vein is formed by the union of two large veins—the **splenic** vein and the **superior mesenteric** vein (Fig. 9-15). They drain the territories supplied by the corresponding arteries, with some additions—the splenic vein usually receives the inferior mesenteric drainage, and the superior mesenteric vein covers not only the primary

Fig. 9-14 Midline sections of the abdomen in the four-month fetus (A) and the adult (B). The dorsal mesenteries of the stomach and transverse colon fuse together in fetal life, leaving the transverse colon adhering to the deep surface of the greater omentum in the adult.

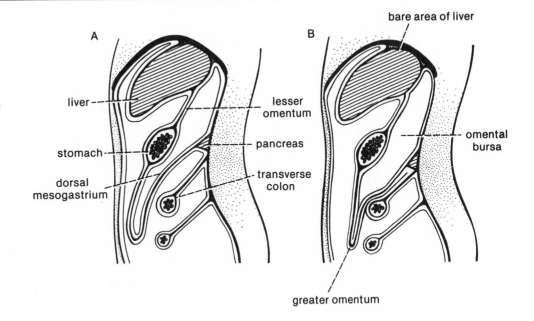

intestinal loop but also the territory supplied by the gastroduodenal branch of the hepatic artery (duodenum and greater curvature). The stomach's lesser curvature has a venous loop, corresponding to the arterial loop formed by the left and right gastric arteries, but emptying at both ends directly into the portal vein.

Almost all the abdominal lymph returns to the veins via the thoracic duct. The lower end of the duct lies below the diaphragm, on the front of vertebral body L.1 or L.2, just alongside the aorta. It is often dilated to form an elongated sac called the **cisterna chyli,** which receives tributaries from the viscera and body wall. Lymph draining into it from the small intestine is frequently milky-looking because it contains emulsified fat. Most of the lymph from the interior of the liver drains back to the same point, along the course of the hepatic artery; but some of it follows the hepatic veins and inferior vena cava up into the thorax—and the whole diaphragmatic surface of the liver drains ventrally upward, via channels in the falciform ligament, into lymphatics accompanying the internal thoracic vessels along the inside of the rib cage and up into the neck. Neoplasms originating in the liver can thus spread along a fearfully wide variety of pathways.

Fig. 9-15 The portal vein and its major tributaries. The inferior mesenteric vein usually ends in the splenic vein, as shown here; but it may join the superior mesenteric vein instead, or all three veins may meet at the same point.

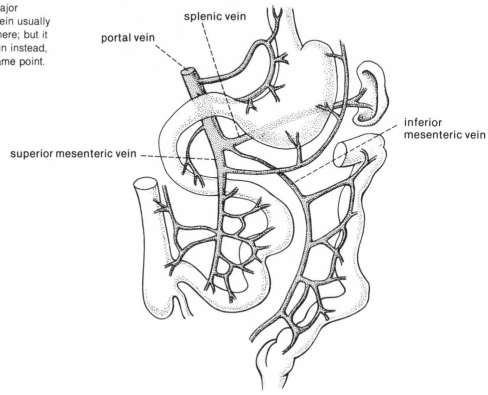

splenic vein

portal vein

inferior mesenteric vein

superior mesenteric vein

■ Gut Muscles and Their Innervation

Most of the gut's fleshy substance is smooth muscle, derived from mesoderm that condenses around the endodermal gut tube of the embryo. Throughout the abdominal part of the gut, this smooth muscle becomes disposed in two layers—an inner, *circular* layer that constricts the gut's contents like a fist squeezing a tube of toothpaste and an outer, *longitudinal* layer that controls gut length and tension. (The stomach has a third, innermost layer, which is also longitudinal.) The outer, longitudinal layer is evenly spread over the outside of the small intestine; but on the stomach and colon, it is concentrated into discrete bands—the three teniae coli on the colon and unnamed bands along the two curvatures of the stomach. The inner, circular layer of gut muscle is primarily responsible for shoving the gut contents along toward the anus with rhythmic waves of contraction (peristalsis). However, it is thickened at various points to form ring-like muscular sphincters that have the opposite effect, squeezing the gut shut and blocking the movement of its contents. The two principal sphincters are the pyloric sphincter and an **internal anal sphincter,** which holds the anus closed between defecations. (The lower end of the esophagus also acts like a sphincter to control movement of food between esophagus and stomach, but there is no anatomical sphincter there.)

The two ends of the gut tube are clothed in striated, voluntary muscle derived from somites. An **external anal sphincter,** formed by a specialized loop of body-wall muscle attached to our vestigial tail bones, surrounds the anus just below the internal sphincter. This voluntary sphincter gives us some control over where and when we expel feces from the rectum; when the internal sphincter relaxes, we can hold the anus closed voluntarily for a short period. At its other end, the gut is enveloped in striated gill-arch musculature, from the lips down through the upper two-thirds or so of the esophagus. The rest of the gut muscle is smooth muscle, derived from unsegmented mesoderm. It is therefore innervated by autonomic motor fibers and not under voluntary control.

Like the heart, the gut's smooth muscles (and glands) receive a dual innervation from both subdivisions of the autonomic nervous system. Sympathetic and parasympathetic impulses have opposite effects on the gut muscles, as they always have in regions where they overlap. The *parasympathetic* nerves are primarily responsible for maintaining and coordinating gut function. Their impulses to the gut promote the secretion of digestive fluids and produce and control the waves of peristaltic contraction that keep the gut's contents moving along. *Sympathetic* impulses do just the opposite: they dry up digestive-fluid secretion, constrict the flow of blood to the gut, close the involuntary sphincters, and inhibit peristalsis. (Anger, anxiety, or anything else that produces a general sympathetic-system stimulation therefore tends to be incompatible with good digestion.) The two autonomic subdivisions also differ in their synaptic arrangement. As in the thorax, parasympathetics synapse on microscopic ganglion cells embedded in the walls of their target organs, whereas sympathetics synapse on cells clustered in large, visible ganglia located in the dorsal wall of the celom.

Sympathetic motor fibers to the abdominal viscera originate from *thoracic* spinal nerves. (This arrangement reflects the fact that the abdominal viscera form in the thoracic region and descend into the abdomen, just as the heart descends from the cervical region into the thorax.) The preganglionic sympathetic fibers to the viscera of the abdomen leave the spinal cord through ventral roots, enter ventral rami, and cross via rami communicantes to the sympathetic trunk—exactly like preganglionic sympathetics to the skin or heart. But unlike those other preganglionic fibers, they do not synapse in the ganglia of the trunk. Instead, they pass through the sympathetic trunk without synapsing and continue medially to clusters of ganglion cells lying on and around the aorta. These **preaortic ganglia** (Fig. 1-11) are grouped at points where major visceral arteries arise from the abdominal aorta. The nerves that connect the sympathetic trunk to the preaortic ganglia are called **splanchnic** nerves (Gk. *splanchna,* "innards"). They are made up of the preganglionic sympathetic motor fibers to the abdominal viscera (and visceral sensory fibers following sympathetic pathways back in the opposite direction). The preganglionic fibers run through the splanchnic nerves to the preaortic ganglia, where they synapse. From there, postganglionic fibers travel with the arterial branches to the viscera.

The principal preaortic sympathetic ganglia and their connections are shown in Fig. 9-16. The largest are the **celiac ganglia** on either side of the celiac trunk. They receive not only the **greater splanchnic** nerves (that carry most of the visceral branches from the thoracic part of the sympathetic trunk) but also the fibers of the vagus nerve that enter the abdomen along with the esophagus. (The vagal fibers, of course, do not synapse in the celiac ganglia.) A web of dense pre- and postganglionic autonomic fibers, including both sympathetics and vagal parasympathetics, ties the two celiac ganglia to each other and to the ganglia adjoining the origin of the superior mesenteric artery, forming a lumpy, stringy network called the **celiac plexus.** Because of its size and complexity, this tangle of ganglia was once known as the *cerebrum abdominale* (L., "abdominal brain"); it was also called the solar plexus, from a fancied resemblance of its radiating fibers to the rays of the sun.

The parasympathetic fibers from the vagus nerve pass through the celiac plexus to accompany the branches of the celiac trunk and superior mesenteric artery. They innervate the parts of the gut that those arteries supply—which is to say, almost the whole abdominal gut, from the lower esophagus down to the left colic flexure.

The rest of the abdominal gut—descending colon, sigmoid colon,

Fig. 9-16 Abdominal sympathetic innervation (schematic).

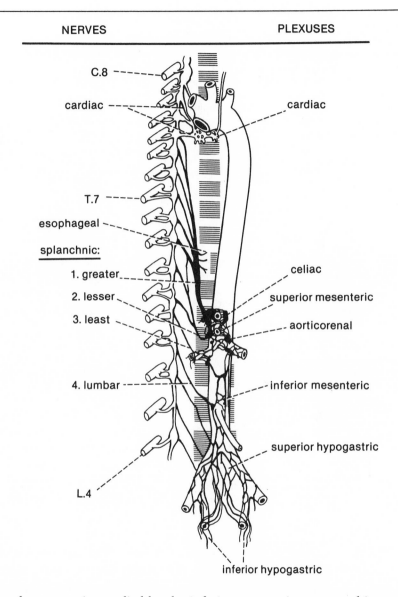

NERVES

PLEXUSES

C.8

cardiac

cardiac

T.7

esophageal

splanchnic:

1. greater

2. lesser

3. least

celiac

superior mesenteric

aorticorenal

4. lumbar

inferior mesenteric

superior hypogastric

L.4

inferior hypogastric

and rectum—is supplied by the *inferior* mesenteric artery and innervated by the *sacral* parasympathetic outflow. Preganglionic parasympathetic fibers emerge from the spinal cord through the ventral roots of spinal nerves S.2–S.4. They leave the ventral rami of those nerves on the front of the sacrum to pass into a network of autonomic nerve fibers surrounding the rectum and the internal iliac vessels on each

Fig. 9-17 The hypogastric plexuses and their connections. Postganglionic sympathetic fibers from the sympathetic trunk (*cross-hatched*) run medially into the plexuses, forming lumbar splanchnic (LSP) and sacral splanchnic (SSP) nerves (*black*). Preganglionic parasympathetic fibers from ventral rami S.2–S.4 enter the inferior hypogastric plexuses as **pelvic** splanchnic nerves (*dark stipple*).

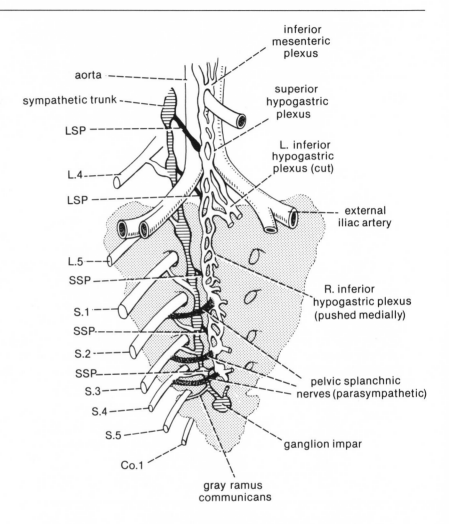

side. The three strands of parasympathetic fibers connecting the ventral rami to these plexuses bear the confusing name of **pelvic splanchnic** nerves. Unlike all the other axon bundles called "splanchnic nerves," these are strictly parasympathetic and have no connection to the sympathetic trunk.

The networks of nerve fibers on either side of the rectum are called the **inferior hypogastric plexuses.** Through them, the sacral parasympathetic outflow is distributed to the rectum and other pelvic viscera. Some of the parasympathetic fibers run upward from the inferior hypogastric plexus on each side to reach the inferior mesenteric plexus on the front of the aorta. They pass through this plexus (without synapsing in its ganglia) and follow branches of the inferior mesenteric artery to supply the sigmoid colon and descending colon. The left colic flexure, where the inferior and superior mesenteric arteries anastomose, therefore marks the approximate boundary between vagal and sacral parasympathetic territory in the abdominal gut.

Postganglionic *sympathetic* fibers (and accompanying visceral sensory fibers) are also distributed to the rectum and other pelvic viscera through the inferior hypogastric plexuses. They reach those plexuses via two routes. Some sympathetic fibers run medially from *paravertebral* ganglia (of the sympathetic trunk) and enter the inferior hypogastric plexuses. Others reach those plexuses from above, descending from the *preaortic* ganglia surrounding the origin of the inferior mesenteric artery. These descending fibers follow the route taken by the sacral parasympathetic fibers that climb out of the pelvis toward those same ganglia. The resulting skein of ascending parasympathetic and descending sympathetic fibers in the midline is called the **superior hypogastric plexus.** It hangs down between the common iliac arteries like a narrow loincloth hanging down between a person's legs (Fig. 9-16), and divides into the two inferior hypogastric plexuses near the upper edge of the sacrum (Fig. 9-17).

The bundles of sensory and postganglionic sympathetic fibers that tie the hypogastric plexuses to the sympathetic trunk are called lower **lumbar splanchnic** and **sacral splanchnic** nerves. After giving them off, the sympathetic trunk continues downward to end on the front of the coccyx. There it unites with the trunk of the opposite side to form a midline **ganglion impar** (L. *impar*, "unpaired"), of uncertain function (Fig. 9-17).

The Evolution and Development of the Urogenital Organs

10

■ History of the Excretory System

Every living thing is chemically different from its surroundings. A living organism must therefore continually work to bring matter in across its boundary, rearrange and sort through it, and eject the unwanted materials while holding back the things that are needed. This process of sorting and ejecting is called **excretion.** Any part of the body surface can serve as an excretory organ. The human body gets rid of many unwanted substances via the skin, the gut, and the lungs, but the bulk of the excretory work is done by two specialized organs that are called **kidneys** and develop in our posterior celom wall.

The kidney's evolutionary history traces a series of major shifts in the habitats of our ancestors. Vertebrates probably evolved from *Branchiostoma*-like lower chordates that left their muddy ocean-bottom homes for a life in fresh water. This move led to several important anatomical changes. Getting around in the strong, variable currents of rivers and streams called for more specialization of the head end of the body (including the development of eyes and a brain) and a more powerful swimming apparatus. The first vertebrates also had to remodel their excretory system. The move out of the salt sea into fresh water placed them in new surroundings that were less salty than their body fluids. Water thus tended to diffuse into their bodies and make them swell up like a soaked prune. To live in fresh water, they needed some way of pumping the water out as fast as it diffused in; and specialized epithelial cells of the sort that serve *Branchiostoma* as excretory organs were just not up to the task.

Life in fresh water was made possible by the appearance of a new excretory system early in vertebrate history. Although we have no fossil kidneys to study, we can get some idea of how this system evolved by looking at its comparative embryology in modern verte-brates.

Lampreys, which are the most primitive living fishes, hatch in fresh water. The larval lamprey gets rid of excess water via a pair of **glomeruli** in each segment. The glomeruli are tangled balls of capil-lary-sized arterioles protruding into the celom. They develop from small arteries that grow out of the dorsal aorta into the adjoining celom-wall mesoderm. This part of each developing body segment, just ventral to the somites, is called the **nephrotome** (Fig. 1-10). The whole series of nephrotomes eventually forms a longitudinal **nephro-genic** (Gk., "kidney-forming") **cord** on each side of the celom's dorsal wall.

The high (arterial) pressure inside the lamprey's glomerular vessels allows water to diffuse out of the blood into the celom while the vessels' cell membranes hold back the salts and macromolecules that the larval lamprey needs. The lamprey hatchling can therefore pump water out into the celom as fast as it diffuses in through the gills and gut. The excreted water is removed from the celom by a tube that runs along the glomerular mass on each side. Through this tube, the water drains into the tail end of the gut, the **cloaca** (L., "sewer").

Glomeruli and the associated drainage system are present in most of the segments of the lamprey's body. The first glomeruli form in the pericardial part of the celom. Their drainage duct grows tailward through the nephrogenic ridge to reach the cloaca and open into it. As it grows, the duct seems to stimulate the formation of a second mass of glomeruli in the abdominal region. The two masses of primi-tive kidney material are known as the **pronephros** and **mesonephros** (Gk., "front kidney" and "middle kidney"). The duct on each side that drains these primitive kidneys into the cloaca is called the **mesonephric duct** (Fig. 10-1).

In human ontogeny, a rudimentary pronephros forms in the cervi-cal region during the third week after conception. A mesonephric duct grows tailward from this rudiment and stimulates the formation of a mesonephros. There is no evidence of any actual mesonephric function in human beings; at this stage of development, the placenta is doing the kidney's job.

Shortly after the mesonephric duct reaches the cloaca of the human embryo and opens into it, the definitive kidney starts to form. Its duct buds off from the tail end of the mesonephric duct. This new duct, which has no equivalent in the lamprey, grows back up headward

Fig. 10-1 A. Schematic cross section through the axial region of a 5-mm human embryo, showing a mesonephric corpuscle (glomerulus + Bowman's capsule). The three series of aortic branches (to somite, mesonephros, and gut) are numbered. B,C. Schematic cutaway view of the left side of the cloacal region, showing development of the mesonephric duct in a typical vertebrate embryo.

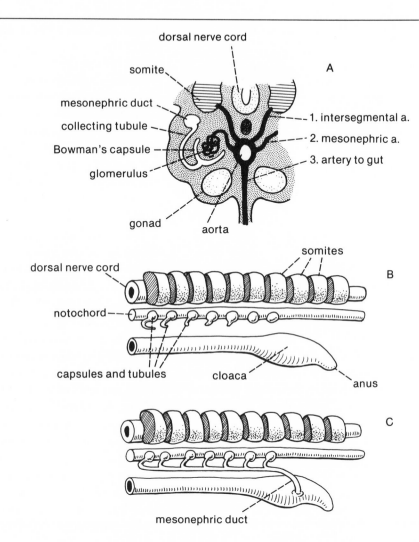

into the nephrogenic cord. As it grows, a cap of nephrotome material condenses around its growing tip. This material differentiates into millions of microscopic glomeruli. The new duct branches as it grows, sending a separate small blind-ended extension to each glomerulus and wrapping around it to form a drainage tubule for that glomerulus. The whole mass of glomeruli and their tubules constitutes the definitive kidney, or **metanephros** (Gk., "rear kidney"). The new duct, which the metanephros trails behind it as it grows and moves cranially up through the abdomen (Fig. 10-5), becomes the **ureter** that drains urine from the adult kidney into the bladder.

The collecting tubule draining each glomerulus is specialized for resorbing water from the glomerular filtrate. This specialization produces a more concentrated urine. It seems to have originated as an adaptation to living in salt water again, when some of the primitive freshwater vertebrates went back to the sea. They found it had become saltier than their blood, so they (like most saltwater fishes today) were confronted with the reverse of their original problem. They had to come up with some means of preventing water from diffusing *outward* and shriveling them up. Some groups of fishes (sharks, hagfishes) just gave up and allowed salt or urea to accumulate in their blood. Doing this raised their blood's ionic concentration to that of sea water and so eliminated the osmotic pressure. But the bony fishes from which we evolved developed a different strategy for living in salt water. Their glomeruli shrank and their collecting tubules elongated; so the total kidney surface available for pumping water out (the glomeruli) was reduced relative to that for pulling water back in. The resulting ability to produce a concentrated urine allows bony fishes to live in the modern sea. It was indispensable for their descendants' conquest of dry land, where desiccation is a constant threat and water is not always at hand.

Many bony fishes, and even some amphibians, retain a mesonephric kidney as adults. Its disappearance in our own ancestors was not simply an excretory adaptation. The replacement of the mesonephros by a metanephric kidney was tied up with the conversion of the mesonephric duct into a duct for the male gonad.

▪ The Gonads and Their Ducts

Like the kidney apparatus, the gonads of vertebrates also develop in the dorsal wall of the celom. The gonads' close association with the kidneys seems to be accidental, but that accident has had important consequences for human evolution and embryology.

In lampreys and other living jawless fishes, eggs and sperm are discharged along with urine into the celomic cavity. They leave the celom, not via the duct system of the mesonephros, but through a pair of little pores that connect the celom with the cloaca. This arrangement is obviously fairly inefficient; some ova are apt to get lost in the crevices of the celom. In female higher vertebrates, including women, eggs are still shed into the celom just as they are in female lampreys, but the pore leading to the cloaca has become specialized into an egg-collecting tube on each side. This tube runs up from the cloaca along the dorsal celom wall and opens into the celom right next to the ovary. As soon as an egg pops out of the ovary into the celom, it is swept into the mouth of this tube and driven on toward the cloaca by cilia lining the tube.

In an embryo, this egg-collecting tube lies just lateral to the mesonephric duct. It is accordingly known as the **paramesonephric duct** (Fig. 10-2). In the human fetus, the tail ends of the two paramesonephric ducts fuse together near their opening into the cloaca, thereby producing a **uterus** and **vagina** in the midline. The unfused parts of the ducts, which lead from the uterus back to the ovaries, are called the **uterine** (or Fallopian) **tubes.**

Unlike eggs, sperm never enter the celom in higher vertebrates. They always reach the outside by passing through some derivative of

Fig. 10-2 Genital ducts of six-week male (*left*) and female (*right*) embryos. The rete system of the ovary soon degenerates and loses its connections with the mesonephric duct. Structures that persist in the adult are shaded in each half of the diagram. G, gubernaculum (of testis or ovary).

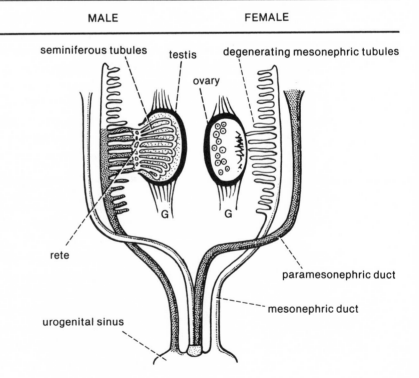

the urinary system. In male amniotes (reptiles, birds, and mammals), the testis develops an early connection with the tubule system of the mesonephric kidney (Fig. 10-2) and soon takes over the mesonephric duct completely. The mesonephros itself degenerates and utterly disappears.

In a female embryo, the ovary also makes a transient connection with the mesonephric duct system. This connection is soon lost in the female, but the mesonephros disappears anyway and is replaced by the metanephros, just as in the male.

■ The Ascent of the Kidneys

The mesonephros of the human embryo receives its blood supply via an irregularly segmental series of vessels, the **mesonephric** arteries. These arteries spring from the descending aorta and run laterally into the nephrogenic tissues on either side (Fig. 10-1), just as they do in a larval lamprey. The gonads, which form in a cleft between the aorta and mesonephros, are also supplied by branches of the neighboring mesonephric arteries. After the third week of development, the human mesonephros begins to degenerate. The ascending kidney, growing upward from the cloacal end of the mesonephric duct, encounters the arteries of the degenerating mesonephros one after another and taps them for its blood supply. For a brief period, each kidney is supplied by several parallel mesonephric arteries. Normally, all but one of these lose their connections with the kidney; only a single mesonephric artery, rechristened the **renal** artery, supplies the kidney after it comes to rest in the upper abdomen. But sometimes multiple renal arteries are found entering a single kidney. In such cases, the kidney has—so to speak—climbed to the top of the "ladder" of mesonephric arteries without letting go of some of the lower rungs.

The kidney normally ascends all the way through the lumbar region and comes to rest against the lower surface of the diaphragm. In the human adult, the kidney lies surrounded by a mass of fat just in front of (ventral to) the Quadratus Lumborum muscle, and its upper end is sheltered from behind by the lowest rib. Figure 10-3 represents a section through the kidney. Its basic form—a fleshy, vascular cap around a branching duct system—reflects its embryonic origins. The kidney's duct system is divisible into several zones, representing finer and finer branches; the single **ureter** ends in a dilated **renal pelvis,** which branches into **major calyces,** which in turn divide into **minor**

Fig. 10-3   Section through an adult kidney. Each conical unit of medullary material is called a **renal pyramid** and has a minor calyx surrounding its urine-secreting tip. The tip of one pyramid is shown diagrammatically enlarged.

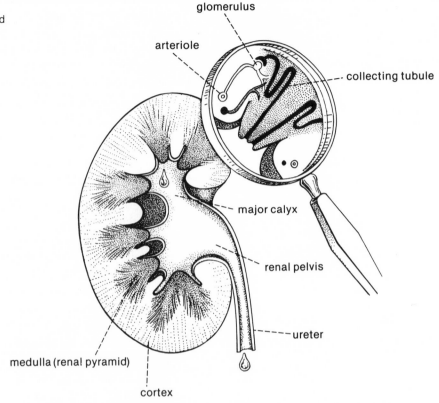

glomerulus

arteriole

collecting tubule

major calyx

renal pelvis

ureter

medulla (renal pyramid)

cortex

calyces, each of which receives the outflow from many microscopic collecting tubules. Those tubules form the **medulla** (inner layer) of the kidney's flesh. The glomeruli are restricted to the outermost layer, or **cortex.** As might be expected, the precise branching pattern of the calyces is variable.

Occasionally, the two embryonic kidneys will ascend together on the same side or fuse together into a shapeless lump and remain down near the pelvic region. Failure to keep an eye out for these striking but harmless anomalies can have catastrophic consequences in surgery; a patient might be killed or condemned to a life of renal dialysis by a surgeon who removed a perfectly healthy fused kidney from the pelvis under the delusion that it was some sort of tumor.

■ The Descent of the Gonads

The testis of vertebrates develops in the dorsal wall of the upper abdominal celom. In nonmammals, it stays there throughout life, in close association with the excretory organs—which is how it managed to steal the mesonephric kidney's duct system in our remote ancestors. But in mammals, the developing testis does not stay put. During fetal development, it moves down the inside of the body wall, slides around ventrally toward the penis, and slips into a protruding body-wall pouch called the **scrotum.** An evagination of the peritoneal cavity grows down into the scrotum before the testis arrives there. After the testis has completed its descent, the connection between this scrotal evagination and the peritoneal cavity is pinched off and lost, leaving each testicle surrounded by its own little celomic sac, the **tunica vaginalis** (from L. *vagina,* "sheath"). Each of these small sacs is a closed bag wrapped around the ventral aspect of the testis; the testis projects into it from behind just as the gut indents the peritoneal cavity (Fig. 8-1).

Why does the testis descend into a scrotum in mammals? For some reason, this descent seems to be necessary to preserve male fertility. Sperm produced by the testis are stored in the testicular end of the mesonephric duct system—the **epididymis.** If the epididymis is not kept relatively cool—cooler than the usual mammalian body temperature—the stored sperm degenerate and lose motility. Elevating the temperature of the testis itself seems to inhibit sperm production as well. Presumably, the testis had to be moved out into a relatively cool location like the scrotum when early mammals became warm-blooded. However, the equally warm-blooded birds seem to get along fine with abdominal testes; and some mammals leave the testis inside the abdomen and just move the epididymis down into the scrotum. All we can say is that the risk and inconvenience involved in having scrotal testes implies that there must be an awfully good reason for it. The mechanisms of testicular descent are just as unclear as its rationale. The descending testis follows a band of soft connective tissue—the **gubernaculum testis**—attached to its lower pole (Fig. 10-2), but the gubernaculum does not seem to exert any actual pull on the testis. Sometimes one or both testes will fail to descend completely in human males, and surgery may be needed to restore fertility.

The ascending kidney takes over the mesonephric arteries it passes in its climb out of the pelvis; but the testis keeps the mesonephric vessels it started out with, and drags them along behind it as it descends. As a result, the testicular arteries and veins spring from the aorta and vena cava in the upper abdomen, where the testis originally formed. From there, they follow a route that traces the path of the testis's descent to the scrotum. In an upright mammal like *Homo sapiens,* the blood returning from the testis therefore has to take a long vertical course up from the scrotum against the pull of gravity. Under the weight of this column of blood, the veins of the testis sometimes become varicose and form a ropy, palpable lump called a **varicocele** in the scrotum. The testis also drags its duct, the **deferent duct** or **ductus deferens** (the old mesonephric duct) down into the scrotum with it. The deferent duct and the accompanying testicular vessels and nerves form a leash of testicular connections in the groin. This leash is called the **spermatic cord.**

The spermatic cord passes through the mouth of the scrotal pouch to reach the testis. If the scrotum were a simple pouch with an open mouth, loops of intestine could slip into it alongside the spermatic cord, with resulting danger of gut injury or strangulation. This danger is guarded against by constriction and elongation of the mouth of the scrotal pouch to form a narrow, tubular **inguinal canal** (L. *inguen,* "groin"). The inguinal canal comprises balloonlike evaginations of three of the four subcutaneous body-wall layers (Fig. 10-4); the scrotal extensions of the body-wall muscles and fascia have special names. The mouths of the three balloons are offset from one another. The innermost balloon, derived from the transversalis fascia on the inside of the body-wall muscles (Fig. 10-4C), starts laterally and runs medially between the deep and superficial layers of those muscles before entering the mouth of the most external balloon (derived from the External Oblique muscle: Fig. 10-4A). This staggered formation of the inguinal canal ensures that contraction of the abdominal muscles or any increase in intraabdominal pressure will squeeze the canal flat and keep gut loops from sliding into the canal or scrotum. This mechanism does not always work; sometimes a loop of gut pops out anyway. The result is an **inguinal hernia.**

The ovary also descends, following a gubernaculum like that of the testis, but it does not ordinarily descend into a subcutaneous position like that of the testis. It ends its descent just below the rim of the bony pelvis, before it reaches the uterus. The ovary's gubernaculum becomes attached to the side of the uterus, and persists in the adult as a

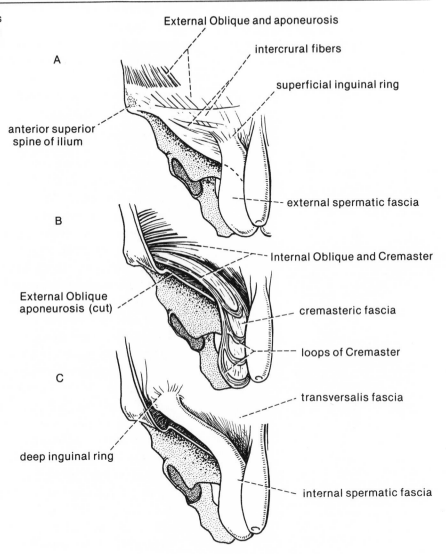

Fig. 10-4 Successively deeper (A, B, C) layers of the scrotum and inguinal canal. These layers are continuous with the lateral body-wall layers indicated in each diagram.

External Oblique and aponeurosis

intercrural fibers

superficial inguinal ring

anterior superior spine of ilium

external spermatic fascia

Internal Oblique and Cremaster

External Oblique aponeurosis (cut)

cremasteric fascia

loops of Cremaster

transversalis fascia

deep inguinal ring

internal spermatic fascia

pair of fibrous cords: one that runs from ovary to uterus and another that runs from the uterus through a vestigial inguinal canal into the labia majora (the hairy "lips" of the vaginal opening), where the ovary would have wound up if it had been a testis.

The ascending kidney drags its duct (the ureter) behind it and taps one mesonephric artery after another as it rises; the descending gonad keeps its own mesonephric artery. When the gonad passes the kidney, it passes to the ventral side of all the structures attached to the kidney. Therefore, in the adult, the duct and vessels of the gonad cross the ventral aspect of the ureter (Fig. 10-5)—but they do not cross the *vessels* of the kidney, which develop from more cranial mesonephric vessels than those destined to supply the gonad.

▪ Division of the Cloaca

In human embryos, as in most nonmammalian vertebrates, the gut and urogenital organs all empty to the outside through a single opening, via the hindgut dilatation called the cloaca. In higher mammals, the cloaca is partitioned during fetal life into several functional subdivisions, and there are multiple openings at the tail end of the trunk.

The mesonephric and paramesonephric ducts of the embryo lie *dorsal* to the gut, in the dorsal wall of the celom. But the urogenital openings of adults lie *ventral* to the anus. Therefore, the mesonephric and paramesonephric ducts have to wrap around the sides of the embryonic gut to reach and open into the ventral part of the cloaca. During the fourth to seventh weeks after conception, that ventral part of the cloaca is partitioned off from the more dorsal, gut-related part. The partition between them is called the **urorectal septum;** it forms as an extension of the mesoderm separating the yolk sac from the allantois (Fig. 10-6). As it grows tailward, the septum divides the cloaca into a gut part in back (continuous with the yolk sac) and a urogenital part in front (continuous with the allantois). The gut part becomes the rectum and anal canal. The urogenital part is called the **urogenital sinus.** In an egg-laying amniote, the urine discharged from the kidneys of an embryo prior to hatching would flow through this sinus to reach the allantois. The primitive function of the allantois as a urine-storage site inside the egg may explain why amniotes' ureters open into the ventral (that is, allantoic) side of the cloaca. In nonamniotes, the urinary ducts have a more direct, dorsal opening into the cloaca.

Most of the human urogenital sinus becomes the **urinary bladder.** In the adult, this is a hollow, muscular sac shaped like a bulging tetrahedron, with a tube attached to each of its four corners (Fig. 10-7). One corner lies behind the top edge of the pubic symphysis (the joint in front between the two hipbones). The tube attached to this front corner of the bladder is the vestigial **urachus,** which connected the urogenital sinus with the allantois (via the navel) in the embryo. A

Fig. 10-5 Descent of gonads. The gonad develops alongside the mesonephros (A) and descends into the pelvis, dragging its duct and a mesonephric artery along with it (B). The kidney climbs out of the pelvis, usurping the arteries of the degenerating mesonephros (*dotted outline*, A).

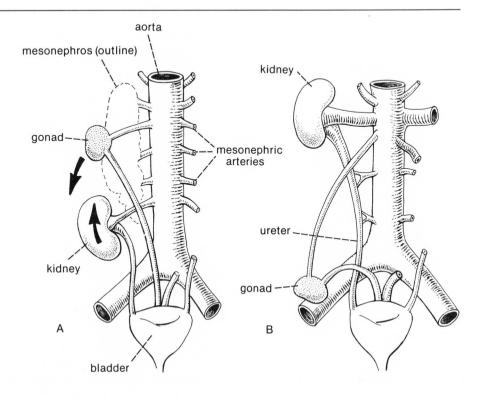

Fig. 10-6 Urorectal septum. The embryonic hindgut (A) is partitioned into a urogenital sinus in front and a rectum in back by the tailward growth of the urorectal septum between yolk sac and allantois (B). Diagrammatic midline sections.

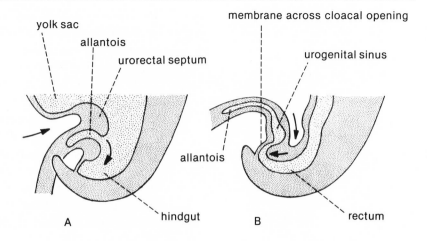

Fig. 10-7 The urinary bladder. A. Left anterior view, showing tetrahedral shape of empty bladder. B. Posterior view of male bladder, showing ductus deferens, seminal vesicles, and the ejaculatory duct through which they empty into the prostatic part of the urethra.

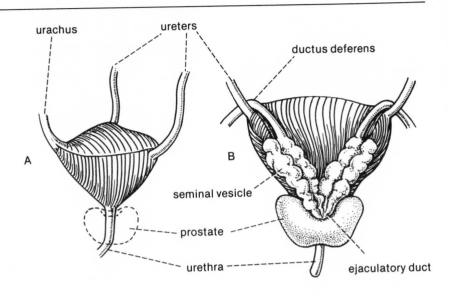

second corner, also in the midline, lies at the bottom (caudal end) of the bladder and points down toward the anal region. The tube leading away from it is the **urethra**. It forms by constriction of the cloacal end of the urogenital sinus, and is the passage through which urine is expelled from the bladder. The other two corners, located dorsally on either side, receive the **ureters** that drain urine into the bladder from the kidneys. The triangle bounded by the ureteric and urethral openings is called the **trigone** of the bladder.

The ureters do not run straight in through the wall of the bladder but traverse it obliquely—so when the bladder is full, the pressure inside it flattens the openings of the ureters and keeps urine from squirting back into them. When this valvelike arrangement fails, the ureters tend to blow up like balloons and kidney damage results.

The urorectal septum grows all the way out to the body surface, thus partitioning the embryo's cloacal orifice into two openings—the anus dorsally, and a urogenital opening more ventrally. While this is going on, the openings of the paired mesonephric ducts slide around tailward toward the dorsal side of the urogenital sinus. The paramesonephric ducts are drawn together between them and fuse in the midline to form a uterus. A midline outpocketing from the urogenital sinus grows out dorsally toward the uterus and forms a tubular **vagina,** which opens at its dorsal end into the uterus and at its ventral end into the urethral part of the urogenital sinus. This fetal condition persists in the male, where the terminal ends of the mesonephric ducts (here rechristened the **ejaculatory ducts**) open into the urethra below the bladder on either side of a little dimple (the **utricle**) that is thought to represent a vestigial vagina.

Although the vagina originally opens into the urethra in the female as well, this condition does not normally persist. Instead, the vagina enlarges, and its lower opening moves tailward along the dorsal surface of the urethra until it reaches the body surface between urethra and anus. (The vagina's upper end also expands, forming a ring-shaped recess, the **fornix,** around the protruding lower end, or **cervix,** of the uterus.) Three separate cloacal openings—urinary, genital, and intestinal—are therefore found in an adult female human being. The male has a more embryonic condition, with urine and gametes being expelled together through the urethra.

Just above the opening of the cloaca in the human embryo, a small lump called the **genital tubercle** forms from the tissues of the cloacal rim. As the cloacal opening becomes subdivided into an anus and a urogenital opening, this tubercle elongates and comes to hang down over the cranial edge of the urogenital aperture (Fig. 10-8). Specialized **erectile tissue** develops from mesoderm in the tubercle and around the entire rim of the urogenital opening.

In the male fetus, the tubercle continues to grow longer, and the erectile-tissue-laden left and right lips of the urogenital opening fuse with the elongated tubercle in the midline. These fused tissues plug up the urogenital opening and form a tubular copulatory organ, the **penis.** The male urethra eventually develops a new outlet onto the tip of the enlarged genital tubercle, which is rechristened the **glans** (L., "acorn") of the penis. In the female, the erectile lips never close over the urogenital opening; and the smaller female "penis," the **clitoris,** retains its early fetal position, hanging down over the aperture of the urethra without enclosing it. (In some mammals—for example, hyenas—the clitoris does grow around the urethra, and male and female external genitals may be virtually indistinguishable.)

Several glands develop as outpocketings from the inner walls of the urogenital sinus. One of these glands, the **prostate,** becomes a sizable structure in the male (Fig. 10-7). It forms as a series of elongated evaginations from the upper end of the urethra, just below the bladder. The adult male's prostate is a mass of glandular tissue and smooth muscle encircling the urethral neck of the bladder like a col-

Fig. 10-8 Early development of external genitals. A. Tail end of embryo with undivided cloacal opening. B. Later stage with cloacal opening partitioned into separate urogenital and anal openings (by growth of urorectal septum: cf. Fig. 10-6). The lateral "lips" of the urogenital opening form the labia majora in females and fuse across the midline to form the skin of the scrotum in males; the phallus develops into the clitoris or penis.

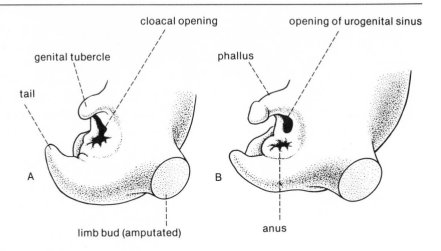

lar. A similar outpocketing from the ejaculatory duct (the distal end of the deferent duct, lying in between the bladder and the rectum) forms a pair of male glands called **seminal vesicles.** The prostate and seminal vesicles add characteristic secretions to the ejaculated semen. More distal outgrowths from the male urethra form a pair of pea-sized **bulbourethral glands,** which are of uncertain function and are embedded in the postpelvic part of the body wall. Their female equivalents, the **greater vestibular glands,** secrete mucous fluids that serve as lubricants during copulation.

▪ The Sympathetic Trunk and the Suprarenals

Just as the parasympathetic division of the automatic nervous system was primitively concerned with digestion, the sympathetic division seems to have been primitively associated with circulation and urogenital functions. This functional difference is reflected in the location of our own ganglion cells. Parasympathetic ganglion cells lie mostly in the walls of the gut. Sympathetic ganglion cells lie in front of the aorta—and alongside it, where the urogenital organs developed.

In a lamprey, most of the sympathetic ganglion cells lie in the walls of blood vessels, where some of them form specialized clusters that secrete neurotransmitterlike substances directly into the bloodstream.

These neurosecretory cells are capable of giving a diffuse sympathetic jolt to the whole body via the blood. In sharks (the most primitive jawed vertebrates living today), the neurosecretory "ganglion" cells have become segmentally arranged glands associated with the segmental kidney. As each mesonephric artery of a shark runs into the mesonephros to supply glomeruli, it is surrounded by a sympathetic-trunk ganglion and a secretory **suprarenal** gland, which is embedded in the dorsal surface of the mesonephric kidney. The suprarenals secrete **epinephrine**, more popularly known as **adrenalin.** Epinephrine is a chemical relative of the norepinephrine released by the axons of postganglionic sympathetic neurons. It produces the same sort of fight-or-flight effects that those neurons produce—speeding up the heart, contracting gut sphincters, and so on. In the shark, the suprarenal glands are clearly segmentally arranged, and it is easy to see that they are related to the ganglia of the sympathetic trunk.

The equivalent of the shark's suprarenal glands in our own bodies is the core, or **medulla,** of our suprarenal glands. (The outer layer, or **cortex,** of our glands secretes metabolic hormones and is the homolog of another gland in the shark.) The human suprarenals are friable, triangular glands that sit atop the kidneys like a pair of cocked three-cornered hats (Fig. 10-9). Although our suprarenals are not segmentally arranged in the adult, accessory suprarenallike glands called **paraganglia** are found at intervals along the sides of the abdominal aorta in the fetus. These organs, which regress after birth, are probably homologous with the segmental suprarenals of sharks. Microscopic remnants of them persist in the adult and may have special but currently unknown endocrine functions. Similar **paraaortic bodies** lying alongside the origin of the superior mesenteric artery continue to enlarge for a while after birth and seem to serve as accessory suprarenal medullae in the infant. They disappear at puberty.

The suprarenal gland is associated with the mesonephros in evolution and development, and this fact is reflected in its blood supply, as noted below. By contrast, its association with the definitive kidney is merely an accident resulting from the fact that the kidney's ascent up the "ladder" of mesonephric arteries ordinarily stops when it runs into the suprarenal gland. When the kidney's ascent is incomplete—say, when the two kidneys fuse together and remain down in the pelvis—each suprarenal gland is still found in the normal position, just above where the kidney ought to be but is not.

Fig. 10-9 Derivatives of mesonephric arteries. At least five arteries (*numbered*) are so derived on each side in the adult.

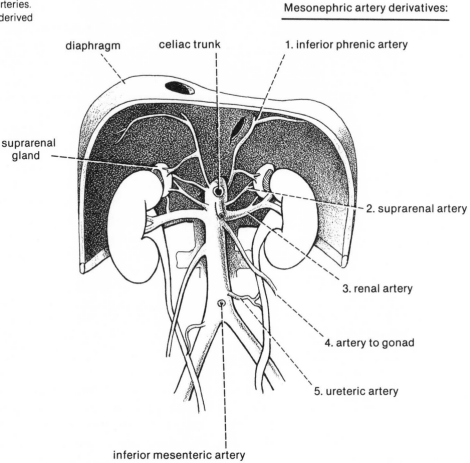

Mesonephric artery derivatives:

diaphragm

celiac trunk

1. inferior phrenic artery

suprarenal gland

2. suprarenal artery

3. renal artery

4. artery to gonad

5. ureteric artery

inferior mesenteric artery

■ The Nerves and Blood Vessels of the Three Paired Glands

The three paired glands that develop in the region of the nephrotome—suprarenals, kidneys, and gonads—are supplied by arteries springing from the sides of the aorta in the upper abdomen. These arteries are all derived from the irregularly segmental series of arteries that supplied the embryo's mesonephros. In the normal adult, three pairs of mesonephric arteries correspond to the three paired glands—**testicular** or **ovarian** arteries to the gonads, **renal** arteries to the kidneys, and **suprarenal** arteries to the suprarenal glands (Fig. 10-9). Two or three lower mesonephric arteries on each side usually persist to supply the ureter that the kidney trailed behind it as it climbed up from the pelvis.

Mesonephric arteries also supply the dorsal edge of the diaphragm. A pair of little **superior phrenic** arteries, which run onto the diaphragm's thoracic face from the thoracic part of the aorta, may be mesonephric-artery derivatives. They remind us that the embryonic urogenital system extended all the way from the pelvis up into the thorax. The larger **inferior phrenic** arteries, on the opposite (lower or abdominal) surface of the diaphragm, betray their mesonephric origins by sending a branch downward to the suprarenal gland. The suprarenals also receive accessory suprarenal branches from the renal arteries on each side, in addition to the suprarenal arteries proper. Thus, each suprarenal gland is ordinarily supplied via *three* of the mesonephric series of arteries.

The suprarenals have a peculiar innervation. The other paired glands (gonads and kidneys) receive postganglionic sympathetic fibers that travel as a plexus along the arteries to those glands and serve mainly to make the arterial walls constrict. Some of the nerve fibers entering the suprarenal gland are nonmyelinated and presumably postganglionic fibers, and probably do the same job of vasoconstriction. But most of the fibers that arrive at the suprarenal medulla are *myelinated* and have apparently not synapsed. They end in the medullary cells and stimulate secretion of epinephrine. The neurosecretory cells of the medulla are in effect themselves ganglion cells—specialized postsynaptic sympathetic "neurons" derived from neural crest; so they, alone of all the body's tissues, receive sympathetic motor innervation directly from the spinal cord, without involving any ganglionic neurons.

■ Venous Drainage of the Urogenital System and Environs

Blood from the abdominal gut returns to the right atrium via remnants of the old yolk-sac drainage system, which are pasted together to form the portal and hepatic veins (and the uppermost bit of the inferior vena cava, between the hepatic veins and the heart) (Fig. 9-5). Blood from the urogenital organs and the adjoining body wall also returns to the heart via a pasted-up system of veins.

The lower half of the inferior vena cava, caudal to the veins of the kidneys, is a body-wall vein. It develops as an abdominal extension of the azygos vein in the thorax, and the two are usually connected in the adult (Fig. 7-11). Like the azygos vein, it receives intersegmental veins (lumbar veins) from the right side.

The rest of the inferior vena cava, from the renal veins on up to the entrances of the hepatic veins, is essentially a mesonephric vein and related to the urogenital organs. It is derived from the right member of a pair of veins (subcardinals) that ran along the ventromedial edges of the mesonephric kidneys and drained blood from them. This mesonephric section of the inferior vena cava receives the veins corresponding to derivatives of the right mesonephric arteries; that is, the right gonadal, renal, suprarenal, and inferior phrenic veins.

The upper half of the inferior vena cava also drains what remains of the left mesonephric venous system, which regressed considerably when the body's venous drainage shifted over to the right side of the heart. As part of that venous shift, the right and left mesonephric venous systems became connected by a midline-crossing anastomosis. In the adult, this anastomosis is considered part of the left renal vein. The left suprarenal, gonadal, and inferior phrenic veins are therefore tributaries of the left renal vein (Fig. 10-10).

The lower (body-wall) half of the inferior vena cava is developmentally *dorsal to the aorta and its paired branches*. The upper, mesonephros-related (urogenital, or subcardinal) half is developmentally *ventral* to those arteries. From this and the preceding paragraph, you can infer the following facts (Fig. 10-10):

1. The left renal vein crosses the aorta ventrally (because it is an anastomosis between the two mesonephros-related systems, which are ventral to the aorta).

2. All mesonephric-artery derivatives that cross the inferior vena cava cross *dorsal* to its urogenital part and *ventral* to its body-wall part; the right inferior phrenic, suprarenal, and renal arteries run behind (dorsal to) the inferior vena cava, but the right gonadal artery runs in front of (ventral to) it. If there is a right accessory renal artery—a lower "rung" of the mesonephric "ladder" that the ascending kidney failed to relinquish—it will lie caudal to the right renal veins and thus will cross the ventral surface of the (body-wall part of the) inferior vena cava.

3. The common iliac arteries and their major branches lie ventral to the corresponding iliac veins.

4. Lumbar veins draining the hypaxial body wall below the level of the renal vein will end in the body-wall part of the inferior vena cava.

Fig. 10-10 Front view of the inferior vena cava. Its lower half (*stippled*) develops from body-wall veins, which lie *dorsal* to the aorta and its branches. Most of its upper half (*white*) develops from mesonephric veins, which lie *ventral* to the aorta and its branches. Note that an accessory renal artery (*dotted line*) persisting below the usual one on the right will accordingly cross the IVC ventrally.

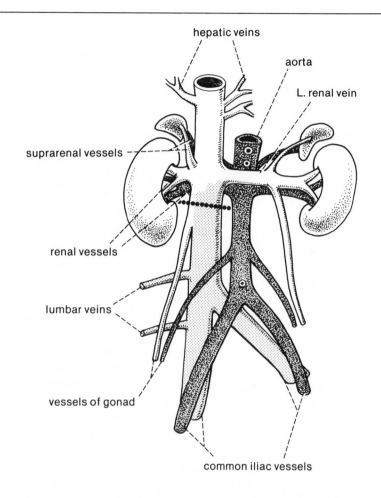

Those from the left side cross behind the dorsal surface of the aorta, as do their hemiazygos counterparts in the thorax. The more cranial half of the inferior vena cava is a urogenital vessel, so it receives no body-wall tributaries. The uppermost one or two pairs of lumbar veins thus drain directly into the azygos and hemiazygos vessels—or down to the lower lumbar region via secondary longitudinal anastomoses.

5. There is usually an anastomosis between the lower left hemiazygos vein and the left renal vein (Fig. 7-11), corresponding to the connection between the azygos vein and the upper (mesonephros-related) half of the inferior vena cava on the right.

The Pelvis and the Perineum

11

▪ The Pelvic Body Wall

A fish's pelvis, like its scapula, is a small flat bone on each side of the trunk, lying in a sheet of hypaxial muscles that overlie (and derive from) the body wall. The plate of bone is called the **hipbone** (L. *os coxae*). In early amphibians, each hipbone grew upward to form a joint with one of the ribs at the base of the tail. This change allowed the hind limb to push directly against the vertebral column in standing and crawling on dry land.

In later land-dwelling vertebrates, still more vertebrae sent ribs down to touch the hipbones on each side. All these vertebrae became fused together into a solid bony mass called the **sacrum** (L. *os sacrum,* "sacred bone"—from its use in Roman animal sacrifice). Our own sacrum normally contains five fused vertebrae. They are still separate at birth but lose their intervertebral joints after puberty.

The hipbones of fishes do not touch the vertebral column, but they usually touch each other in the midline of the belly, in front of the cloacal opening. This contact of the two hipbones across the belly was preserved and firmed up in land-dwelling vertebrates. In human beings, the joint in front between the hipbones takes the form of a pubic **symphysis,** a disk of fibrocartilage surrounded by ligaments that bind the two hipbones tightly together.

The bony ring formed by the sacrum and the two ossa coxae is the **pelvis** (L., "basin"). This ring completely encircles the tail end of the gut, replacing the muscular body wall. Deep to the pelvic ring, the body wall proper becomes fascial; the abdominal muscles end by attaching to the cranial edge of the pelvis and do not continue on underneath it the way their thoracic counterparts do beneath the scapula. However, other hypaxial muscles envelop every available surface of the bony pelvis, because the os coxae is the base of the hind limb.

From the outer face of the fish's os coxae, small muscles arise and run out laterally to attach to the bones inside the pelvic fin. When fish came out on land and started walking on their fins, the fin muscles had to take on the work of propelling the body—and also of supporting the body's weight, since it was no longer buoyed up by water. The muscles of the pelvic fin thus had to become much larger, and the os coxae expanded to provide attachments for them. It did this by developing three flat bony lobes radiating outward from the hip socket. The part of the hipbone that went up dorsally (to meet the sacrum) expanded into a broad blade called the **ilium.** The part that curved ventrally across the belly (to meet the hipbone of the opposite side) became a similar blade called the **pubis.** A third expansion stuck out tailward behind the hip socket, thus affording increased origins for the big propulsive muscles that pulled the hind limb backward and downward in crawling along. This third expansion is called the **is-chium.** In primitive land-dwelling vertebrates (Fig. 11-1), these three lobes were separate bones. They still form separately in the human fetus, and remain separated after birth by bands of persistent cartilage. These bands meet in the center of the hip joint, forming a Y-shaped cartilaginous joint between ilium, ischium, and pubis. The bands of cartilage are gradually replaced by bone after birth, and

Fig. 11-1 Right hipbones of an early reptile (A) and human (B), showing their three constituent bones. Lateral aspect.

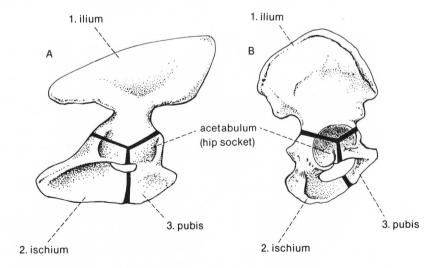

disappear by the age of twenty or so as the three bones fuse together into a single os coxae. Limb muscles arise from both the inner and outer faces of all three parts of the os coxae and run out to attach to the long bones of thigh and leg.

The transversalis fascia lying against the inside of the abdominal body wall does not end at the pelvis's upper rim, as the body-wall muscles themselves do. It continues tailward along the deep surfaces of the limb muscles that arise from the inner face of the pelvis and gets renamed for the limb muscles it touches there. It is called the **iliac fascia** where it lies against the Iliacus muscle arising from the inside of the ilium. It is rechristened the **obturator fascia** where it clothes the Obturator Internus muscle that arises from ischium and pubis. Halfway down over the inner surface of Obturator Internus, muscle fibers spring from the obturator fascia, and the body wall reappears. This postpelvic part of the body wall forms a thin muscular cone with the anus at its apex. It is called **Levator Ani**—the anus-raiser. In a quadrupedal mammal like a dog or a cow, this muscle is not so much an anus-raiser as a flyswatter; its main function is wagging and depressing the tail, to keep pesky insects off the anal region (and to express emotions with tail gestures). We have delegated the fly-swatting (and gesturing) functions to our hands and converted our old caudal body-wall muscles into a **pelvic diaphragm** that helps keep our viscera from sliding down and out through the pelvic ring when we walk around balancing on our hind limbs. However, most of the fibers of the pelvic diaphragm are still attached directly or indirectly to our vestigial tail, the coccyx.

■ The Bony Pelvis and Its Ligaments

Seen from the medial side (Fig. 11-2), the human hipbone looks something like a doughnut standing on edge with a Japanese fan stuck into the top of it. The fan is the broad blade of the ilium. The doughnut is the ischium and pubis, separated from each other by the doughnut's hole, the **obturator foramen**. The hip socket, or **acetabulum** (L., "vinegar cup"), lies just above this hole on the outer surface of the hipbone (Fig. 11-1). Ilium, pubis, and ischium meet each other in the depths of the socket; and the pubis and ischium also meet around the lower edge of the obturator foramen.

Why is there a big obturator foramen in the lower part of the hip bone? In early reptiles (Fig. 11-1), this hole was just a little aperture

Fig. 11-2 Medial surface of left hipbone.

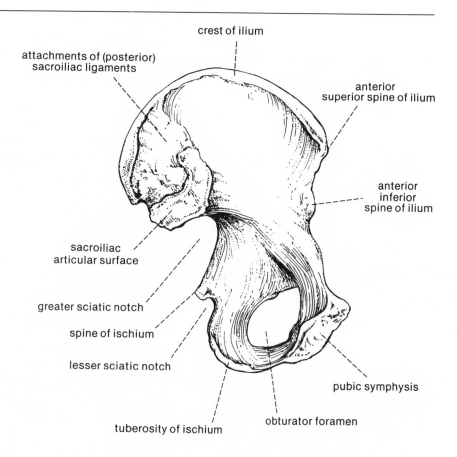

that transmitted nerves and blood vessels to muscles arising from the outer face of the pelvis below the acetabulum. That lower part of the pelvis does not bear any weight in a standing animal; and in later reptiles, it tended to become very thin or to be replaced by a sheet of tough fascia, with a bony frame remaining around it to keep it taut. In our own reptilian ancestors, this fascial "hole" in the bone expanded until it took in the original foramen for the nerve and vessels. The fascia that replaces the bone here is called the **obturator membrane.** Limb muscles still arise from both surfaces of the membrane.

The blade of the ilium also bears no weight, and it is made up of a thin sheet of bone with a thicker bony frame around its margins—much like the obturator-foramen area. But the weight-bearing parts of the hipbone are thick and robust. They form stout bony columns extending downward from the **sacroiliac joint** between ilium and sacrum. When we stand, weight is transmitted from the vertebrae via these bony columns to the hip joint and thence to our lower limbs. This thick columnar part of the bone is easily seen in a medial view (Fig. 11-2).

When we sit, our weight is carried on the backward-projecting ischium. The weight-bearing end of the ischium is a blunt, roughened projection called the **ischial tuberosity** (Fig. 11-2). (You can feel your own ischial tuberosities easily when sitting; they are the two hard bumps that press against your chair at the lower edge of your buttocks.) The body of the ischium, between the tuberosity and sacroiliac joint, is thickened to form a second column of bone, which transmits weight from the sacrum down to the ischial tuberosities when we sit. In front of this weight-bearing region, the ischium becomes abruptly thinner around the edges of the obturator foramen.

Unlike the rest of the human vertebral column, the sacrum is not even approximately vertical. It slopes dorsally away from the lumbar vertebrae. The sacroiliac joint thus lies dorsal to the lumbar vertebrae; so the weight of the body tends to depress the front end of the sacrum and cause the sacrum to rotate forward around the sacroiliac joints. If our sacroiliac joints were ball-and-socket joints, our lumbar vertebrae would drop into our pelvis and our coccyx would fly up in the air whenever we stood or sat up.

As might be expected, the sacroiliac joint is not a ball-and-socket joint. In fact, it is the most immobile synovial joint in the body. Rotation at this joint is prevented by three mechanisms.

1. The L-shaped sacroiliac joint surface (Fig. 11-2) has a helical twist in it. Its front end (the vertical stroke of the L) slopes *laterally* upward; its back end slopes *medially* upward. The space between the two ilia, where the sacrum sits, is V-shaped in front, but lambda-shaped (Λ) in back. Thus the front end of the sacrum acts like the keystone of an arch, and the back end acts like an inverted keystone—resisting downward movement in front and upward movement in back.

2. At the upper end of the sacrum, powerful **sacroiliac** ligaments (Fig. 11-3) tie the sacrum to the crest of the ilium on each side. They keep the anterior part of the sacrum from descending between the two ilia. As more pressure from above is put on the sacrum, these ligaments get tenser. Their tension draws the two ilia closer together, thus clamping the sacrum even more tightly between them.

Fig. 11-3 Rear view of human pelvis, showing ligaments binding the hipbone to the vertebral column. The more superficial ligaments are removed on the left to reveal both ends of the sacrospinous ligament.

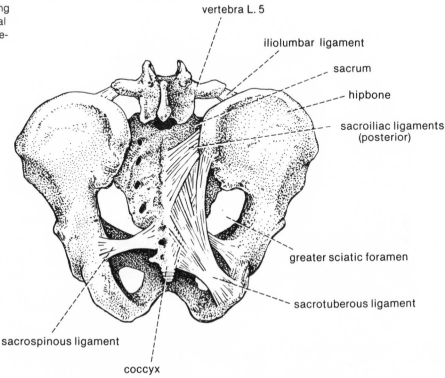

vertebra L. 5

iliolumbar ligament

sacrum

hipbone

sacroiliac ligaments (posterior)

greater sciatic foramen

sacrotuberous ligament

sacrospinous ligament

coccyx

3. Two important ligaments tie the tail end of the sacrum down to the ischia below it, so it cannot swing upward. By far the more powerful of the two is the **sacrotuberous** ligament, which fans out from the tuberosity to attach to the sacrum and coccyx (Fig. 11-3). The other ligament tying the sacrum's back end to the ischium is the **sacrospinous** ligament. It has a broad medial attachment to the sacrum and a somewhat narrower lateral attachment to the body of the ischium. The lateral attachment raises a sharp projection on the ischium, known as the **ischial spine** (Fig. 11-2).

The concavities in the os coxae above and below the spine of the ischium are called the **greater** and **lesser sciatic notches** respectively. The sacrospinous ligament separates the two notches from each other, and the sacrotuberous ligament closes both off medially, thus converting them from mere concavities into complete apertures—the **greater** and **lesser sciatic foramina** (Figs. 11-3 and 11-5A). These are important openings. The greater sciatic foramen is the main gateway through which veins, arteries, and nerves enter and leave the pelvis;

the lesser sciatic foramen is a similar gateway to the external genitals and other superficial structures in the crotch.

■ The Pelvic Diaphragm

The old tail muscles that form our pelvic diaphragm are conventionally divided into two named muscles. The feeblest and simplest is the wispy little **Coccygeus** (Fig. 11-4), which runs across from the ischial spine to the front of the sacrum and coccyx. In a dog, Coccygeus is a powerful muscle that acts to tuck the tail down between the legs. In a human, this sheet of tail-tucking musculature has become almost wholly tendinous and has turned into the sacrospinous ligament. Our Coccygeus just represents a few vestigial muscle fibers remaining on the ligament's deep surface.

The other muscle of the pelvic diaphragm is the **Levator Ani.** This muscle consists of two thin U-shaped slings that loop back around behind the gut and are attached at either end to the pelvis and obturator fascia in front. The obturator fascia is thickened and collagenous where Levator Ani fibers arise from it. This condensation forms a tendinous arch stretching from the inner side of the pubis in front to the ischial spine in back (Fig. 11-4). Fibers of Levator Ani arise along the whole length of this arch.

The deeper of the two slings composing Levator Ani originates far forward, from the pubis and the pubic end of the tendinous arch, and is accordingly called the **Pubococcygeus.** Its fibers run horizontally backward to attach to the sacrum and coccyx in back—and to the anal end of the gut tube itself. In front and in back of the anus, the Pubococcygeus fibers converging from each side toward the midline simply attach to their counterparts from the opposite side (Fig. 11-4). Between coccyx and anus, the juncture of left and right fibers is marked by a tendinous seam, the **anococcygeal** ligament, that ties the anus loosely to the tip of the coccyx.

Immediately in front and in back of the anus, the Pubococcygeus is thickened slightly, and these thickenings have special functions. The one passing behind the anus—the so-called puborectal sling—pulls forward on the back side of the gut tube and puts a kink into it. This kink is the dividing point between the rectal and anal parts of the gut. Contracting, the puborectal sling probably squeezes the anorectal junction closed and so acts as a supplementary voluntary sphincter for the tail end of the gut. The other pubococcygeal thickening, in

Fig. 11-4 The pelvic diaphragm (Levator Ani + Coccygeus). A. Medial view of the diaphragm and its constituents. Elements of Pubococcygeus form distinct thickenings behind and in front of the anal canal (An). P, puborectal sling. B. Inferior surface of Levator Ani.

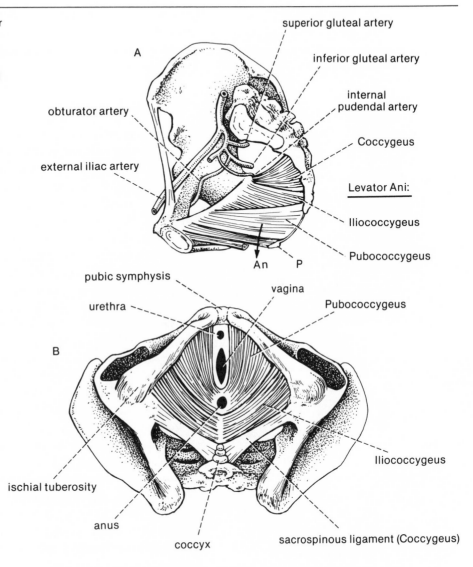

front of the anus, has a similar sphincteric action on the vaginal opening.

The Pubococcygeus contains most of the muscular fibers in Levator Ani. The rest of the muscle—the more superficial sheet that arises from the rear half of the tendinous arch—is much feebler and may be almost wholly aponeurotic. Its fibers slant down and back to insert into the anal end of the gut, the coccyx, and the anococcygeal ligament. Although it has no attachment to the ilium, it is called **Iliococcygeus** because the homologous tail muscle in four-footed mammals does arise from part of the ilium.

■ The Perineum

The pelvic diaphragm is part of the body wall. The *inner* surface of this diaphragm encloses gut-derived viscera innervated by autonomic nerves. The diaphragm's *outer* surface is in contact with subcutaneous fat and other body-wall structures, which are innervated (like the diaphragm itself) by ventral rami. The back edge of the pelvic diaphragm is the sacrospinous ligament, representing the tendinous part of Coccygeus. It follows that anything running forward through the greater sciatic foramen (above the ligament) passes over the upper edge of the diaphragm and thus enters the visceral regions of the pelvis. Conversely, anything running forward through the lesser sciatic foramen (below the ligament) passes into a body-wall space underneath and external to the diaphragm. This lowermost region of the body wall, below the pelvic diaphragm and between the projecting ischia, is called the **perineum.** It contains the external genitalia and several specialized hypaxial muscles that anchor and move the genitalia and anus.

The Levator Ani is shaped like a cone, stuffed into the pelvis with its apex pointing downward. The space on each side between the cone and the bony pelvis is filled in with a mass of fat and is called the **ischioanal (or ischiorectal) fossa** (Fig. 11-5). It provides a conduit for the nerves and vessels of the perineum. The **pudendal** nerve and **internal pudendal** blood vessels leave the pelvis through the greater sciatic foramen, curve around the back of the sacrospinous ligament, and enter the ischioanal fossa through the lesser sciatic foramen. Within the fossa, they run forward on the fossa's lateral wall (that is, the fascia on the inner surface of Obturator Internus), sending branches to all the structures of the perineum.

The muscular slings that make up the Levator Ani are U-shaped; so there is a gap in the pelvic diaphragm in front (between the two arms of the U). Through this gap, the urogenital ducts—the vagina in the female and the urethra in both sexes—pass out of the pelvis toward the body surface. The anterior gap in Levator Ani needs to be guarded to prevent pelvic viscera from pressing down through it. It is

Fig. 11-5 The ischioanal fossa. A. Rear view of pelvis, showing the pudendal nerve and internal pudendal vessels entering the fossa; ligaments as in Figure 11-3. B. Diagrammatic vertical section through pelvis and postpelvic body wall.

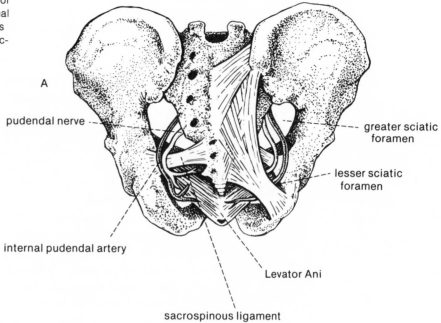

A

pudendal nerve

greater sciatic foramen

lesser sciatic foramen

internal pudendal artery

Levator Ani

sacrospinous ligament

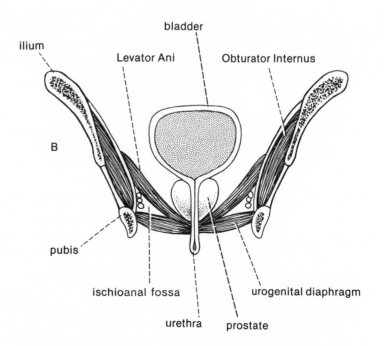

bladder

ilium

Levator Ani

Obturator Internus

B

pubis

ischioanal fossa

urogenital diaphragm

urethra

prostate

blocked by another sheet of hypaxial muscle, the **Transversus Perinei Profundus** (Fig. 11-6) that stretches transversely across between the two hipbones in front, from the pubis back to the ischial tuberosities. This transverse muscle sheet provides a thin floor under the front end of the ischiorectal fossa, in addition to guarding the gap in Levator Ani. Where the urethra passes through it, some of the sheet's muscle fibers wrap around the urethra, thus forming a voluntary sphincter (**Sphincter Urethrae**).

In males, the urethra emerges in the center of the well-developed Transversus Perinei Profundus, and the Sphincter Urethrae is a simple sphincter with circularly arranged fibers. The arrangement is somewhat different in females, because the vaginal opening displaces the urethra cranially (up toward the pubic symphysis) and also cleaves the Transversus Perinei Profundus into right and left halves. This muscle tends to be correspondingly wispy and fascial in females. Its best-developed part is the Sphincter Urethrae, which takes the form of a muscular sling in the fascia. The sling curves over the top of the female urethra and pinches it shut when it contracts.

The Transversus Perinei Profundus, together with the tough fascias enclosing it, is known as the **urogenital diaphragm** (Figs. 11-5B and 11-6). This diaphragm anchors the urogenital openings in place and helps support them. Because the urogenital diaphragm does not extend backward beyond the ischial tuberosities, it has a posterior free edge. This free edge is tied to the anus behind it by a loop of hypaxial muscle fibers that form the **external anal sphincter** (Sphincter Ani Externus) mentioned in Chapter 10. Behind the anus, the fibers of this voluntary sphincter attach to the coccyx; in front of it, they attach to each other and intertwine with fascial and muscular fibers of the urogenital diaphragm.

The fibrous condensation in the midline where the Sphincter Ani Externus and urogenital diaphragm are attached to each other is an important anchorage for many of the pelvic structures. Fibers of Levator Ani's preanal thickening (the vaginal-sphincter part of Pubococcygeus) also tie into this tangled mass, as do fibers from the internal (involuntary) anal sphincter and from the fascias surrounding the prostate or vagina. The resulting wad of connective tissue is called the **central tendon of the perineum,** or perineal body (Fig. 11-9C). It keeps all the visceral and body-wall structures of the perineal region tied together, fixed in place by their connections to each other—and to the bony pelvis, via the pelvic and urogenital diaphragms.

Fig. 11-6 Muscles of the urogenital diaphragm. A. Male. B. Female. The Levator Ani, which lies deep to the urogenital diaphragm, is added in A.

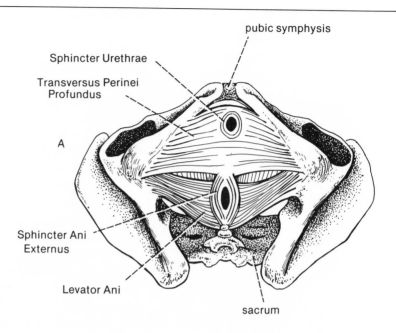

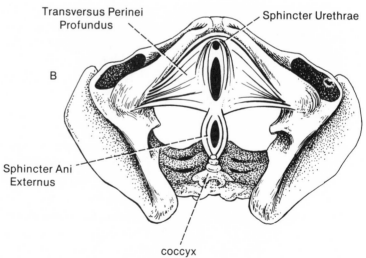

■ The External Genitalia

Another, still more superficial layer of body-wall structures lies plastered against the underside of the urogenital diaphragm, on either side of the urogenital openings. These structures are the erectile organs and associated musculature of the external genitalia. They have no equivalent in the typical body segment.

There are two masses of erectile tissue here on each side—the **bulb** near the midline, and the **crus** (pl. **crura**) more laterally. The bulb is attached to the underside of the urogenital diaphragm; the crus is attached to the bony "frame" under the lower edge of the obturator foramen. In the male, the bulbs and crura are drawn out cranially to form a pendulous copulatory organ, the **penis** (L., "tail"), that hangs down from the superficial fascia of the lower belly. When the lips of the urogenital sinus close over the urethral opening in the male fetus (see Chapter 10), the erectile bulbs on either side of the opening fuse across it to form a single **bulb of the penis** in the midline (Fig. 11-7). The adult male's urethra emerges into this bulb after passing through the urogenital diaphragm, and runs upward and forward to end at the tip of the penis. This penile part of the urethra is enclosed within a tubular prolongation of the bulb called the **corpus spongiosum.** At its tip, the corpus spongiosum expands into a bulbous, acorn-shaped dilatation called the **glans** (L., "acorn"), which surrounds the urethra's opening. The crura (L., "legs") arising from the pubis on either side are similarly prolonged into stout cylindrical **corpora cavernosa,** which have blunt distal ends that fit into hollows in the back of the glans. The corpora cavernosa are bound tightly to each other—and to the corpus spongiosum and glans—by a dense white fascia called the **tunica albuginea.**

The relaxed penis can be compared to a limp balloon hanging through a sling. The sling in this case is a band of dense superficial fascia, the **fundiform** ligament, which descends from the region of the navel to the front of the pubis and splits to form a loop. All three penile shafts of erectile tissue (the corpus spongiosum plus the two corpora cavernosa) run up the underside of the urogenital diaphragm, thread this loop, and then dangle downward. The flaccid penis thus has a sharp bend in it. In erection, the spongy vascular spaces inside the erectile tissue fill with pressurized arterial blood, and the penis swells and stiffens like a balloon inflated with water. The bend at the fundiform sling straightens out and disappears; so the erect organ

Fig. 11-7 Erectile-tissue masses (A) and overlying slips of body-wall muscle (B) in the male perineum. The right corpus cavernosum in (A) has been removed to show the hollows in hipbone and glans, where its ends attach.

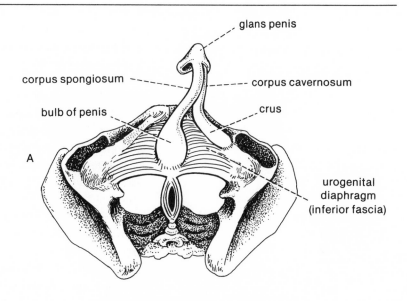

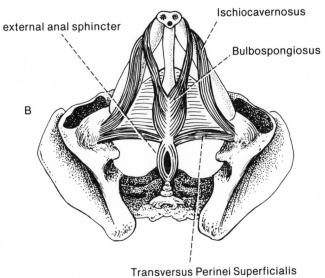

curves up headward as its pendulous part lines up with the attachments of the crura to the pubis.

The female arrangements (Fig. 11-8) are similar, with two conspicuous exceptions. (1) The vagina opens onto the body surface right through the middle of the urogenital diaphragm, so the female's bulbs do not fuse in the midline. Instead, they form two separate masses of erectile tissue, the **bulbs of the vestibule,** on either side of the vaginal opening. (2) As a result, the female urethra is not enclosed in a corpus spongiosum, and the glans of the clitoris is connected to the bulb on each side only by wispy little bands of erectile tissue. The crura and corpora cavernosa are much like those of the male, but considerably smaller.

In both sexes, each mass of erectile tissue is overlain by a thin sheet of hypaxial musculature (Fig. 11-7). The **Ischiocavernosus** arises on each side from the ischium, behind the crus of the penis or clitoris, and wraps laterally around the crus to insert into the tunica albuginea of the corpus cavernosum. The **Bulbospongiosus** muscle similarly overlies the bulb of the penis (or vestibule). It arises from the central tendon in the back (and from a midline raphe in the male) and wraps up around the base of the corpus spongiosum to insert into the tunica

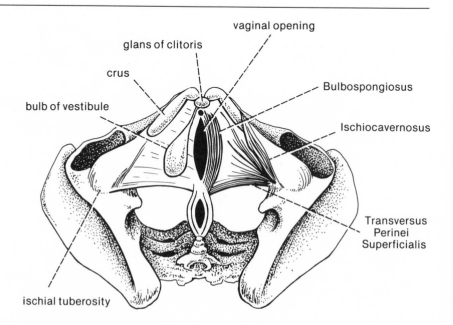

Fig. 11-8 Superficial perineal structures in the adult female. The superficial muscles are omitted on the left of the diagram to expose the crus and the bulb of the vestibule.

glans of clitoris

vaginal opening

crus

bulb of vestibule

Bulbospongiosus

Ischiocavernosus

Transversus Perinei Superficialis

ischial tuberosity

albuginea (or into the fascia of the clitoris). The origins of the two muscles in back are connected by a feeble slip of transverse fibers (**Transversus Perinei Superficialis**) on the anal edge of the urogenital diaphragm; so these three superficial perineal muscles on each side form a little triangle with its rear apex in the central tendon of the perineum.

The functions of these muscles are debated. Some authorities insist that the ones overlying the erectile tissues aid in producing erection, by compressing the veins and causing blood to accumulate in the vascular spaces of the erectile tissue. If this story were correct, erection ought to be voluntary—because these are hypaxial muscles, under voluntary control. It is not. (It can, of course, be controlled to some extent, like salivation and various other autonomic responses, if you have a sufficiently vivid imagination.) In males, the Bulbospongiosus contracts reflexly after urination or ejaculation of semen, thereby squeezing the last few drops of liquid out of the lowermost part of the urethra (inside the bulb of the penis). The female Bulbospongiosus has a slight sphincteric action on the vaginal opening.

There are several peculiar specializations of the skin and superficial fascia at the tail end of the body wall. We shall describe four of them.

1. The skin on either side of the vaginal opening is elaborated into two concentric pairs of vertical "lips"—the hair-covered, fatty **labia majora** laterally and the hairless **labia minora** more medially. The labia minora meet over the top of the clitoris, forming a hood, or **prepuce,** for the female "penis." The labia majora are the female equivalent of the scrotum (minus the gonads and all the body-wall outpocketings that form the coverings of the spermatic cord).

2. The tube of skin enclosing the pendulous part of the penis is underlain by extremely elastic fascia that permits the skin to slide easily back and forth over the tunica albuginea. This is presumably a sort of internal lubricatory mechanism that reduces frictional irritation to both sexes during copulation. This mobile skin is homologous with that forming the prepuce of the clitoris. Like that prepuce, it is tacked down to the underside of the glans by a band called (in both sexes) the **frenulum.**

3. Supplementing the fundiform ligament, a smaller condensation of superficial fascia in the midline—the **suspensory ligament of the penis** (or clitoris)—anchors the penis (or clitoris) directly to the pubic symphysis and helps support the bend in the corpora cavernosa.

4. The fatty superficial fascia on the front of the abdomen contains membranous septa, which fuse into a deep membranous sheet in the perineum. This deep perineal sheet (Colles's fascia) is attached to the rear and side edges of the urogenital diaphragm (Fig. 11-9C). As a result, if the bulb of the penis or the enclosed part of the male urethra (the *bulbous* urethra) are torn open by a traumatic injury, blood and urine leaking from the tear will not spread into the thighs or backward toward the anus because the attachments of Colles's fascia bar the fluids from entering those regions. The pocket in which the leaking fluids may accumulate below the urogenital diaphragm is called the **superficial perineal pouch.**

Is there a *deep* perineal pouch? Yes; this name is given to the space bounded by the fascias enclosing Transversus Perinei Profundus. Ordinarily, the deep pouch contains nothing but the Transversus and the Sphincter Urethrae (and the bulbourethral glands in the male). However, if an injury tears the part of the male urethra that runs through this pouch (the *membranous* urethra), extravasated blood and urine are unable to spread out of the deep pouch, which thus becomes painfully engorged.

■ The Pelvic Celom and the Pelvic Viscera

The peritoneal sac is a closed bag indented by viscera. In the typical body segment, the peritoneal sac is deeply indented on its dorsal aspect by the gut. The dorsal reflections of the peritoneum to the left and right of the gut form a dorsal mesentery, through which the gut's nerves and blood vessels travel to reach their target organs.

Things are different in the pelvis because the peritoneal cavity does not extend down below the level of the pubic symphysis. The bladder, uterus, rectum, and other pelvic viscera thus do not have a dorsal mesentery. Although the lower end of the peritoneal bag is draped over these viscera from above, their lower surfaces have a broad direct contact with the body wall. Thus nerves and blood vessels can reach the pelvic viscera more directly than in the abdomen, by running in various directions through the thick extraperitoneal fascia.

The lower half of the pelvic part of the gut—the rectum and anal canal—is immersed in this fascia. The upper two-thirds or so of the rectum, however, is clothed in peritoneum. It differs from the sigmoid colon above it only in lacking a dorsal mesentery. After a downward

197 THE PELVIS AND THE PERINEUM

Fig. 11-9 Diagrammatic midline sections through the pelvis. In the adult male (A) and female (B), the pelvic end of the peritoneal cavity dips down between the pelvic viscera, forming named pouches of peritoneum. The fold of peritoneum draped over the uterus is called the broad ligament (cf. Fig. 11-11). C. Fascias and enclosed structures of the postpelvic body wall in the male. The bladder and rectum are shown as distended in the male, empty and collapsed in the female.

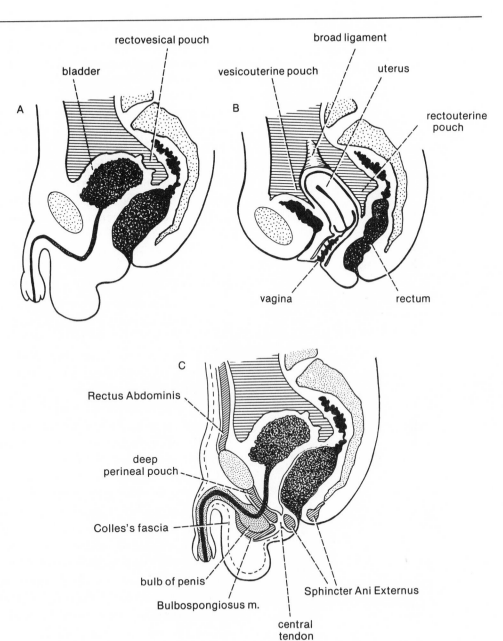

course of about ten centimeters along the front of the sacrum, the rectum ends at the **perineal flexure** (the intestinal kink produced by the Pubococcygeus muscle). There is usually a bulbous dilatation of the rectum, the **rectal ampulla,** just above the flexure. The short length of gut between the flexure and the anal opening (about three centimeters long) is known as the **anal canal.**

In males, the peritoneal sac is reflected off the rectum onto the back of the bladder. The part of the peritoneal cavity that dips down between rectum and bladder is called the **rectovesical pouch** (Fig. 11-9). From the upper surface of the bladder, the peritoneum simply continues ventrally and sideways onto the inside of the body wall.

The female arrangement is not quite so simple because the uterus sticks upward and forward between bladder and rectum, indenting the bottom of the peritoneal cavity (Fig. 11-9). The cavity dips in deeply in front and in back of the uterus, thereby forming **recto-uterine** and **vesicouterine pouches.** The rectouterine pouch (between rectum and uterus) reaches down as far as the upper end of the vaginal wall, contacting the vagina's posterior fornix just behind the uterine cervix. This fact has good and bad implications. The good news is that surgeons can drain blood and foreign matter from the bottom of the peritoneal cavity here easily, by making an incision from the vagina into the rectouterine pouch. The bad news is that objects thrust up into the vagina—for example, a coathanger in the hands of an amateur abortionist—can also pierce through the thin vaginal wall into the rectouterine pouch and cause a life-threatening infection of the peritoneum.

The peritoneal cavity surrounds the uterus in front and in back, but not on its sides. The left and right surfaces of the uterus are connected to the body wall by mesenterylike folds called the **broad** ligaments. You can get a graphic idea of their arrangement by draping a napkin over an upside-down water glass (representing the uterus). Pinch the two layers of the napkin between a thumb and forefinger on either side of the glass and raise the pinched folds straight up to the height of the glass. The folds to the left and right of the glass represent the broad ligaments; the cloth covering the front of the glass is the uterine side of the vesicouterine pouch and that on the back of the glass represents the uterine side of the rectouterine pouch.

The ovary hangs from the rear surface of the broad ligament suspended by its own tiny "mesentery" of peritoneum, the **mesovarium** (Fig. 11-11). The uterine tube runs sideways in the upper edge of the broad ligament and opens through a hole into the peritoneal cavity, directly in front of the ovary. In ovulation, an ovum pops out through the peritoneum clothing the ovary and is swept down the tube to the uterus.

The extraperitoneal fascia surrounding a woman's pelvic viscera is condensed in places to form "ligaments" of thickened connective tissue and smooth muscle fibers. These condensations fan out forward, backward, and sideways from the lower end of the uterus and help to support it and keep it from everting into the vagina. The laterally running **transverse cervical** ligaments (also known as the cardinal ligaments) anchor the cervix and the top part of the vagina to the fascia on the inner surface of Levator Ani on each side. Other condensations, the **uterosacral** ligaments, run dorsally from the cervix and vagina around either side of the rectum to attach to the sacrum. They indent the bottom of the peritoneal sac and produce a pair of **rectouterine folds** of the peritoneum. Yet other condensations tie the mouth of the uterus to the bladder and pubic bone in front.

It is not clear how much all these fascial condensations contribute to keeping the uterus in place. Much of the job seems to be done by the Levator Ani; at any rate, paralysis of the Levator Ani is often followed by uterine *prolapse,* in which the uterus sinks down into the vagina, turning the vagina's upper end inside out like the partly inverted finger of a shucked-off glove. Presumably the weight of the uterus is normally borne indirectly by Levator Ani, via the support it gives to the rectum (which presses against the back of the cervix) and the bladder (which supports the body of the uterus from underneath; Fig. 11-9B). Repeated childbirth, which stretches and weakens the Levator Ani, is the main factor predisposing women to prolapse of the uterus.

▪ The Blood Supply to the Pelvic Viscera

As noted in Chapter 9, the artery that grows out into the hind limb has taken over the job of supplying the pelvic gut and its derivatives. This greatly enlarged intersegmental vessel, the **common iliac** artery, divides into **internal** and **external iliac** arteries on the front of the sacroiliac joint. The external iliac, which is the major artery of the lower limb in the adult, continues down into the thigh. The internal iliac artery curves downward and dorsally into the pelvis and breaks up into a spray of vessels. These provide blood to the pelvic viscera and also to the surrounding parts of the body wall. In general, the body-wall branches arise first, and the visceral branches come off further down; but the branching pattern is variable.

Figure 11-10 shows a common pattern of branches of the internal iliac artery. Near its origin, it gives off a series of arteries that fan out to supply the body wall. The **iliolumbar** and **lateral sacral** arteries, arising high up, are longitudinal anastomoses that have taken over the intersegmental branches of the vestigial sacral part of the aorta (median sacral artery). The **internal pudendal** artery supplies the perineum, as described earlier. Three other body-wall branches, the **obturator, superior gluteal,** and **inferior gluteal** arteries, supply regions of the hind limb near the pelvis. (Remember that the limbs are specialized outgrowths of the body wall.) The two gluteal arteries leave the pelvis in back, through the greater sciatic foramen; the obturator artery exists ventrally, through the upper edge of the obturator foramen (Fig. 11-4).

After giving off all these body-wall branches, the internal iliac commonly splits into two terminal branches that supply the pelvic viscera. The lower of these two visceral branches is a common trunk for the **middle rectal** and **inferior vesical** arteries. The distributions of the two correspond roughly to the division of the embryonic hindgut into rectum and urogenital sinus. As its name implies, the middle rectal artery reaches the middle part of the rectum and is supplemented by two other arteries: a **superior rectal** branch from the inferior mesenteric artery and an **inferior rectal** branch of the internal pudendal that runs up out of the anal region. Like the abdominal part of the gut, the rectum has a highly anastomotic blood supply, and blood passing through any of these vessels can supply the whole rectum if necessary.

The inferior vesical artery on each side courses downward and forward to supply most of the bladder. Its branches also supply most of the reproductive organs in the pelvis—the uterus, uterine (fallopian) tubes, and vagina in females and the deferent and ejaculatory ducts, prostate, and seminal vesicles in males. The female arteries run in the base of the broad ligament. Their equivalents in males simply run directly to their target organs.

The ovary is the only major pelvic organ that does not get its principal blood supply from a branch of the internal iliac artery. Its blood vessels run down into the pelvis from high up in the abdomen (Chapter 10), following the trail taken by the ovary when it de-

Fig. 11-10 Branches of the internal iliac artery in the male (schematic). The arteries (numbered) of the right side and the pelvic viscera lying medial to them are seen here from the lateral aspect.

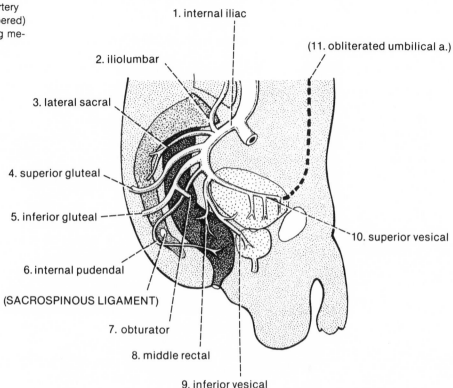

1. internal iliac

(11. obliterated umbilical a.)

2. iliolumbar

3. lateral sacral

4. superior gluteal

5. inferior gluteal

6. internal pudendal

(SACROSPINOUS LIGAMENT)

10. superior vesical

7. obturator

8. middle rectal

9. inferior vesical

scended. They reach the ovary through the lateral end of the broad ligament (Fig. 11-11). The surrounding fascia is thickened to form a **suspensory ligament of the ovary** that ties the ovary to the inside of the bony pelvis.

The trail that the ovary *would* have followed down into the labia majora if it had been a testis is marked by two fibromuscular cords, remnants of the ovary's gubernaculum: the **ligament of the ovary** and the **round ligament of the uterus.** The ligament of the ovary runs just below the uterine tube inside the broad ligament, connecting the ovary to the upper corner of the uterus. Branches of the ovary's blood vessels run with it, anastomosing with the internal iliac's uterine branches coming up from below. The round ligament of the uterus curves back laterally through the broad ligament, onto the inside of the body wall, to hook around the inferior epigastric artery and run back medially through the inguinal canal. This course is the same as

Fig. 11-11 Uterus and ovaries seen from behind. The peritoneum has been removed on the right to disclose the contents of the broad ligament. Note the anastomosis of ovarian and uterine vessels. The ligament of the ovary and the round ligament of the uterus are fibrous cords derived from the ovary's gubernaculum.

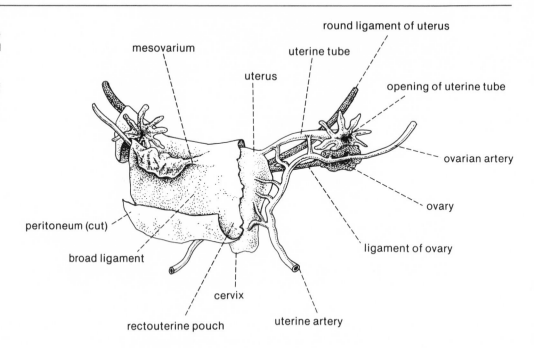

that of the deferent duct, which the fetal testis drags along with it when it moves down its gubernaculum into the scrotum.

In the fetus, the most important branch of the internal iliac artery is the one to the allantois—the **umbilical** artery that vascularizes the placenta. In the adult, most of this vessel is an atrophic cord, but its proximal end persists to supply a cluster of small **superior vesical** arteries to the upper front corner of the bladder—where the urachus persists as a reminder of the embryonic connection here between bladder and allantois.

▪ Pelvic Veins and Portal Anastomoses

Most of the blood from the pelvic organs drains back through tangled, plexiform tributaries of the internal iliac veins, which correspond to branches of the internal iliac artery. From there, the blood flows on into the inferior vena cava. Blood from the rectum can also drain up through the portal system of veins, however, because the inferior, middle, and superior rectal veins are all connected with each other, and the superior one drains into the portal vein's inferior mesenteric tributary.

Because there are no valves in the portal system, blood from the portal vein can also flow in the other direction—that is, down through the inferior mesenteric vein to reach the venous plexus around the rectum. This fact has clinical importance. If the flow of blood through the liver is obstructed by disease—by cancer, for instance, or by alcoholic cirrhosis—then the veins around the rectum provide a path back to the heart for blood that cannot get through the diseased liver. As liver obstruction becomes increasingly complete, more and more blood from the intestines will flow backward through the few portal-vein tributaries that anastomose with veins outside the portal system. Besides the veins of the rectum, these include esophageal veins around the upper end of the stomach, portal-vein twigs that communicate with the renal veins (in the gut mesenteries that fuse to the peritoneum across the front of the kidneys), and even little portal branches in the liver's falciform ligament, which anastomose with the epigastric veins around the navel. Swollen with an overload of portal-system blood, the anastomosing veins become bloated and varicose. The protruding anal varicosities called **hemorrhoids** are a common result. Ugly, tortuous epigastric varicosities—known as the **caput Medusae** ("Medusa's head") after the snake-haired Gorgon of Greek myth—may pop out in serpentine coils under the skin of the belly. Varicose esophageal veins can become so engorged and weakened that they tear open and gush blood, sometimes with fatal results.

■ Nerves of the Pelvic Viscera: Review of Autonomics

The innervation of the pelvic viscera is complicated, and the effects that the motor nerves have on some of those viscera—especially the reproductive apparatus—are still largely a mystery. Because autonomic motor fibers reach the pelvic organs by three distinct pathways, it seems worthwhile to repeat here a fair amount of what was said in earlier chapters about the autonomic nervous system.

All *sympathetic* motor pathways begin in the intermediolateral column of the spinal cord, in segments T.1 to L.2. Sympathetic fibers targeted for the pelvic viscera start from the lower segments of that column and follow the usual course (ventral root, ventral ramus, white ramus communicans) into the sympathetic trunk. They run down to the pelvis by two routes—via the trunk itself, or via splanchnic nerves that enter the chain of mesenteric ganglia on the front of the abdominal aorta. They synapse in the ganglia they encounter along either route. The fibers that enter the pelvis are all postsynaptic.

They form **lumbar** and **sacral splanchnic** nerves running medially from the sympathetic trunk and a **superior hypogastric plexus** running down from the aorta. All these fibers feed into two tangled skeins of autonomic nerves, the **inferior hypogastric plexuses,** lying on either side of the rectum (Figs. 9-16 and 9-17).

The *parasympathetic* motor pathways to the pelvic viscera also begin in the spinal cord, in the sacral equivalent of the intermediolateral column. They emerge with the ventral rami of spinal nerves S.2 and S.4 and form parasympathetic bundles (the **pelvic splanchnic** nerves) that enter the inferior hypogastric plexuses. Like the sympathetic fibers in those plexuses, the parasympathetics follow the branches of the adjacent internal iliac artery to their target organs. (Some of them also run up the superior hypogastric plexus to supply the distal colon.)

The innervation of the rectum and anal canal follows the usual gut-tube pattern. Parasympathetic impulses synapse on ganglion cells buried in the rectum's muscular walls, causing peristalsis and relaxing the internal anal sphincter. The result is an urge to move one's bowels. (The bowel movement itself has to wait for the voluntary *external* anal sphincter to relax as well.) Sympathetic stimulation has the opposite effect, relaxing the walls of the rectum and contracting the involuntary sphincter. The arteries of the rectum, like those of the rest of the gut, also contract under sympathetic stimulation. This rechannels blood into the striated muscles, which are needed more than the gut in fight-or-flight situations.

The bladder is derived from the embryonic hindgut, and its innervation is much like that of the rectum. Parasympathetics empty it; sympathetics constrict its outlet and keep it from being emptied. The smooth muscles of the bladder are thickened at the top of the urethra to form an involuntary sphincter of sorts. This **Sphincter Vesicae** is thought to contract under sympathetic stimulation, but it may not actually be powerful enough to hold back urine without help from the surrounding voluntary muscles. The slow peristaltic waves in the ureters that "milk" urine from the kidneys down into the bladder appear to be independent of nerve impulses; they keep on going even in cases where the ureter has had its innervation stripped off.

Still less is known about the innervation of the gonads. When the gonads descend into the pelvis, they drag not only their blood vessels along behind them, but also their sympathetic nerves. These probably act to constrict the accompanying arteries. It is not clear whether there are any parasympathetic nerves that reach the gonads. Parasympathetic postsynaptic fibers do reach the uterus and uterine tubes—their cell bodies form recognizable ganglia near the uterine cervix—but nobody knows what purpose these nerves serve. The smooth muscles in the walls of these female reproductive organs seem to be mostly or entirely controlled by hormones circulating in the bloodstream.

The male reproductive apparatus is another story. Erection of the penis and ejaculation of semen both depend on autonomic nerve impulses. The penis is normally kept limp by sympathetic impulses that constrict the arteries supplying the erectile tissue. During sexual excitation, *parasympathetic* impulses reaching these vessels (from the autonomic plexus around the prostate) cause their walls to dilate, thus engorging the erectile tissue with blood and making the penis stiffen. Ejaculation is produced by intense *sympathetic* discharges that cause the ductus deferens, seminal vesicles, and prostate to contract and squirt their contents into the urethra. As might be expected, this sympathetic stimulation also causes the Sphincter Vesicae to contract, preventing semen from backing up into the bladder. Reflex contractions in the Bulbospongiosus help to empty the urethra inside the bulb of the penis, just as they do following urination. A renewed predominance of sympathetic over parasympathetic impulses following orgasm constricts the arteries of the erectile tissue and thus causes the penis (or its female equivalents) to become flaccid again.

THE
LIMBS

PART IV

Fundamentals
of Limb Anatomy

12

■ Limb Origins and Ontogeny

The first vertebrates, like today's lampreys and hagfishes, lacked jaws and paired fins. They also had only two semicircular canals. Jaws, fins, and a third semicircular canal all appeared together as a suite in early bony fishes some 400 million years ago. All three features may have originated as adaptations for feeding on actively swimming prey, instead of grubbing around on the sea bottom as most primitive fishes seem to have done.

The paired fins of jawed fishes are specialized flaps of the body wall that serve as steering organs in swimming. The base of a fish's fin is a flat plate of bone attached to the muscles of the body wall. The fin itself is a flexible fan of smaller bones that sticks out sideways from the plate. This bony fan is moved by two little masses of muscle—a dorsal group of **elevators** that pull it upward and a ventral group of **depressors** that pull it downward. These little muscles adjust the angle at which the fin meets the water, thus causing the fish to turn, climb, or descend as it swims forward propelled by its tail.

The "fins" of land-dwelling vertebrates are usually much larger and stouter than fish fins. The basic arrangement and developmental pattern of the limbs of amphibians, reptiles, birds, and mammals is nevertheless still the same as in fishes. In a human embryo, just as in a fish embryo, the limbs form from hypaxial (body-wall) mesenchyme that streams off the ventral and lateral surface of the somites and proliferates under the skin. The resulting lump of skin-covered mesenchyme is called the **limb bud** (Fig. 12-1). The limb-bud mesenchyme splits into dorsal and ventral masses, corresponding to the elevator and depressor muscles. Bones form in between these two masses. As the limb bud increases in size, the two primitive muscle

Fig. 12-1 Diagrammatic section along the axis of a limb bud, showing fundamental dorsal–ventral division in muscles and nerves.

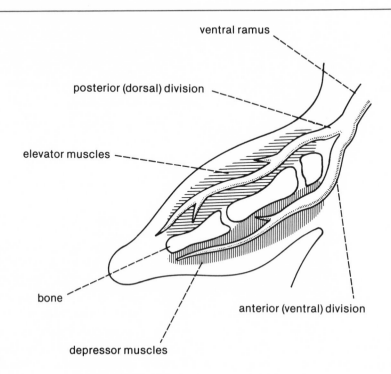

ventral ramus

posterior (dorsal) division

elevator muscles

bone

anterior (ventral) division

depressor muscles

masses subdivide and differentiate into many independent muscles crossing the various joints between the limb bones.

The distinction between elevators and depressors is reflected in the innervation of the limb muscles. Like all other hypaxial structures, the limbs are innervated by ventral rami of the segmental nerves. Each limb bud is invaded by several ventral rami (from the segments that contributed mesenchyme to it). As each ventral ramus grows down into the limb bud, it splits into two branches—an **anterior** (or ventral) **division** that innervates the depressor muscles, and a **posterior** (or dorsal) **division** that innervates the elevator muscles.

Hold your upper limb straight out sideways from the body, with the palm facing ventrally. This position approximates the posture of one of your fishy forebears, lying belly down on a Devonian mud flat. All the muscles on the ventral surface of your limb in this position, from the edge of your sternum out to the tips of your fingers, are depressor muscles, derived from the ventral mass of premuscle mesenchyme in your embryonic limb bud. They are innervated by the anterior divisions of the ventral rami that supply the upper limb. Similarly, all the muscles on the back side of your limb, from your shoulder blade down to your fingertips, are elevator musculature, derived from the dorsal mass of mesenchyme and innervated by posterior divisions of those same ventral rami. Similar remarks apply to the lower limb (although the posture is harder to assume).

Obviously, people do not move around on their bellies with their arms and legs sticking out sideways; and so our "elevator" and "depressor" muscles do not produce the movements that these names imply. We are going to use these terms in describing human limb musculature; but it is important to note that they refer only to the fundamental dorsal–ventral division in our limb muscles and nerves and imply *nothing* whatever about muscle *function*.

The ventral rami that grow out into the limb bud do not simply split into anterior and posterior divisions and keep on growing and branching like a row of separate trees in an orchard. Instead they swap fibers back and forth, thus forming a nerve plexus at the base of the limb. Each of the nerves that emerges from this plexus and streams out into the limb usually contains fibers from more than one ventral ramus. This intermingling of the ventral rami obliterates the anatomical boundaries between body segments in the limbs.

■ Muscle Groups

Although the body's segmentation is obscured in the limbs, a new organizing principle comes into the picture. The embryonic masses of premuscle mesenchyme in the limb bud go on subdividing after their nerves have grown into them. As a result, *several muscles in the adult limb will usually share a single nerve,* because they all developed from a single mass of mesenchyme supplied by that nerve. For the same reason, they will usually lie close together in a cluster and will frequently have similar attachments and actions.

Such a cluster of "sibling" muscles, sharing a common developmental history and a single motor nerve, is called a **muscle group.** There are far fewer muscle groups than muscles in the limbs. For example, there are fifty-eight muscles in the human forelimb, but they can be conveniently lumped into fourteen basic muscle groups. Learning the fundamental arrangement of these fourteen groups makes it easier to go on and learn the facts about the fifty-eight muscles.

Muscle groups are not mere theoretical constructs cooked up as aids to memory. Because they develop from separate masses of mesenchyme, the muscle groups are separated from each other in the adult by sheets of connective tissue called **intermuscular septa,** which condensed out of the tissues left between the premuscle masses. Anyone who eats mammal flesh is familiar with intermuscular septa. For example, in a ham steak (which is a cross section through a pig's thigh), the septa appear as curved partitions of tough, inedible tissue running from the ham bone out to the steak's circumference. The major intermuscular septa in the limbs form the boundaries between the major muscle groups (Fig. 15-8). The limbs thus come apart into their constituent muscle groups physically, not just theoretically. Major nerves and blood vessels also help to demarcate muscle groups; they tend to grow into the limb bud along intermuscular septa, where they can avoid the tugging and squeezing they would be subjected to if they ran right through the flesh of a contracting muscle.

▪ The Limb Skeleton

Fish fins are flexible paddles full of small bones. Turning these pliant flippers into limbs suitable for getting around on land involved transforming them into jointed rods with a few much larger bony elements. The basic pattern of the early amphibian limb skeleton is retained in our limbs (Fig. 12-2). Each limb has three major joints in it, dividing it into four pieces or **limb segments** (not to be confused with body segments). The most *proximal* limb segment (that is, the one closest to the body) is the basal plate buried in the body-wall muscles. In our upper limb, this is the shoulder blade (scapula); the lower limb's basal plate is the hipbone (os coxae). The next segment out (the upper arm or thigh) has a single large bone in it. The one after that (the forearm or calf) has two parallel bones in it. The most *distal* limb segment (the one farthest from the body) is a fan of jointed bony rays—the hand or the foot. This fan has a cluster of small wrist bones (**carpals**) or ankle bones (**tarsals**) at its proximal end. From this base sprout five **digital rays,** forming the bones of the fingers or toes. Each digit contains a large proximal "meta" bone—**metacarpals** in the hand, **metatarsals** in the foot—and a chain of shorter distal bones called **phalanges.** The hand and foot of land vertebrates typically retain some of the many-jointed flexibility of the ancestral fish limb.

The bony plates at the base of each limb are called **limb girdles** in land-dwelling vertebrates. They are much larger than their homologs

Fig. 12-2 The limb skeleton and its serial homologies in land-dwelling vertebrates.

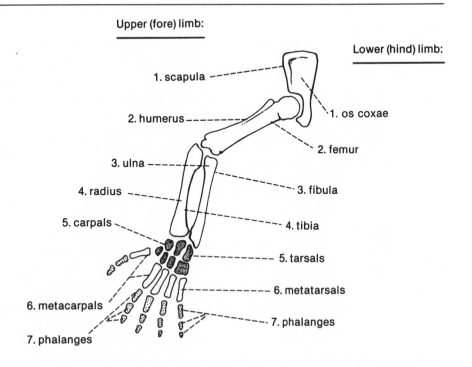

Upper (fore) limb:

Lower (hind) limb:

1. scapula

2. humerus

3. ulna

4. radius

5. carpals

6. metacarpals

7. phalanges

1. os coxae

2. femur

3. fibula

4. tibia

5. tarsals

6. metatarsals

7. phalanges

in fish because they have to bear the body's weight and provide attachment for the enlarged elevator and depressor muscles. In early land dwellers, the left and right hind-limb girdles joined the sacral vertebrae dorsally to produce a complete bony ring embedded in the body wall all around the tail end of the abdomen. This composite ring, the pelvis (Chapter 11), provides a stable base for the hind limb.

The human forelimb girdle (or **shoulder girdle**) has a more complicated structure and history. The basal plate of a fish's front fin is attached to the back end of the head. When land-going fishes started walking on their fins, the forelimb girdle needed to be liberated from the skull so that the animals' heads did not, say, automatically turn left whenever they brought the right forelimb forward. This need was met by shoving the girdle tailward and leaving a short flexible neck between the girdle and the back of the skull. When the limb girdle moved aft, however, some of the head's dermal armor and gill muscles stayed attached to it. Our own shoulder girdle is still attached to the skull by a couple of those old gill muscles (Trapezius, Sternocleidomastoideus)—which are the only limb muscles not innervated by ventral rami.

The forelimb girdle of our primitive reptilian ancestors was a complicated and unwieldy contraption, solidly jointed onto the sternum and looking something like a pelvis with no sacrum. It incorporated both dermal and cartilage-replacement bones. Our own shoulder girdle is simpler and more mobile. In today's mammals (except for the Australian egg-layers), three primitive cartilage-replacement bones have fused together to form the shoulder blade or **scapula,** which bears the socket for the ball-and-socket shoulder joint. Only one of the dermal elements remains—the **clavicle,** or collarbone, which is an S-shaped rod running from the sternum to the "point" of the shoulder. That "point" is formed by a projection (the acromion process) on the scapula just above the shoulder joint's socket. The clavicle acts as a strut to keep the scapula and the shoulder socket it carries sticking out laterally, away from the rib cage (Fig. 12-3). The clavicle holds the acromion process at a constant distance from the sternum. But the scapula is otherwise free to slide and rotate around on the back of the rib cage. It does so whenever we raise or lower our shoulders or move them forward and backward.

In mammals, the long cylindrical limb bones typically form as cartilaginous rods and then ossify in three pieces—a central **diaphysis** and two terminal **epiphyses.** Until growth ceases, these three ossification centers are separated by intervening **epiphyseal** (or **growth) plates** of persisting cartilage (Fig. 12-4). During growth, these plates deposit new cartilage on the ends of the diaphysis. The cartilage is replaced by bone, and the process continues until the bone reaches adult length. The three bony pieces fuse together and growth stops.

There are some exceptions to this general pattern of limb-bone development. The bones of the digital rays have only a single epiphysis. The clavicle is a dermal bone and thus is not preformed as a rod of cartilage. It does develop an epiphysis and epiphyseal plate at its medial end, however; so the adult clavicle includes some cartilage-replacement bone. The tarsal and carpal bones mostly ossify from single centers. (However, some represent fusions of primitively separate bones, which still ossify independently and then grow together.) Secondary **traction epiphyses** develop at several places where muscles attach to the limb bones (Fig. 12-4). An example is the crest of the ilium, which forms as a separate little bony crust along the top of the ilium where the body-wall muscles are attached. It fuses with the iliac

Fig. 12-3 The human thorax and shoulder girdle, seen from the head end. Compare with Fig.
13-1.

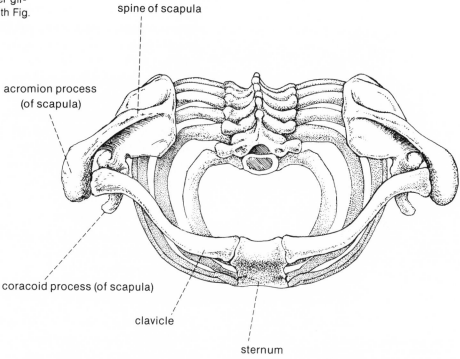

spine of scapula

acromion process
(of scapula)

coracoid process (of scapula)

clavicle

sternum

blade following puberty. All these epiphyses allow the chief stress-
bearing parts of a child's bones (joint surfaces or muscle attachments)
to ossify solidly without giving up the cartilage plates involved in
bone growth.

■ Limb Movements and Their Terminology

Any connection between two separate bones is called a **joint.** All of
an adult's limb joints are mobile joints of the synovial type (Fig.
2-6)—that is, where two limb bones come into contact, the contacting surfaces of both bones are covered with slick hyaline cartilage and
surrounded by a synovial membrane oozing lubricant fluid into a
joint cavity between the two surfaces. (The only exception is the joint
between the tibia and fibula at the bottom of the calf, which is usually
a fibrous joint with no articular cartilage, synovial membrane, or
joint cavity.)

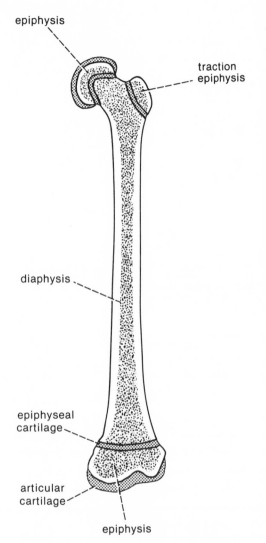

epiphysis

traction
epiphysis

diaphysis

epiphyseal
cartilage

articular
cartilage

epiphysis

Fig. 12-4   The parts of a developing limb bone.

The movements that are possible at a synovial joint are limited both by the shape of the articular surfaces and by the anatomy of the fibrous capsule surrounding the joint. Take two coins and place one directly on top of the other, representing two articular cartilages of a synovial joint. The coins' flat contact surfaces restrict their movements. As long as the upper coin lies flat atop the lower one, it can move only by spinning around a vertical axis or sliding horizontally. This restriction still leaves a lot of mobility, because there are an infinite number of possible vertical axes and horizontal paths. But if you tape the two coins together at one point on their edges, only one possible movement remains—rotation around a vertical axis passing through the taped points. The tape imitates a tight part of the joint's fibrous capsule. If the "capsule" were tight everywhere—if both coins' edges were encircled with a band of tape—no movement of one coin on the other would be possible. This simple model shows how joint-surface shape and capsular anatomy both contribute to limitation of mobility.

There are always limitations on any joint's mobility. The most mobile type of joint surface is a ball-and-socket configuration like that of the hip joint, in which one articular cartilage is a sphere and the other is a spherical cup. Such a joint allows rotation and swinging in all directions. But even in a ball-and-socket joint, the fibrous capsule always checks any movement after a certain point. Most of the joints in our limbs are not ball-and-socket joints, but something more like hinges, with narrowly limited mobility around a single axis. Whenever limitations on movement do not interfere with function, *evolution works to limit joint mobility*. Fewer axes of movement at a joint mean that fewer muscles are needed to control that joint; so more and more of the job of keeping the joint stable can be shifted over from muscles to capsular ligaments. This shift is desirable because ligaments use up a lot less food and oxygen than muscles do.

The terms used in describing movements at our joints are somewhat arbitrary. Every axis of movement permits rotation or sliding in two directions (to and fro); so there are at least two named movements for every joint. Where there are an infinite number of possible axes of rotation at a joint, the usual convention is to define two or three perpendicular axes and then describe other rotations as combinations of those terms (like describing a 45° vector on a map as north plus east). The common terms for describing human limb-joint movements are presented in the following paragraphs.

1. **Flexion.** This term comprises most of the movements ordinarily called bending: bending the knee, elbow, fingers, or toes. Applied to the ball-and-socket joints at the base of our limbs (the shoulder and hip joints), flexion has a special meaning: rotation through a transverse axis that swings the limb *ventrally*—that is, bringing the knee or elbow up in front.

2. **Extension.** The opposite of flexion, in any sense: that is, straightening out the fingers or knee, swinging the elbow backward, and so on.

3. **Abduction.** Movement away from the midline. Usually, the midline referred to is the body's midline. Abduction at the shoulder or hip means swinging the limb out sideways. Abduction at the wrist means swinging the hand out sideways from a special reference position (the so-called "anatomical position") in which the hand dangles alongside the thigh with the palm facing ventrally. Wrist abduction, then, is the same thing as swinging the hand toward its thumb side; the term "radial deviation" is coming to be preferred over "abduction" for describing this movement. ("Radial" refers to the **radius,** the forearm bone on the thumb side.) In the special case of the fingers and toes, the midline axis to which "abduction" refers is the midline of the hand or foot, not of the body. Abducting your fingers or toes is the same thing as spreading them apart.

4. **Adduction.** The opposite of abduction, in any sense. Drawing the elbow medially down against the thorax, pressing the extended fingers together, and so on. The preferred term for wrist adduction is "ulnar deviation," referring to the **ulna** (the other bone in the forearm, on the little-finger side).

5. **Volarflexion.** Flexion at the ankle or wrist: a hinge movement that carries the whole hand in the direction of the palm or the foot toward the sole. Sometimes called simply *flexion.*

6. **Dorsiflexion.** The opposite of volarflexion: extension of the wrist or ankle. Why is this special term used? Because extreme dorsiflexion of the wrist or ankle does not *straighten* the limb; like volarflexion, it puts a 90° bend between the hand and the forearm, or between the foot and the leg.

7. **Medial rotation.** Any rotation that carries the *ventral* surface of some limb segment medially. Bring your elbow down to your side and flex it to a 90° angle, so that your hand sticks out in front of you; then fold your arms across your chest. Your humerus (the bone in your upper arm) rotates medially when you do this; the movement takes

Fig. 12-5 The forearm bones and hand in pronation and supination. A right forearm, anterior view.

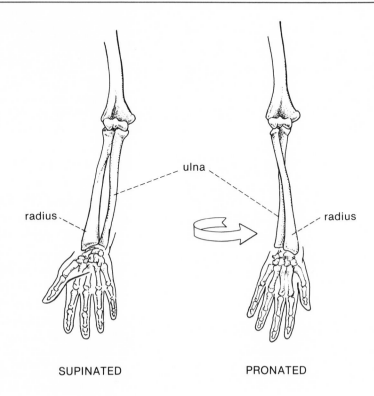

ulna

radius

radius

SUPINATED

PRONATED

place at the shoulder joint. Likewise, pointing your knees inward involves medial rotation at the hip joint.

8. **Lateral rotation.** The opposite of medial rotation, in any sense.

In addition to the general terms that can be used to describe movement at any joint, there are a few that have a more restricted application. Medial rotation of the radius across the ulna, which flops the hand into a palm-down position (Fig. 12-5), is called **pronation** (prone = "face down"). The reverse movement—bringing the two forearm bones back into parallel and turning the palm upward—is **supination.** Volarflexion of the ankle is also called **plantarflexion** (L. *planta*, "sole of the foot"). Turning the sole of the foot inward, so that it faces medially, is **inversion** of the foot; the reverse movement is **eversion.** These two foot movements involve coordinated movements at the joints between the tarsal bones (see Chapter 16).

The Shoulder
and the Arm

13

■ **The Bones and Joints of the Shoulder Region**

The human upper limb is much more mobile than the lower limb, chiefly because the scapula is not jointed solidly onto the vertebral column as the hipbone is. When the upper arm bone moves in its socket, the socket-bearing scapula at the base of the limb can itself slide and rotate against the underlying rib cage to enhance the movement. The ball-and-socket shoulder joint is called the **glenohumeral** joint, a name combining those of the upper arm bone (**humerus**) and its socket (the **glenoid fossa**) at the lateral edge of the scapula.

The bones of the shoulder region are shown in Figure 13-1. The humeral "ball" or **head** is considerably larger than its glenoid socket and has a more extensive articular surface. This disproportion between the two articular surfaces is typical of highly mobile joints. Whenever the humerus swings in any direction, parts of the spherical humeral head that were not previously touching the scapula rotate into the glenoid socket. Great mobility thus requires a large "spare" joint surface on the humerus. In general, you can tell how mobile a joint is by looking at the excess articular surface left over when the bones are articulated together.

The scapula is a flattened plate, roughly the shape of a right triangle with its hypotenuse lying alongside the vertebral spines. The glenoid lies at the scapula's right-angled (upper lateral) corner. The spine of the scapula projects from its dorsal surface and ends laterally in the **acromion process,** which sticks out behind (dorsal to) the glenoid, looking something like the handle of a misshapen trowel (Fig. 13-1). In front, medial and a bit ventral to the glenoid, the **coracoid process** projects forward from the scapula's cranial edge like a fingertip reaching sideways toward the head of the humerus. These two bony pro-

Fig. 13-1 The thorax (*dashed lines*) and right shoulder girdle. Front (A) and back (B) views.

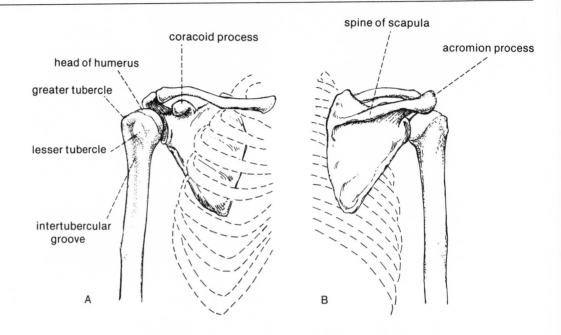

jections from the scapula provide attachments for muscles—and for ligaments that help limit the mobility of the scapula.

Most of the limitation on scapular movement is due to the clavicle, not to ligaments. The clavicle holds the scapula at a fixed distance from the sternum; so the scapula can only swivel around at the end of the clavicle like a trowel nailed by its handle to the end of a gearshift. Strong **coracoclavicular** ligaments (Fig. 13-2) run laterally from the scapula's coracoid process to the lateral end of the clavicle and prevent the scapula from being driven medially (by a blow to the side of the humerus, for instance). These ligaments are stronger than the clavicle itself—a fall on the shoulder is more likely to break the collarbone than to tear the ligaments. Because the capsule of the **acromioclavicular** joint between the scapula and clavicle is not very strong, the coracoclavicular ligaments are also largely responsible for keeping the two bones from separating under stress.

The capsule of the glenohumeral joint is also rather weak. Moreover, it has to have a lot of slack in it because the joint is so mobile. (If the capsule of any joint had no slack in it, that joint could not be moved without tearing the capsule; remember the coin-and-tape

Fig. 13-2 Ligaments of the right shoulder. Anterior view.

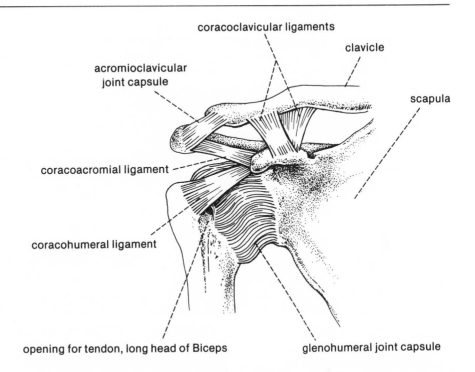

coracoclavicular ligaments

clavicle

acromioclavicular joint capsule

scapula

coracoacromial ligament

coracohumeral ligament

opening for tendon, long head of Biceps

glenohumeral joint capsule

model in Chapter 12.) As a result, the glenohumeral joint capsule offers little resistance to dislocation, and so the shoulder is one of the most easily dislocated joints in the body. A thick **coracoacromial** ligament (Fig. 13-2), binding the coracoid and acromial processes of the scapula together, forms a tough, flexible arch over the top of the humeral head (without attaching to it) and thus helps prevent upward dislocation. A thinner **coracohumeral** ligament guards against downward dislocation. The acromion itself prevents dislocation of the humeral head in a backward (dorsal) direction. In all other directions, the muscles that move the glenohumeral joint are the only real defense against dislocation of the shoulder.

The spherical humeral head is one of three bony masses at the upper end of the humerus. The other two are the **greater** and **lesser tubercles** of the humerus (Fig. 13-1). These tubercles, and the ridges or crests that run downward away from them on the front of the humerus, are the sites of attachment for almost all the muscles that control the glenohumeral joint and guard it against dislocation.

▪ Movements of the Scapula

The two kinds of shoulder movements (movement at the glenohumeral joint and movement of the whole shoulder girdle) add up to a lot of mobility. The humeral ball can rotate in any direction in the glenoid socket, and the scapula can slide in any direction across the back of the rib cage. The four basic movements of the scapula are **elevation** (raising the shoulder, as in shrugging), **depression** (the opposite of elevation), **protraction** (thrusting the shoulder forward) and **retraction** (the opposite of protraction, that is, throwing the shoulder back). The clavicle also swings up, down, forward, or backward with the scapula. During elevation or depression, the scapula not only slides upward or downward across the back, it also **rotates.**

Most movements of the humerus are accompanied by sliding and rotation of the scapula. Swing your arm sideways from your body until your hand is pointing straight up in the air. This may feel like a single simple rotation of 180° to you, but you can easily prove (by using your other hand to palpate the greater tuberosity and acromion) that it is not. Abduction of the humerus alone can go no further than about 90°. The rest of this movement is produced by a combination of protraction and elevation of the scapula, which starts rotating as soon as the humerus begins to swing away from its vertical rest position. Anything that damages the muscles producing these scapular movements may produce significant and surprising defects in upper-limb function.

▪ The Brachial Plexus

Although the human upper limb is attached to the thorax, the limb is mostly innervated from the *cervical* part of the spinal cord, because the embryonic limb bud formed alongside the lower cervical somites. This is another example of the general tailward slippage of body segments relative to spinal-cord segments.

The ventral rami that grow into the upper limb bud form the **brachial plexus.** Five ventral rami, from C.5 to T.1, feed into this plexus. (These rami are known, confusingly enough, as the "roots" of the plexus; do not confuse these with the dorsal and ventral roots of a spinal nerve!) The upper and lower pairs of these five ventral rami fuse, forming three parallel nerve **trunks.** Each trunk then divides into **anterior** and **posterior divisions** (Fig. 13-3). From this point on down the limb, elevator and depressor innervation are wholly separate.

Fig. 13-3 Simplified schema of the right brachial plexus. Posterior-division nerves (to elevator musculature) are shaded.

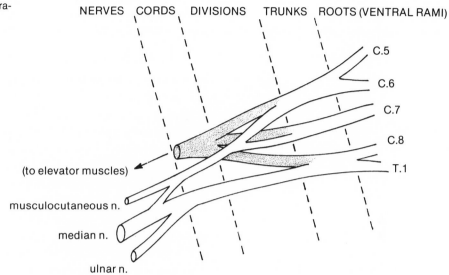

NERVES · CORDS · DIVISIONS · TRUNKS · ROOTS (VENTRAL RAMI)

C.5
C.6
C.7
C.8
T.1

(to elevator muscles)

musculocutaneous n.

median n.

ulnar n.

The three *posterior* divisions of the plexus are destined to supply the elevator muscle groups. They fuse to form a single **posterior cord** of the plexus, which divides into the nerves to the elevator musculature. Most of the fibers in this cord go into the **radial** nerve, which supplies all the elevator muscles below the shoulder area.

The three *anterior* divisions of the brachial plexus do not form a single anterior cord; the two upper ones join to form a **lateral cord,** and the lowermost anterior division simply gets rechristened the **medial cord.** (The three cords of the plexus—posterior, lateral, medial—are named for their relationship to the big **axillary** artery, the continuation of the subclavian artery, which runs through the midst of the plexus.) The lateral and medial cords then bifurcate, and the adjoining pair of branches fuse, producing an M-shaped arrangement that ends in three major nerves. These three nerves, reading from lateral to medial, are the **musculocutaneous, median,** and **ulnar** nerves. They provide most of the motor innervation to the depressor muscles in the arm, forearm, and hand, respectively.

The muscles surrounding the shoulder joint, and some of the specialized body-wall muscles that connect the shoulder girdle to the vertebrae and ribs, receive smaller branches from various parts of the plexus. We will fit them into the picture as we deal with the muscles involved. The attachments, actions, and innervations of all the limb muscles supplied by the brachial plexus are detailed below and sum-marized in the accompanying tables.

■ Trapezius

Almost all the muscles that attach to the bones of the upper limb are innervated by the brachial plexus. (A few minor limb muscles are innervated from higher cervical ventral rami.) But there is one impor-tant limb muscle that is not supplied by spinal nerves at all, but by a cranial nerve. This muscle, **Trapezius** (L., "diamond-shaped"; cf. *trapezoid*) is a made-over branchial (gill) muscle. It is the most superficial muscle on the back and the largest branchiomeric (gill-arch-derived) muscle in the human body.

The Trapezius of terrestrial vertebrates seems to be derived from a muscle sheet in fish that runs down from the back of the head to the tops of the gill-arch bones (Fig. 21-1). In a fish, this muscle lifts the whole set of gills up dorsally when it contracts. The tail end of this gill-lifting (Trapezius) sheet attaches to the forelimb girdle bones, which lie directly behind the gill arches. When the head and forelimb girdle parted company in early amphibians, the Trapezius sheet lost its connection with the gill-arch bones; but it remained stretched between the skull and scapula, acting to pull the scapula dorsally and cranially when it contracted. It still does this in our own bodies.

The Trapezius has improved its efficiency in the course of our evolution by extending its origin from the skull down onto the spines of the thoracic vertebrae. The upper fibers of Trapezius still originate from the skull (and from the upper cervical spinous processes; Fig. 13-4) and stream down to the shoulder, inserting into the acromion and the lateral third or so of the clavicle. Obviously, these upper fibers of Trapezius act to pull the point of the shoulder up toward the skull. The lower fibers, coming *up* to the scapula from the lower thoracic spinous processes, insert on the *medial* end of the scapula's spine, which they pull *downward*. Together, the upper and lower fibers of Trapezius thus produce a torque that can rotate the glenoid upward (Fig. 13-5B) without sliding the whole scapula up toward the head. This arrangement allows for more powerful and more finely controlled elevation of the glenoid than would be possible with just the upper fibers of Trapezius alone.

Being a branchial muscle, Trapezius is innervated by a cranial nerve. But this nerve, the **spinal accessory** nerve (cranial nerve XI),

Fig. 13-4 Limb muscles on the back.

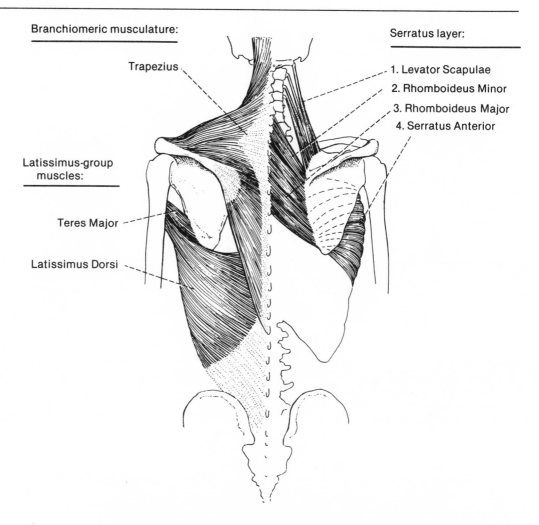

Branchiomeric musculature:

Trapezius

Latissimus-group muscles:

Teres Major

Latissimus Dorsi

Serratus layer:

1. Levator Scapulae
2. Rhomboideus Minor
3. Rhomboideus Major
4. Serratus Anterior

differs from all other cranial nerves in having its motor cell bodies in the cervical part of the spinal cord, not in the brain itself. The nerve follows the spinal cord up into the skull, exits the braincase, and runs back down the neck, sending motor fibers into the deep surface of Trapezius (Chapter 22).

■ The Serratus Layer

The scapula is held against the thorax by a specialized lamina of the body-wall muscles. This sheet of hypaxial muscles (Fig. 13-4) is at-

Table 13-1   Serratus layer.

Muscle	Origin	Insertion	Action	Nerve
Serratus Anterior	Outer surfaces of the first 8 or 9 ribs	Medial edge of scapula's deep surface	Draws the scapula forward; holds its medial edge down when the arm is raised	Long thoracic n.
Rhomboideus Major	Spines of thoracic vertebrae 2 to 5	Medial edge of scapula (below the spine of the scapula)	Retracts the scapula; aids in depressing the glenoid	Dorsal scapular n.
Rhomboideus Minor	Spines of vertebrae C.7 and T.1	Medial edge of scapula (at medial end of the scapula's spine)	Retracts the scapula; aids in depressing the glenoid	Dorsal scapular n.
Levator Scapulae	Transverse processes of cervical vertebrae 1 to 4	Upper end of scapula's medial edge	Retracts the scapula; aids in depressing the glenoid	Branches from ventral rami of C.3 and C.4 (see Fig. 22–5)

Fig. 13-5 Scapular rotation. Arrows indicate the directions of pull of the named muscles, which act together either to depress the shoulder (A) or to elevate it (B).

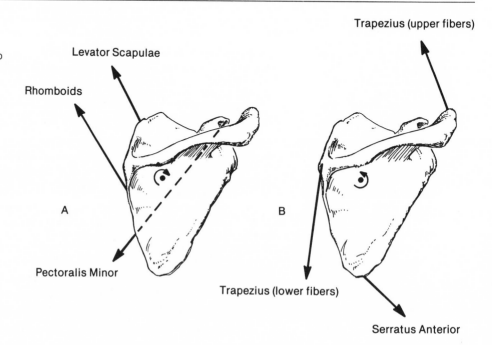

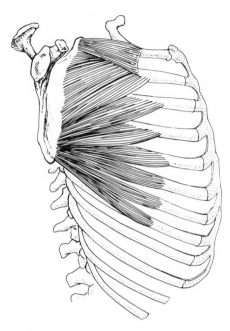

Fig. 13-6 The right Serratus Anterior.

tached to the *medial* edge of the scapula, from which it stretches away in both directions: forward (ventrally) beneath the scapula to attach to the ribs and backward (dorsally) beneath Trapezius to attach to the vertebral spines. The muscles in this sheet are innervated from high up on the roots of the brachial plexus, above the point where the plexus sorts itself out into its anterior and posterior divisions. They are therefore neither elevators nor depressors, but a transitional layer intermediate between the limb muscles and the underlying body wall.

This sheet of slightly specialized body-wall muscles may be called the **Serratus layer** of the forelimb musculature (Table 13-1). It has two major components:

1. **Serratus Anterior** (Figs. 13-4 and 13-6) arises along a zigzag line (L. *serratus,* "sawtoothed") from the upper eight or nine ribs by muscle slips that interdigitate with the origin of Obliquus Externus Abdominis. (Serratus is an evolutionary derivative of the External Oblique.) These slips fuse and run around onto the back beneath the scapula, attaching all along the scapula's medial (or *vertebral*) border.

2. **Rhomboideus Major** and **Minor** (Fig. 13-4) pick up where Serratus Anterior leaves off and continue medially headward from the scapula to the spines of the upper thoracic vertebrae (and C.7).

Serratus Anterior and the Rhomboids together form a mobile belt of muscle around the thorax, to which the scapulae are attached like a pair of shoulder holsters. This belt can contract to pull the scapulae forward or backward. Because the Rhomboids run medially upward (craniad) from the scapula's medial edge, they tend to pull that edge up and thus rotate the scapula so that the shoulder is depressed and the glenoid points more downward (caudad). Serratus Anterior (especially its lower part) has the opposite direction and effect, so it can assist Trapezius in elevating the shoulder (Fig. 13-5).

The original function of Serratus Anterior is easier to understand in a four-footed mammal (Fig. 13-7). The Serratus of a typical quadruped such as a dog acts like a hammock slung between the two shoulder blades, cradling the thorax and supporting its weight. In ourselves, the main function of Serratus Anterior is to thrust the scapula forward or resist a backward push against the shoulder—say, in punching or shoving. When we get down on our hands and knees, Serratus resumes its old function. Abduction of the arm also requires the help of Serratus to prevent the medial edge of the scapula from rising; without Serratus, Trapezius cannot keep the weight of the

Fig. 13-7 Configuration of thorax, scapula, and Serratus Anterior in a quadruped (A) and *Homo* (B). Schematic cross sections.

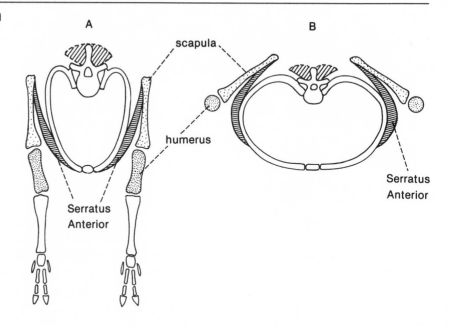

abducted arm from twisting the scapula and depressing the glenoid. In a patient with a paralyzed Serratus Anterior, the force that the partly abducted arm exerts on the scapula causes the vertebral border of the scapula to jut out dorsally under the skin of the back. This "wing scapula" is a diagnostic sign of Serratus Anterior paralysis.

In primitive four-footed mammals, the origins of Serratus Anterior extended all the way from the bottom of the rib cage up onto the transverse processes of the cervical vertebrae. In *Homo,* the lower cervical slips of the Serratus have been lost. An upper cervical remnant of this muscle sheet remains, however. This detached cranial edge of the Serratus Anterior is called **Levator Scapulae** (Fig. 13-4). Like Serratus Anterior, it runs from "ribs" to the medial edge of the scapula—but, of course, the vestigial cervical "ribs" from which it arises are just bumps on the front of the cervical transverse processes (Fig. 2-3A). Functionally, Levator Scapulae acts like the Rhomboids (Fig. 13-5A).

Figure 13-8 shows the finer details of the brachial plexus. The nerves to the Serratus layer arise from the roots of the plexus and run down from the neck to supply Serratus Anterior and the Rhomboids. The two muscles have separate nerves. (Unfortunately, these are not just called "the nerve to the Rhomboids" and "the nerve to Serratus

Fig. 13-8 Diagram of the right brachial plexus.
Posterior-division nerves are shaded.

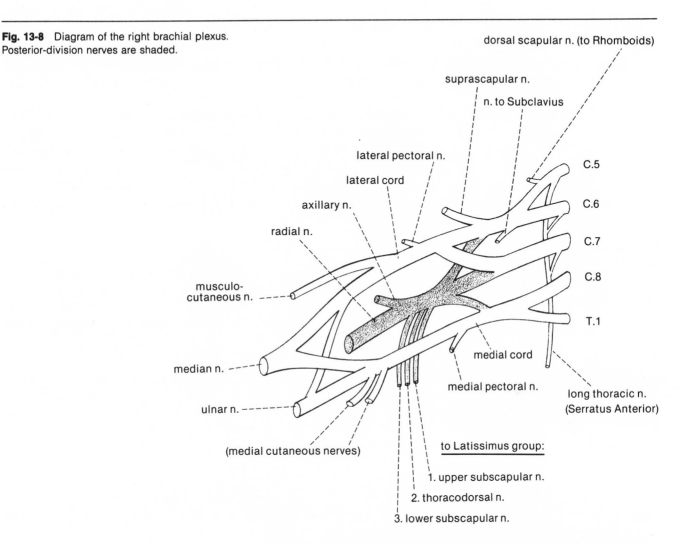

Anterior." The nerve to the Rhomboids is the **dorsal scapular nerve**
and that to Serratus Anterior the **long thoracic nerve.**) The Levator
Scapulae is supplied from ventral rami further up in the neck (C.3–
C.4), not from the brachial plexus.

■ The Axilla and Its Walls:
The Latissimus and Pectoral Groups

Axilla is Latin for "armpit"; but in anatomical usage the word refers
to the whole space between the upper end of the humerus and the rib

cage, not just the hairy concavity under the arm. This space is complex and important because the major vessels and nerves that enter the limb from the root of the neck pass through it.

Thrust your fingers into your own armpit. You will find it to be a four-sided hollow (Fig. 13-9). The medial wall is Serratus Anterior, through which you can feel the underlying rib cage. The lateral wall is the muscle-covered shaft of the humerus. The front (ventral) and back (dorsal) walls are formed by sheets of muscle running from the back and chest to the upper humerus. These four walls converge at their upper ends, coming to a point near the head of the humerus and thus enclosing a pyramid-shaped space. This space is the axilla. (The pyramid's base is the hairy skin of the armpit.)

The front and back walls of the axilla belong to different muscle groups. As might be expected, the dorsal wall is a sheet of elevator musculature and the ventral wall is a depressor muscle. Both attach to almost the same point on the front of the humerus (Fig. 13-9).

The dorsal sheet comprises three muscles, which form the **latissimus** group of elevators—Latissimus Dorsi, Teres Major, and Subscapularis (Table 13-2). **Latissimus Dorsi** (L., "broadest muscle of the

Fig. 13-9 Diagrammatic cross section of axilla. The muscles forming its front and back walls act as medial rotators (*arrow*) of the humerus.

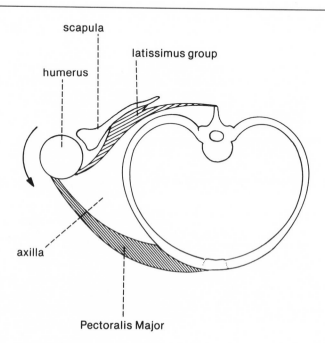

scapula

latissimus group

humerus

axilla

Pectoralis Major

Table 13-2 Elevator muscles of the shoulder region.

Muscle	Origin	Insertion	Action	Nerve
Latissimus group (three parallel nn. from posterior cord)				
Latissimus Dorsi	Spines of vertebrae T.7–T.12; thoracolumbar fascia (slips from iliac crest, the lower 3–4 ribs, and the lower corner of the scapula)	Lesser tubercular crest (crest leading downward from lesser tubercle), and floor of intertubercular groove (bicipital sulcus)	Extends, adducts, medially rotates humerus; aids in depressing the glenoid	Thoracodorsal n.
Teres Major	Lower edge of scapula	Lesser tubercular crest	Extends adducts, medially rotates the humerus	Lower subscapular n.
Subscapularis	Deep surface of scapula	Lesser tubercle	Medially rotates humerus	Upper AND lower subscapular nn.
Deltoid group (axillary nerve)				
Deltoideus	Lateral ⅓ of clavicle; scapular spine and acromion process	Deltoid tuberosity of humerus	Abducts humerus; can also flex, extend, or rotate in either direction (and even adduct)	Axillary n.
Teres Minor	Lower edge of scapula	Back of greater tubercle	Laterally rotates humerus	Axillary n.

back") originates by a big fan-shaped aponeurosis from the lower thoracic vertebral spines and the thoracolumbar fascia overlying the epaxial muscles (Fig. 13-4). Its fleshy fibers run *between* the humerus and the rib cage and converge on a ribbonlike tendon, which inserts into the humerus high up in front on the ridge leading downward from the lesser tubercle (Fig. 13-1). **Teres Major** (L., "big round one") is a slip of the latissimus sheet that has shifted its origin from the thorax onto the lateral edge of the scapula. (A few fibers of Latissimus itself originate right next to it.) Its insertion is just medial to that of Latissimus. **Subscapularis,** the third member of this group, has a large fleshy origin from the whole of the scapula's *deep* surface; it inserts higher up, into the lesser tubercle itself (Fig. 13-13).

All of the latissimus group of elevator muscles can rotate the humerus medially (Fig. 13-9). Latissimus and Teres Major, because their insertions lie some distance below the glenohumeral joint, also have enough leverage around that joint's center to act as powerful adductors (pulling the humerus medially) and extensors (pulling it backward). Subscapularis neither adducts nor extends, because it inserts so close to the joint that its line of pull passes almost directly through the axes of adduction and extension. By pulling downward on the humerus, Latissimus also acts as a powerful depressor of the glenoid.

The front wall of the axilla is formed by a single depressor muscle, **Pectoralis Major,** which arises along a sweeping arc running from the medial part of the clavicle down onto the sternum (and the upper six or so costal cartilages). There is usually a gap between the clavicular and sternocostal parts of the muscle. The fibers of Pectoralis Major insert on the **greater tubercular crest** on the front of the humerus—the one leading downward from the *greater* tubercle (Fig. 13-1). They do so in what might seem like a peculiar way: the lowest (sternocostal) fibers go to the upper end of this crest and the *highest* (clavicular) fibers go to the *lower* end, so the muscle's fibers cross each other and form a complex U-shaped tendon of insertion (Fig. 13-10). This arrangement means that all parts of the muscle get stretched to about the same degree when the arm is abducted, so they can all be equally effective in pulling it back into the adducted position again. A little experimentation with your own arm will show you that Pectoralis Major also can act as a medial rotator (Fig. 13-9) and a flexor of the shoulder—and can also help to retract (that is, extend) the arm from a flexed position, pulling it back down toward the front of the rib cage.

The Pectoralis Major is the biggest and most important of three depressor muscles on the front of the thorax (Table 13-3). These three can be thought of as constituting a muscle group, the **pectoral** group (L. *pectorem,* "chest"). The other two are **Pectoralis Minor** and **Subclavius.** These two run from the rib cage up to the bones of the shoulder girdle. Pectoralis Minor, a fan-shaped muscle that arises from the ribs underlying Pectoralis Major, inserts into the scapula's coracoid process. The little Subclavius runs from the first rib to the clavicle (Fig. 13-10). Pectoralis Minor and Subclavius both act to pull the girdle bones downward and forward.

The muscles that form the front and back walls of the axilla enclose the brachial plexus and are innervated by branches from its three cords. Three or four little nerves arise from the posterior cord and run downward and backward to supply the back wall of the axilla—that is, the latissimus group. (The nerve to Latissimus Dorsi is called the

Fig. 13-10 Pectoral muscles. Pectoralis Major is shown on one side, the underlying Pectoralis Minor and Subclavius on the other.

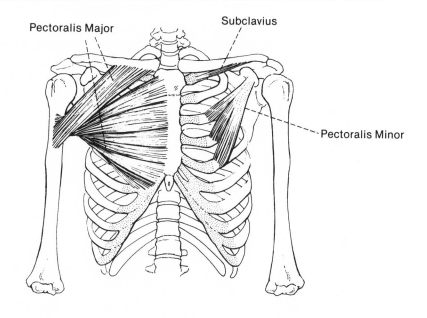

Table 13-3 Depressor muscles of the shoulder region.

Muscle	Origin	Insertion	Action	Nerve
Pectoral group (pectoral nn: n. to Subclavius)				
Pectoralis Major	Medial ½ of clavicle; sternum and costal cartilages 1–6	Greater tubercular crest (crest leading downward from greater tubercle)	Medially rotates, flexes, and adducts humerus	Lateral and medial pectoral nn.
Pectoralis Minor	Anterior ends of ribs 3–5	Coracoid process	Protracts and depresses glenoid end of scapula	Lateral and medial pectoral nn.
Subclavius	Anterior end of 1st rib	Underside of clavicle	Protracts and depresses the clavicle	Nerve to Subclavius
"Spinatus" group (suprascapular n.)				
Supraspinatus	Supraspinous fossa of scapula	Top of greater tubercle	Abducts humerus	Suprascapular n.
Infraspinatus	Infraspinous fossa of scapula	Back of greater tubercle	Laterally rotates humerus	Suprascapular n.

thoracodorsal nerve; the **subscapular** nerves to either side of it supply Teres Major and Subscapularis.) The two anterior-division (depressor-muscle) cords of the plexus each give off a **pectoral** nerve, and both pectoral nerves (lateral and medial) send branches anteriorly into the Pectoralis Major and Minor. (Subclavius has its own little nerve from the ventral rami of C.5 and C.6 and could equally well be called a muscle group of its own.)

■ The Deltoid Group

The lateral aspect of the shoulder is surrounded by a short but powerful muscle, called **Deltoideus** because it looks like a triangle (a capital Greek letter delta) standing on its apex. Its fibers originate from the spine of the scapula and the lateral third or so of the clavicle. They converge on several little tendons within the muscle, all of which fuse and insert on a vague bump (the deltoid tuberosity) about halfway down the lateral side of the humerus.

The Deltoid is the major abductor of the arm. However, because it surrounds the glenohumeral joint on all sides except medially, it can also help to rotate the humerus in every other direction. Its front (clavicular) fibers can pull the humerus forward (flexion) or rotate it medially, and its rear fibers (from the scapula's spine) can pull it back dorsally again or rotate it laterally. Its most medial fibers, both in front and in back, run *below* the axis of abduction and adduction, so they can actually act to hold the arm in an adducted position (Fig. 13-11)—thus making Deltoideus an adductor as well.

The Deltoideus is innervated by the **axillary** nerve, which is one of the two terminal branches of the posterior (elevator-muscle) cord of the brachial plexus (Fig. 13-8). This nerve loops backward and sideward around the upper end of the humerus, running along deep to the Deltoideus and supplying it. The axillary nerve also sends a branch to the **Teres Minor,** which is the other member of the **deltoid** group of elevators. Teres Minor is connected with Deltoideus by its history and innervation; but its position and function make it easier to consider Teres Minor along with the Infraspinatus muscle.

■ The "Spinatus" Muscles and Teres Minor

In reptiles and amphibians, the scapula is a large, flat, vertically oriented blade (Fig. 13-12A). From its lateral surface, elevator mus-

Fig. 13-11 Deltoideus, back (A) and front (B) views.

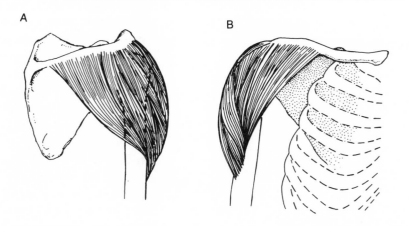

cles arise above and depressor muscles arise below. In mammals, the lower part of the plate, down near the coracoid process, is reduced. The depressor muscle (Supracoracoideus) that occupied this part of the plate in reptiles has thus had to find new origins; and it has done so by creeping onto the dorsal surface of the scapula, into what used to be elevator territory. The original cranial edge of the scapula is

Fig. 13-12 Evolution of Supraspinatus and Infraspinatus. A. The homologous muscle (Supracoracoideus) in a reptile. B. The migration of the muscle from the reptilian to the mammalian position in the pouch young of an opossum. C. An adult opossum. All views from the left.

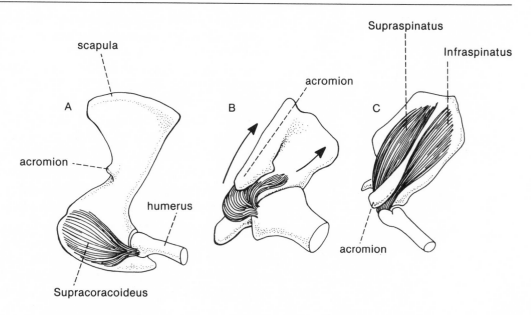

bent backward to become the scapular spine and acromion; a **su-praspinous fossa** spreads out cranially from the blade to provide a new cranial edge. The reptilian muscle, spreading dorsally onto the expanded scapula, is split by the spine of the scapula into two parts—**Supraspinatus** and **Infraspinatus**. This phylogeny is recapitulated during ontogeny (Fig. 13-12B, C). Although Supraspinatus and Infraspinatus lie on the back of the limb girdle in elevator territory, they are innervated like the depressors they really are, via a nerve (the **suprascapular** nerve) containing anterior-division fibers from the upper trunk of the plexus (Fig. 13-8).

As it spread up onto the scapula, Infraspinatus pushed its way in between Deltoideus and Teres Minor and shoved Teres Minor's origin down to the lower (axillary) edge of the scapula. Teres Minor now runs from that edge to the back of the greater tubercle (Fig. 13-13) and acts as a lateral rotator of the humerus. Infraspinatus, just above it, has similar attachments and actions. Supraspinatus also inserts on the greater tuberosity but has to run directly over the top of the glenohumeral joint to get there. It therefore rotates neither medially nor laterally; instead, it abducts the arm. The four short muscles running from the scapula to the upper end of the humerus—the two "spinatus" muscles, Teres Minor, and Subscapularis from the latissimus group—are sometimes called the rotator cuff (Fig. 13-13). Together, they constitute a sort of active "capsule" for the glenohumeral joint, contracting en masse to pull the humerus and scapula more tightly together whenever any dislocating forces threaten the joint's integrity.

▪ The Muscles of the Arm

After dealing with the shoulder and the sixteen muscles that affect its movements, the anatomy of the arm comes as a considerable relief. There are only four muscles in the arm—one elevator and three depressors (Table 13-4).

The elevator muscle is **Triceps Brachii** (L., "three-headed [muscle] of the arm"). It is the mass of flesh on the back of the arm. As its name suggests, it has three heads of origin (Fig. 13-14). The **long head** arises from the lower edge of the glenoid socket on the scapula; the other two heads arise from the shaft of the humerus. All three heads insert together on the olecranon process of the ulna (the bony lump at the point of the elbow; Gk. *olekranion*, "elbow-head"). Triceps ex-

Fig. 13-13 The short muscles running laterally from the scapula to the upper end of the humerus. A. Ventral (anterior) view. B. Dorsal view.

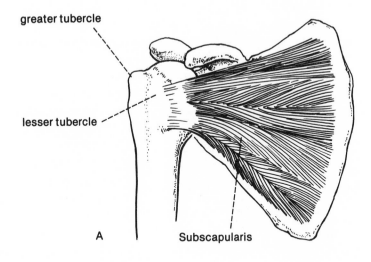

greater tubercle

lesser tubercle

A   Subscapularis

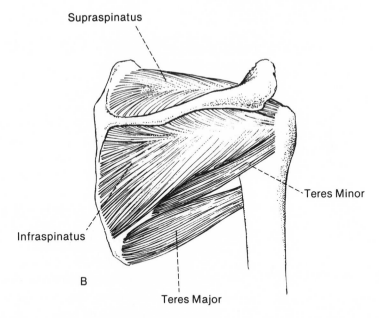

Supraspinatus

Teres Minor

Infraspinatus

B

Teres Major

tends the elbow joint when it contracts, bringing the forearm into line with the shaft of the humerus.

The radial nerve, the largest branch of the posterior cord of the brachial plexus (Fig. 13-8), supplies Triceps. In fact, it innervates *all the elevator muscles of the arm and forearm*. It enters the elevator-

Table 13-4 Muscles of the arm.

Muscle	Origin	Insertion	Action	Nerve
Depressors (brachial group: musculocutaneous n.)				
Coracobrachialis	Coracoid process	Middle of humerus, on the medial edge	Adducts and flexes arm	Musculocutaneous n.
Brachialis	Lower ½ of the front of the humerus; lateral and medial septa between depressors and elevators	Proximal ulna (coronoid process)	Flexes elbow	Musculocutaneous n.
Biceps Brachii	Coracoid process (short head); upper edge of glenoid fossa (long head)	Proximal radius (bicipital tuberosity)	Flexes elbow; supinates	Musculocutaneous n.
Elevators (triceps group: radial n.)				
Triceps Brachii	Lower edge of glenoid fossa (long head); posterior surface of humeral shaft (medial and lateral heads)	Olecranon process of ulna	Extends elbow	Radial n.

muscle mass by running backward below the lower edge of the latissimus group—that is, below Teres Major (Fig. 13-14). As it runs down the arm toward the elbow, it winds laterally backward around the humeral shaft. Because the radial nerve lies in direct contact with the bone, it interrupts the humeral origin of Triceps and splits it into two heads—a **lateral head** high up and a much larger **medial head** that occupies most of the back of the humerus.

The three depressor muscles on the front of the arm (Fig. 13-15) constitute the **brachial** group (L. *brachium,* "arm"). They include muscles capable of moving both shoulder and elbow joints. One of them crosses only the shoulder joint; one crosses only the elbow joint; and one crosses both joints.

The one that crosses both joints is **Biceps Brachii;** it produces the prominent bulge above the crook of the elbow that children display when they ask someone to "feel their muscle." As its name (L. *biceps,* "two heads") implies, Biceps has two heads of origin—one from the coracoid and another from the upper rim of the glenoid fossa. The one arising from the glenoid rim is distinguished as the **long head,** but

Fig. 13-14 Triceps Brachii, viewed from behind. A. The intact muscle. B. Origins (*shaded*) of its three heads and relationships of the radial nerve. Stipple in B shows where Triceps inserts into the ulna's olecranon process.

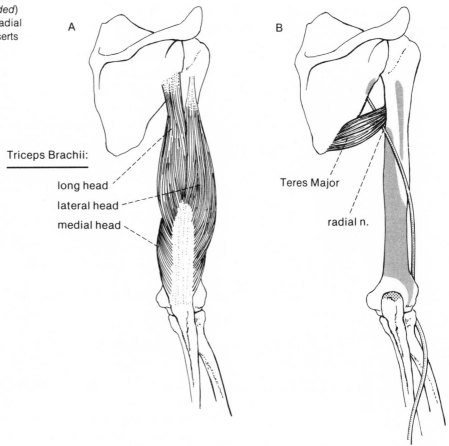

A

B

Triceps Brachii:

long head

lateral head

medial head

Teres Major

radial n.

the two are about the same length. The long head arises by a slim, cordlike tendon that runs directly over the top of the glenohumeral joint (inside the joint capsule; Fig. 13-2) and courses down the front of the humerus in the groove between the two tubercular crests—hence the old name of "bicipital sulcus" for this groove. The long head develops a fleshy belly on the front of the arm, where it is joined by the belly of the short head; the two fuse and insert into the radius. (Some of the fibers of Biceps also insert via a fibrous band into the deep fascia covering the flexor muscles in the forearm.) Biceps flexes the elbow; and (as we shall see later) it is also a powerful supinator.

The other two muscles in the brachial group are shorter, lie deeper,

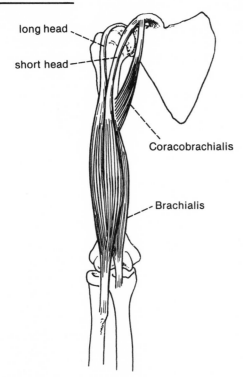

Biceps Brachii:

long head

short head

Coracobrachialis

Brachialis

Fig. 13-15 The three muscles of the brachial group. Front view of right arm.

do not produce any prominent bulges when they contract, and have simpler attachments and actions. **Brachialis** comes off the whole lower half of the front of the humerus and inserts into the ulna just below the elbow. It flexes the elbow when it contracts. It is a bigger and more powerful muscle than Biceps and is more important in elbow flexion—though of course it cannot help Biceps in supinating the radius, because it does not attach to the radius. Finally, **Coracobrachialis** is a smaller muscle running from the coracoid to an insertion on the humerus (medial to the upper end of Brachialis); it flexes the shoulder joint, pulling the humerus forward. It can also adduct the arm. (It is not very important in producing either movement.) Its name reflects its attachments.

■ **Some Obvious Principles**

The three muscles of the brachial group exemplify three self-evident principles of muscle anatomy.

1. *Muscles cannot move joints that they do not cross.* Is Brachialis a medial rotator of the shoulder, or a lateral rotator? Neither; it runs from the humerus to the ulna, does not cross the glenohumeral joint, and therefore has no effect on the shoulder. When learning the mechanical facts about a muscle, notice which joints it crosses, figure out what effects it has on those joints, and stop. In general, a muscle will produce *some* movement at every joint it crosses, though it may be only a feeble movement. If a muscle's line of pull crosses a joint but passes very close to the joint's axis of rotation, the muscle usually will not be very effective at moving that joint around that axis—for the same reason that it is not effective to try to slam a door by pushing on it right next to its hinges.

2. *Two-joint muscles are superficial to one-joint muscles.* In general, the more joints a muscle crosses, the more superficial it has to be. The epaxial muscles (Chapter 4) illustrate this principle. The most superficial back muscles cross many intervertebral joints, whereas the deepest ones are short and run from one vertebra to its neighbor. If the shortest ones were superficial, they would have to make holes in the longer ones to reach their attachments. Likewise in the arm: Biceps Brachii has to lie superficial to Brachialis, because it arises much further up the limb (from the scapula instead of the humerus) but inserts right alongside Brachialis.

3. *Bones are harder than meat.* This means that wherever a muscle's tendon slides back and forth across a bony surface, it has to be lubricated to keep the bone from chafing the softer tissue. Tendons sliding against bone are always surrounded by outpouchings of synovial membrane from some nearby joint—or else enclosed in little separate bags of synovial membrane called **bursae** (L. *bursa,* "purse"). We see this in the long head of Biceps. Its tendon moves back and forth in the intertubercular groove and therefore is surrounded there by a tubular extension of synovial membrane from the lining of the shoulder joint.

■ The Arteries of the Axilla and Arm

The anterior or pectoral fins of fish are hooked on to the back end of the head, and so the artery to the anterior fin on each side comes off from the collecting vessel that drains oxygenated blood from the top of the gill arches. After giving off the arteries to the fins, these paired vessels fuse to form the dorsal aorta in the midline.

The same arrangement is seen in the human embryo (Fig. 7-10). The arteries to the upper limbs therefore do not emerge from the sides of the *descending* aorta as do the typical body-wall arteries; instead, they arise from the *arch* of the aorta, which represents a persistent part of the old gill-vessel system. The origins of these vessels were sketched in Chapter 7.

The primary artery of the upper limb (Fig. 13-16) curves out of the upper opening of the rib cage, over the top of the first rib, and plunges down into the axilla between the axilla's front wall (the Pectoralis Major) and back wall (the latissimus sheet). It changes names twice as it runs along. Before it crosses the first rib, it lies behind the clavicle and is known as the **subclavian** artery. When it crosses the first rib and enters the axilla, it is called the **axillary** artery. As it crosses the lower edge of the latissimus sheet (that is, the caudal edge of Teres Major), it leaves the axilla, enters the arm proper, and is rechristened the **brachial** artery. All three are one continuous vessel, derived from the specialized intersegmental artery that grew out along the axis of the embryonic limb bud.

We would expect the axial artery of a limb bud to lie in the limb's central plane, between the elevator and depressor masses, and this is exactly what we find. The axillary artery lies in the axilla with elevators behind it and depressors in front of it. The roots and trunks of

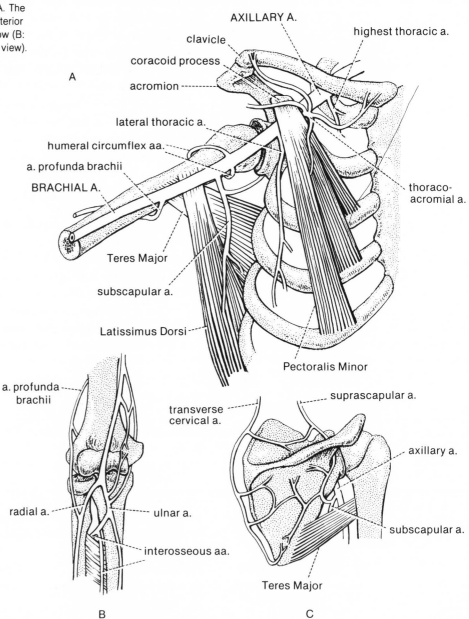

Fig. 13-16 Arteries of the upper limb. A. The right axillary artery and its branches. Anterior view. B,C. Anastomoses around the elbow (B: anterior view) and scapula (C: posterior view).

A

AXILLARY A.

highest thoracic a.

clavicle

coracoid process

acromion

lateral thoracic a.

humeral circumflex aa.

a. profunda brachii

BRACHIAL A.

thoraco-acromial a.

Teres Major

subscapular a.

Latissimus Dorsi

Pectoralis Minor

a. profunda brachii

transverse cervical a.

suprascapular a.

axillary a.

radial a.

ulnar a.

interosseous aa.

subscapular a.

Teres Major

B

C

the brachial plexus lie behind the upper end of the axillary artery, thereby reflecting the fact that the spinal cord (from which the nerves grew down into the limb) is more dorsal than the arch of the aorta (from which the artery is coming). But when the growing brachial plexus of the embryo invaded the axillary region and split up into anterior and posterior divisions, the anterior divisions of the plexus grew around to the ventral side of the limb to reach the depressor musculature. The *lower* half of the axillary artery therefore winds up being surrounded by the brachial plexus (Fig. 13-17).

The axillary artery's continuation, the brachial artery, stays in between the elevator and depressor masses as it runs down into the flesh on the medial side of the arm. As is usually the case, the elevator–depressor division here is marked by a septum of deep fascia, the **medial intermuscular septum**. This septum separates the brachial group from the triceps group, and muscles of both groups (Triceps, Brachialis, Coracobrachialis) have fibers that attach to it. The brachial artery lies on the septum's ventral aspect, gradually curving laterally as the elbow flexors narrow toward their tendons of insertion. Following their medial edges, it arrives at the hollow of the elbow and splits into the two major vessels (**radial** and **ulnar** arteries) that supply the forearm. The axial artery of the limb bud continues

Fig. 13-17 Relationship of the axillary artery to the brachial plexus. Compare with Fig. 13-8.

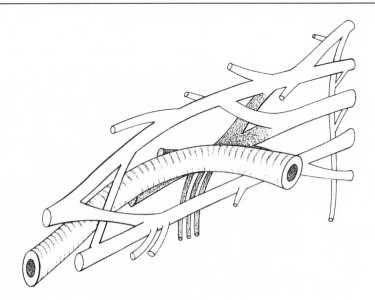

into the forearm as a much-reduced vessel, the anterior interosseous artery (Fig. 13-16).

Each of the three named sections (subclavian, axillary, brachial) of the arterial trunk to the upper limb sends off branches to the surrounding muscles:

Subclavian Artery   Most of the subclavian artery's branches supply the head, neck, and thorax; but one of its branches, the **thyrocervical trunk** (Fig. 21-19), helps supply the base of the upper limb. This trunk comes off the subclavian artery just before it reaches the Scalenus Anterior. Two of the trunk's three branches run backward across the neck and supply muscles attaching to the scapula. The **suprascapular** branch of the thyrocervical trunk goes laterally and winds around backward under the scapula's acromion process, sending branches into Supraspinatus and Infraspinatus (Fig. 13-16C). The **transverse cervical** branch of the trunk runs more medially back toward the *vertebral* edge of the scapula, sending branches into the surrounding muscles—Trapezius, Levator Scapulae, and the Rhomboids. (The thyrocervical trunk's third branch, the inferior thyroid artery, supplies the thyroid gland in the neck.)

In about half of all cases, the transverse cervical artery supplies only Trapezius and is called the **superficial cervical** artery. The branch to Levator Scapulae and the Rhomboids then originates directly from the subclavian artery and is called the **dorsal scapular** artery.

Axillary Artery   The axillary artery runs behind (dorsal to) the depressor muscles; so it runs behind the tendon of Pectoralis Minor as it traverses the axilla (Fig. 13-16A). The part of the artery that lies behind this tendon is conventionally labeled the *second* part of the artery; the parts above and below are (naturally) the *first* and *third* parts respectively. Conveniently enough, the first part has one branch, the second two branches, and the third three branches:

1. The first part of the artery gives off a little **superior thoracic** branch to the body wall.
2. The second part gives off the **thoracoacromial** artery, which ramifies between and supplies Pectoralis Major and Minor (the *anterior* wall of the axilla), and the **lateral thoracic** artery, which runs downward along the lateral edges of the two Pectorales and supplies Serratus Anterior (the *medial* wall of the axilla). The

lateral thoracic artery anastomoses with the intercostal arteries it passes and can be thought of as another longitudinal anastomosis between intersegmental arteries. (Compare it with the *internal* thoracic artery.)

3. The third part of the axillary artery gives off three branches—two **humeral circumflex** arteries, which form a loop around the neck of the humerus under cover of Deltoideus (running along with the axillary nerve), and the **subscapular** artery. The subscapular artery sends muscular branches to the latissimus muscle group and thus supplies the *posterior* wall of the axilla. It also gives off a **circumflex scapular** branch that wraps around the lateral edge of the scapula to anastomose with the transverse cervical and suprascapular arteries on the back of the scapula. There is a very extensive network of anastomotic arteries around the scapula (Fig. 13-16C), and blood can get to the limb through these if anything occludes the axillary artery.

Brachial Branches The brachial artery has only one major branch, the **profunda brachii** artery, which follows the radial nerve's spiral course through the Triceps group. After supplying Triceps, the profunda brachii artery ends on the lateral side of the elbow in a couple of parallel **radial collateral** branches. These anastomose with corresponding **recurrent** branches from the arteries in the forearm. Similar **ulnar collateral** and **recurrent** branches connect the arteries on the medial side of the elbow. Like the scapula, the elbow is thus surrounded by a network of arterial anastomoses (Fig. 13-16B).

▪ The Cutaneous Veins and Nerves

In many areas of the body, the veins have roughly the same names and courses as the arteries. In others—especially the viscera and the inside of the skull—the veins and arteries have different names and pathways. The limbs present an intermediate case. Some of the veins in the limbs are deep veins that follow the arteries, but others are large superficial vessels that lie directly under the skin and are not accompanied by arteries. In the upper limb, the superficial veins are bigger than the deep ones.

Why should the limbs have such large superficial veins? A limb is a column of solid muscle and bone wrapped in tough, inelastic deep fascia. When the limb muscles contract, the nerves and vessels run-

Fig. 13-18 Cutaneous veins and cutaneous innervation of the upper limb. Posterior (A) and anterior (B) views.

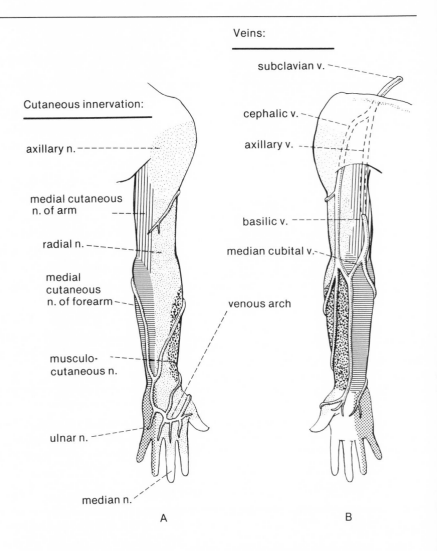

Cutaneous innervation:

axillary n.

medial cutaneous n. of arm

radial n.

medial cutaneous n. of forearm

musculo-cutaneous n.

ulnar n.

median n.

A

Veins:

subclavian v.

cephalic v.

axillary v.

basilic v.

median cubital v.

venous arch

B

ning through those muscles are compressed. The arteries contain blood under high pressure and have thick, contractile walls, so they can still deliver blood despite being compressed. But the thin-walled veins that run with them are likely to be squashed flat by the surrounding muscles. Prolonged contraction of the limb muscles thus can interfere with deep venous drainage. To help compensate for this, the deep veins are connected through many anastomoses to enlarged superficial veins, which lie outside the muscles and deep fascia and provide an alternative channel for the return of blood to the heart. When the muscles of the upper limb contract, blood runs from the deep veins into the superficial ones and flows through them back toward the heart. (The pattern in the lower limb is different; see Chapter 15.)

The superficial veins are very variable, especially in the distal parts of the limbs. One constant feature is a subcutaneous **venous arch** that runs across the dorsal surface of the hand or foot. In the embryo, each end of this arch empties into a major superficial vein that follows the boundary between the elevator and depressor masses. This embryonic arrangement tends to get obscured later in ontogeny, but it is retained in the arm (Fig. 13-18). The **basilic** vein (Gk. *basileus,* "king") on the medial side of the arm and the **cephalic** vein (Gk., "head") on the lateral side both run roughly along the elevator–depressor boundary. The basilic vein plunges into the medial intermuscular septum and becomes the axillary vein. It is joined higher up by the cephalic vein, which dives in between Deltoideus (elevator) and Pectoralis Major (depressor) to reach it. The two are joined across the crook of the elbow (or **cubital fossa**) by a variable anastomosis usually involving a **median cubital** vein. This is a favored site for intravenous injections or the removal of blood.

The subcutaneous fascia that contains the superficial veins also carries major sensory nerves to the skin of the arm and forearm (Fig. 13-18). Anterior-division nerves supply most of the cutaneous innervation; however, the radial nerve sends named cutaneous branches to a strip down the back of the limb, and the skin over the flesh of Deltoideus is supplied by that muscle's nerve (axillary nerve). The musculocutaneous nerve innervates the skin on the lateral aspect of the forearm. Above the wrist, the medial aspect of the limb is supplied by purely sensory cutaneous nerves (medial cutaneous nerves of arm and forearm) from the medial cord of the plexus.

14

The Hand and the Forearm

Human beings are unique among mammals—in fact, among living vertebrates—in having converted their forelimbs into purely manipulatory organs. The business end of our upper extremity is the hand. All the anatomical features of our upper limbs are as they are because they have some functional value in manipulating things. The details of the hand's anatomy and actions are thus crucial to an understanding of our upper limbs. Because almost all the muscles in the forearm attach to hand bones and act to move them in various ways, we shall treat the forearm here as an appendage of the hand rather than the other way around.

▪ Bones and Joints of the Hand

The skeleton of the hand (Fig. 14-1) consists of five digital rays springing from a cluster of short, blocky **carpal** (wrist) bones. The thumb ray is counted as the first digit, and so on over to the little finger, which is the fifth. Each ray consists of a proximal **metacarpal** and a string of **phalanges.** There are two phalanges in the thumb and three in the other, longer digits.

The joints between the phalanges of every digit are hinge joints, with roughly cylindrical articular surfaces and a single axis of rotation. Their fibrous capsules have **palmar** and **collateral** ligamentous thickenings (Fig. 14-2). The palmar ligaments of the interphalangeal joints are slack in the flexed position; they are drawn tighter as the finger is extended and check extension when they become taut. The collateral ligaments, lying at the sides of the joint, pass through the axis of joint rotation and remain tight throughout the range of extension and flexion. They do not check normal (hinge) movements, but they help prevent other movements. (For example, you cannot wiggle your thumb's distal phalanx much from side to side while

248

Fig. 14-1 Skeleton of right hand. Palmar aspect.

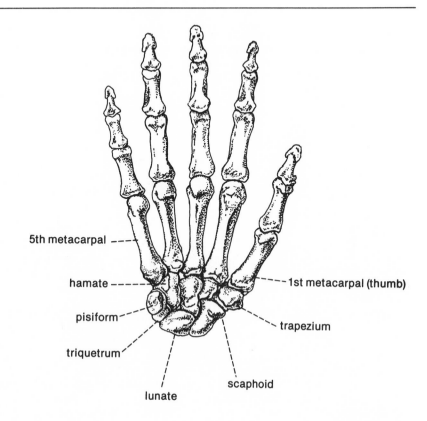

5th metacarpal

hamate

pisiform

triquetrum

lunate

1st metacarpal (thumb)

trapezium

scaphoid

holding the proximal phalanx still, because you would have to tear the collateral ligaments of the interphalangeal joint to do so.) All the other hinge joints in the limbs have a similar ligamentous arrangement: a check ligament limits extension, while collateral ligaments on the sides prevent abduction, adduction, and rotation.

The metacarpophalangeal joints (between the metacarpal and the proximal phalanx of each digit) have looser collateral ligaments and more ellipsoidal articular surfaces. This arrangement allows for a fair degree of abduction of the proximal phalanges (spreading the fingers apart) as well as flexion and extension. But abduction is limited when these joints are flexed, because of the eccentric attachments of their collateral ligaments (Fig. 14-2).

The "knuckles" or heads of metacarpals 2 to 5 are bound together by deep, transversely running ligaments (Fig. 14-3), so these metacarpals cannot be abducted from each other. The metacarpal of the

Fig. 14-2 Collateral and palmar ligaments of interphalangeal and metacarpophalangeal (M-P) joints. The eccentrically attached collateral ligaments of the M-P joints are slack in the extended position, thereby allowing the extended fingers to be abducted and adducted.

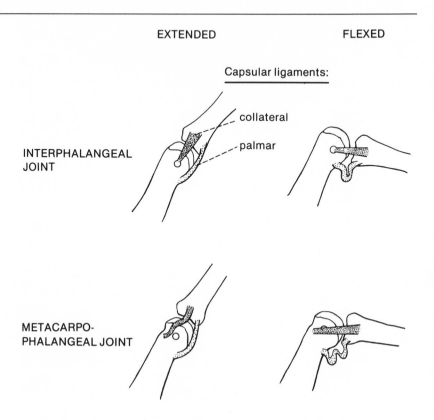

thumb is not bound to the head of the neighboring metacarpal and can therefore be abducted from the other metacarpals. The base of the thumb's metacarpal has a saddle-shaped surface that articulates with a similar surface on the wrist bone called the **trapezium.** A joint like this—known as a **sellar** joint (L. *sella,* "saddle")—is almost as mobile as a ball-and-socket joint, permitting rotation around all three perpendicular axes. However, it does not allow as much rotation around the metacarpal's long axis as a ball-and-socket joint would (Fig. 14-4).

Look at the nails of your extended fingers and note that the thumbnail is set almost at right angles to the others. The thumb's named *movements* are also perpendicular to the similarly named movements of the other digits. Whereas flexion of the second digit (index finger) carries it directly into the palm, flexion of the thumb sweeps it *across* the palm, at right angles to the plane of index-finger flexion. (*Exten-*

Fig. 14-3 Carpal and metacarpal bones of right hand, palmar view. The heads of metacarpals 2–5 are bound together by transverse ligaments. The wrist joint is shown in an exploded view to display the radius's articular surface and the disk that intervenes between the ulna and the proximal carpals.

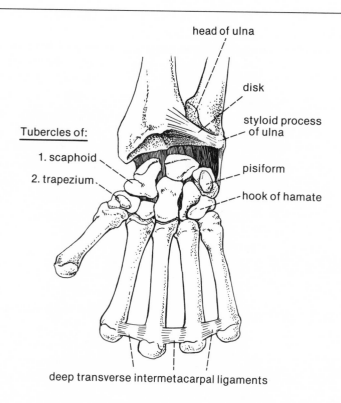

head of ulna

disk

styloid process of ulna

Tubercles of:

1. scaphoid

2. trapezium

pisiform

hook of hamate

deep transverse intermetacarpal ligaments

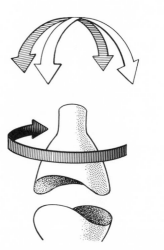

Fig. 14-4 A saddle-shaped (sellar) joint like that between thumb and trapezium allows swinging in any direction (*upper arrows*) but restricts rotation (*lower arrow*).

sion of the thumb sweeps it back again, toward the thumb position used in thumbing a ride.) Similarly, abduction and adduction of the thumb move it in a plane perpendicular to the plane in which the index finger abducts and adducts.

Abducting the thumb (that is, swinging it in a ventral direction toward the wrist) tends to rotate it around into a position of *opposition*, in which the thumbnail faces almost in the opposite direction to the nails of the other digits. This automatic rotation is produced mainly by capsular ligaments in the joint between the thumb's metacarpal and the trapezium. The opposability of our thumb affords us two principal and different gripping positions. In holding and working a screwdriver, the thumb stays in its nonopposed position, 90° out of phase with the other digits. In holding a baseball bat, the thumb swings into 180° opposition. We unconsciously shift from one grip to the other, depending on the heft and shape of the object being grasped.

■ The Intrinsic Muscles of the Hand

Most of the force in our grip comes from forearm muscles that send tendons down across the wrist to insert on the bones of the digits. These *extrinsic* hand muscles include both elevators and depressors. The elevators extend the fingers and dorsiflex the wrist; the depressors do the opposite.

The hand also has *intrinsic* depressor muscles, which lie wholly within the palm (Table 14-1). They produce three sorts of movement that the extrinsic muscles are not well-positioned for producing: (1) abduction and adduction of the fingers; (2) special movements of the thumb and little finger; and (3) simultaneous flexion of some joints and extension of others. There are four groups of intrinsic hand muscles.

Interossei The Interossei are the most dorsal of the hand's intrinsic muscles. They are stuffed in between the metacarpals and take their name from that fact. The Interossei originate from the metacarpals and insert on the proximal phalanges of the digits (Fig. 14-5). Their main function is to abduct and adduct the fingers. They are divisible into two groups—a **dorsal** group and a ventral or **palmar** group— that have different positions, attachments, and actions.

Abduction is the job of the **Dorsal Interossei.** The thumb and little finger have their own special abductors, and no Dorsal Interosseus muscle is provided for these two digits. The third digit, which sits in the midline of the hand, can be abducted away from the midline in either direction, so it needs (and gets) *two* Dorsal Interossei. There are therefore four Dorsal Interossei—one each for digits 2 and 4 and two for digit 3. Their attachments to the phalanges are shown in Figure 14-5. Their bellies can be felt as soft spots in between the metacarpals on the back of your hand. The largest and most important is the one for the second digit. You can test its function by pinching your thumb and index finger together hard. As you do, use your other hand to palpate the back of the fleshy web between the thumb and index finger. The bulging you feel as you pinch is the first Dorsal Interosseus contracting to exert an abduction force on the index finger. This force keeps the thumb from pushing the index finger toward the little finger.

There are also four **Palmar Interossei,** one for every digit except the third (which requires no adductor because it already lies in the mid-

Table 14-1   Intrinsic muscles of the hand.

Muscle	Origin	Insertion	Action	Nerve
Thenar group (median n.)				
Flexor Pollicis Brevis	Flexor retinaculum and trapezium (plus a variably present deep head, from the distal carpal bones)	Lateral sesamoid of thumb	Flexes proximal phalanx of thumb; helps rotate thumb into opposition	Median n. (deep head commonly by ulnar n.)
Abductor Pollicis Brevis	Flexor retinaculum	Lateral side of thumb's proximal phalanx	Abducts thumb	Median n.
Opponens Pollicis	Flexor retinaculum and trapezium	Lateral side of 1st metacarpal	Rotates thumb into opposition	Median n.
Hypothenar group (ulnar n.)				
Flexor Digiti Minimi Brevis	Flexor retinaculum and hook of hamate	Medial side of little finger's proximal phalanx	Flexes proximal phalanx (metacarpophalangeal joint)	Ulnar n.
Abductor Digiti Minimi	Pisiform (and attached tendons)	Medial side of little finger's proximal phalanx	Abducts little finger	Ulnar n.
Opponens Digiti Minimi	Flexor retinaculum and hook of hamate	Medial side of 5th metacarpal	Rotates metacarpal into opposition with thumb	Ulnar n.
Palmaris Brevis	Flexor retinaculum and palmar aponeurosis	Skin over hypothenar muscles	Deepens hollow of palm	Ulnar n.
Other intrinsic muscles				
Adductor Pollicis	Distal carpals, proximal ends of metacarpals 2 and 3 (oblique head); shaft of 3rd metacarpal (transverse head)	Medial sesamoid of thumb	Adducts thumb	Ulnar n.
Lumbricals	Tendons of Flexor Digitorum Profundus	Tendons of Extensor Digitorum	(See Fig. 14-16)	Median n. (1st 2 Lumbricals) Ulnar n. (2nd 2)
Interossei	(See Figs. 14-5 and 14-15)		(See Fig. 14-5)	Ulnar n.

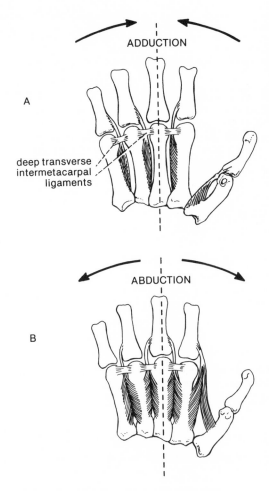

A

ADDUCTION

deep transverse
intermetacarpal
ligaments

B

ABDUCTION

Fig. 14-5 Palmar (A) and Dorsal (B) Interossei of the hand and the movements they produce (*arrows*). Palmar view.

line of the hand). They lie on the palmar aspect of the Dorsal Interossei. The Palmar Interossei draw their digits toward the third digital ray. This movement is called *adduction* of digits 2, 4, and 5—but *flexion* of the thumb. The thumb's Palmar Interosseus muscle is therefore sometimes described as part of Flexor Pollicis Brevis, in the thenar muscle group.

Thenar and Hypothenar Muscles The two digits at the margin of the hand (digits 1 and 5) have special functions and movements, and each has developed a cluster of specialized Interossei at its base to enhance its independent mobility (Fig. 14-6). There are three muscles in each cluster—an *opponens* that inserts into and rotates the metacarpal, and a *short flexor* and an *abductor* that both attach to the proximal phalanx and move the metacarpophalangeal joint.

The three muscles at the base of the thumb, which form its fleshy "ball," are called **thenar** muscles. They all originate from the trapezium (the carpal bone at the thumb's base) and the ligaments attached to it, and they tend to be more or less inseparable at those origins. The superficial **Abductor Pollicis Brevis** (L. *pollicis,* "of the thumb") wraps around the thumb's metacarpal to insert near the dorsal side of the proximal phalanx. This near-dorsal insertion allows Abductor Pollicis Brevis to pull that phalanx in a ventral direction—and thus to abduct the thumb. The **Opponens Pollicis** lying deep to it attaches to the whole shaft of the metacarpal and acts to twist the metacarpal around and pull it into the opposed position. **Flexor Pollicis Brevis** lies on the edge of the thenar mass, toward the center of the palm. It has a second, deep head that arises from the center of the cluster of carpal bones. There is a small bony nodule developed in its tendon of insertion into the proximal phalanx (which it flexes). Such bones in tendons are called **sesamoids;** there are usually several in each hand and foot.

The **hypothenar** muscles, which form the "ball" of the little finger, have attachments and actions comparable to those of the thenar muscles, but they are smaller and weaker (Fig. 14-6) because their digit has only a slight rotatory mobility and cannot be moved into a fully opposed position. Their names are similar to those of the corresponding thenar muscles (with *Digiti Minimi* [L., "of the little finger"] substituted for *Pollicis*)—**Abductor Digiti Minimi, Opponens Digiti Minimi, Flexor Digiti Minimi Brevis.** In the skin over the hypothenar muscles, there is a wisp of depressor-muscle fibers called

Fig. 14-6 Thenar, hypothenar, and Lumbrical muscles. Palmar view after removal of skin and palmar aponeurosis.

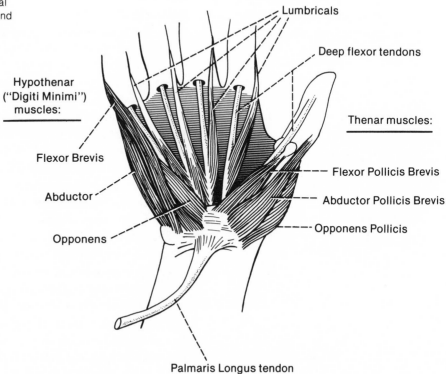

Lumbricals

Deep flexor tendons

Hypothenar ("Digiti Minimi") muscles:

Thenar muscles:

Flexor Brevis

Flexor Pollicis Brevis

Abductor

Abductor Pollicis Brevis

Opponens

Opponens Pollicis

Palmaris Longus tendon

Palmaris Brevis, which produces a characteristic wrinkle in the "heel" of the hand when it contracts. It may help to deepen the cupped palm in grasping something like a softball.

Adductor Pollicis   Plastered across the palmar surface of the Palmar Interossei in primitive reptiles was a sheet of small **adductor** muscles. These muscles arose from the central (third) digital ray and fanned out to insert into the other digits. Contracting, they drew those digits toward the midline of the hand. Our own Palmar Interossei have taken over this job, so we have lost most of the adductor sheet. But we have kept the thumb's adductor because it strengthens the grip of our opposable thumb. Our **Adductor Pollicis** (Fig. 14-17) arises from the whole length of the third metacarpal and from the carpals at its base. It inserts into the thumb's proximal phalanx via a tendon (and sesamoid) that it shares with the first Palmar Interosseous muscle. It does what its name implies.

The *Lumbrical* muscles (Fig. 14-6), which attach to the tendons of the hand's extrinsic flexors and extensors, are intrinsic muscles because they lie wholly within the palm; but we shall discuss them later, along with the extrinsic tendons that they tie together.

▪ Radius, Ulna, and Wrist

The two forearm bones—the **radius** on the thumb side and the **ulna** on the little-finger (medial) side of the limb—are rough inverted reflections of each other (Fig. 14-7A). The radius has a small *proximal* end with a cylindrical joint surface that fits into a notch in the ulna, and its distal end is large; the ulna's proximal end is large, and it has a small, pointed *distal* end with a cylindrical joint surface that fits into a notch in the radius.

The elbow joint has a single capsule and joint cavity (Fig. 14-8), but three very different articular surfaces. The joint between humerus and *ulna* is a simple hinge. Its notched, pulleylike articular surface limits the ulna's swing almost completely to a single plane during flexion and extension. (The ulna can also rock laterally a bit during pronation.) The joint between the humerus and *radius* is more mobile, resembling a ball-and-socket joint. But the mobility of the radius at this joint is severely limited by a stout **interosseous membrane** that binds the radius to the ulna (Fig. 14-7B). This ligamentous partition between the elevator and depressor muscles ties the radius's swinging movements to those of the ulna. However, it leaves the radius free to spin on its long axis—or rather, on an axis passing through its proximal end and the ulna's distal end.

The proximal end of the radius articulates with the ulna at the third elbow-joint surface, the **proximal radioulnar joint.** The radius is held tightly against the ulna here, not by the loose capsular fibers connecting the two, but by an **anular** ligament (Fig. 14-8) that encircles the neck of the radius without attaching to it. Within this ligamentous collar, the head of the radius is free to spin against the ball-shaped **capitulum** of the humerus and the concave radial notch of the ulna; and it does so in pronation and supination. (Although the elbow has collateral ligaments like those of other hinge joints, the one on the radial side does not attach to the radius—because that would interfere with pronation and supination. Instead, it runs from the humerus to the anular ligament.)

The *distal* radioulnar joint (near the wrist) is also built to allow free

Fig. 14-7 A. The axis (*dashed line*) around which the radius rotates in pronation. Compare with Fig. 12-5. B. Interosseous membrane binding the radius to the ulna.

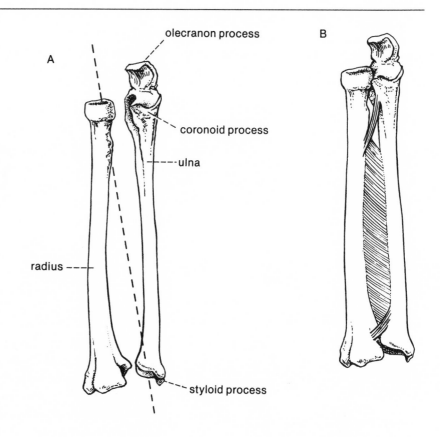

rotation of the radius. But here it is the ulna that has the convex cylindrical articular surface and the radius that has the reciprocal notch. As a result, the axis of radial rotation passes *through the distal ulna;* so the radius flops across the ulna in pronation (Fig. 14-7)—instead of just spinning in place alongside the ulna as it would if both ends of the ulna bore a concave radial notch.

The hand articulates with the radius via the cluster of carpal bones. Three of the proximal carpals (Fig. 14-1) fit together to form a smooth, egg-shaped articular surface that articulates with a reciprocal hollow in the distal end of the radius (Fig. 14-3). Because this radiocarpal joint surface is ellipsoidal rather than spherical, the carpal cluster and the attached hand can be flexed and extended on the radius and also abducted and adducted—but not rotated. When the radius rotates, the hand therefore rotates with it around the tip of

Fig. 14-8 Principal ligaments of the elbow joint. Anterior view. C, capitulum of humerus.

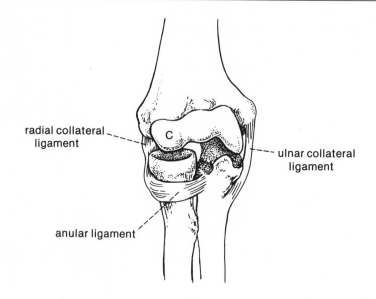

radial collateral ligament

ulnar collateral ligament

anular ligament

the ulna: palm up in supination, palm down when the radius swings across the ulna into the pronated position.

In primitive mammals, both forearm bones articulated with the proximal carpals. In our own wrist, the ulna has withdrawn from its carpal contacts, thereby allowing freer rotation of the hand and radius around the ulna. The rounded ulnar head is separated from the carpals by a **disk**, a triangular band of fibrocartilage that fans out from the tip (**styloid process**) of the ulna to attach to the edge of the carpal socket on the radius (Fig. 14-3). One side of this disk rotates against the ulnar head when the radius rotates; the other extends the concave surface against which the carpals slide when the wrist is bent in various directions (flexion, abduction, and so on). The disk thus provides two differently shaped articular surfaces, allowing for two types of otherwise incompatible movements at the same joint. Other such articular disks are found in the knee and jaw joints.

From the radial and ulnar edges of the carpal cluster, bony bumps stick out ventrally into the palm (Fig. 14-3). One of these is a separate bone—the little **pisiform** (L., "pea-shaped") bone. The other three are projections from other carpals—the hook of the **hamate** on the ulnar side and the tubercles of the **scaphoid** and **trapezium** on the thumb side. These four bony prominences are tied together by a thick ligamentous band called the **flexor retinaculum** (Fig. 14-17). This band retains the hand's extrinsic flexor tendons against the wrist, preventing them from popping out like taut bowstrings when the wrist is flexed. Together, the flexor retinaculum and the carpal bones enclose a passageway—the **carpal tunnel** (Fig. 14-9). The extrinsic flexor tendons pass through this tunnel from the forearm into the palm of the hand.

■ The Extrinsic Flexors of the Hand and Wrist

In primitive reptiles, the palm of the hand was crammed with a complex mass of intrinsic flexor muscles. Superficial to these, just under the scaly skin of the palm, lay a big, flat tendon—the **palmar aponeurosis**. All the finger-flexing muscles in the reptilian forearm inserted into this aponeurosis. There were two layers of those extrinsic flexor muscles—a superficial layer arising from the humerus's medial epicondyle (the bony lump you can feel on the medial side of

Fig. 14-9 The extensor tendons and retinaculum. A. Dorsal view showing synovial tendon sheaths. B. Schematic section through wrist.

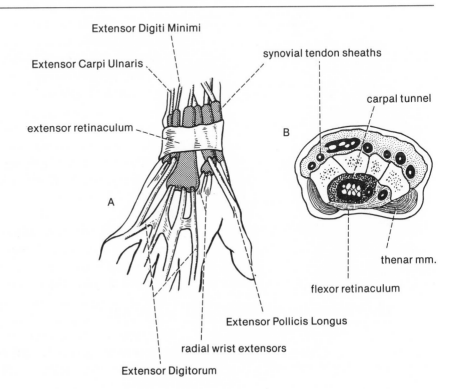

Extensor Digiti Minimi

Extensor Carpi Ulnaris

synovial tendon sheaths

carpal tunnel

extensor retinaculum

B

A

thenar mm.

flexor retinaculum

Extensor Pollicis Longus

radial wrist extensors

Extensor Digitorum

your elbow), and a deeper layer arising from the radius and ulna (and the interosseous membrane stretched between them). Through the palmar aponeurosis, these finger flexors pulled on five smaller tendons that ran from the aponeurosis to the tips of the five digits. Any pull on the aponeurosis caused all five digits to curl toward the center of the palm.

We still have the palmar aponeurosis just under the skin of our palms. But the finger-flexing muscles and the five fingertip tendons no longer attach to it. The only remnant of the old reptilian setup is a vestigial and sometimes absent little muscle—**Palmaris Longus** (Fig. 14-6)—that runs down from the humerus's medial epicondyle to insert on the palmar aponeurosis. In early mammals, the five digital tendons attached to the fingertips became detached from the underside of the palmar aponeurosis and gained direct attachments to the finger-flexing muscles in the forearm. The proximal edge of the old palmar aponeurosis was thickened to form the flexor retinaculum, underneath which our liberated digital flexor tendons slide in and out of the palm. In our monkeylike ancestors, the forearm musculature attached to those tendons became more finely subdivided, thus making it possible to flex one digit without flexing all of them.

There are two flexor tendons, one superficial and one deep, for each of our digits—except the thumb, which lacks a superficial tendon. The five deep tendons are the old fingertip tendons that were attached to the reptilian palmar aponeurosis. In humans, their muscle bellies arise from the forearm bones and the interosseous membrane (Fig. 14-10; Table 14-2). The muscle belly pulling on the thumb's deep flexor tendon is a wholly separate muscle, **Flexor Pollicis Longus**; the other four tendons have only partly separable bellies and so are lumped together as **Flexor Digitorum Profundus,** the deep flexor of the digits. Each of the five deep flexor tendons inserts on the distal phalanx of its digit. These deep flexors can flex all the joints they cross—including the wrist joints (the radiocarpal joint and the fairly mobile joints between the proximal and distal rows of carpal bones) and the knuckle joints of the five digital rays.

The other, more superficial set of digital flexor tendons has a more complex arrangement and history. In early reptiles, these superficial flexor tendons were attached to intrinsic muscles of the hand. During the course of our evolution from primitive mammals, those intrinsic hand muscles gradually shifted their origins up through the carpal tunnel into the forearm, where they stole the whole superficial,

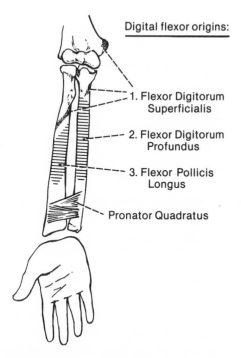

Digital flexor origins:

1. Flexor Digitorum Superficialis

2. Flexor Digitorum Profundus

3. Flexor Pollicis Longus

Pronator Quadratus

Fig. 14-10 Pronator Quadratus and the origins of the digital flexors in the forearm.

Table 14-2 Depressor muscles in the forearm.

Muscle	Origin	Insertion	Action	Nerve
Superficial layer				
Flexor Carpi Ulnaris	Medial epicondyle of humerus; medial edge of upper ⅔ of ulna	5th metacarpal (and hamate) via pisiform	Flexes and adducts wrist	Ulnar n.
Palmaris Longus	Medial epicondyle	Flexor retinaculum and palmar aponeurosis	Flexes wrist	Median n.
Flexor Digitorum Superficialis	Medial epicondyle, plus a strip across the ventral surfaces of radius and ulna (see Fig. 14-10)	Middle phalanges of digits 2–5	Flexes wrist and fingers	Median n.
Flexor Carpi Radialis	Medial epicondyle	Base of 2nd metacarpal (with a slip to 3rd metacarpal)	Flexes and abducts wrist	Median n.
Pronator Teres	Medial epicondyle (plus a slip from the coronoid process of the ulna)	Lateral edge of proximal radius	Pronates	Median n.
Deep layer (cf. Fig. 14-10)				
Flexor Digitorum Profundus	Upper ¾ of ulna and adjoining ½ of interosseous membrane	Distal phalanges of digits 2–5	Flexes wrist and fingers	Ulnar n. (medial half) Median n. (lateral half)
Flexor Pollicis Longus	Middle ⅓ of radius and adjoining part of interosseous membrane	Distal phalanx of thumb	Flexes joints of thumb	Median n.
Pronator Quadratus	Medial edge of distal ulna	Distal radius	Pronates	Median n.

epicondylar layer of finger-flexing musculature away from the deep flexor tendons. Not content with that, they also took over a thin superficial layer of the deeper flexor musculature arising from the bones of the forearm.

The result of this shift of attachments is our **Flexor Digitorum Superficialis.** It arises mostly from the humerus's medial (flexor) epicondyle, but partly from a thin strip along the proximal edge of the deep flexor origins in the forearm (Fig. 14-10). Its four tendons pass through the carpal tunnel and insert on the *middle* phalanges of the four fingers. (The thumb has no middle phalanx and does not receive a superficial flexor tendon.) Each finger's superficial flexor tendon forks into two flat bands, which wrap around the sides of the deep tendon and attach to the middle phalanx. The bony phalanx and its (forked) superficial flexor tendon thus form a loop through which the deep flexor tendon slides independently back and forth (Fig 14-11).

Besides Flexor Digitorum Superficialis (and the little Palmaris Longus that overlies it, when present), three other superficial flexor muscles fan out from the medial epicondyle of the humerus (Fig. 14-12A). Two of them are wrist flexors—**Flexor Carpi Radialis** and **Flexor Carpi Ulnaris**. These two muscles lie respectively on the radial and ulnar sides of the digital flexors. They insert on the bases of the metacarpals of the radialmost (index) finger and ulnarmost (little) finger, respectively.

The ulnar wrist flexor can be, and often is, described as inserting into the pisiform, not the fifth metacarpal. But the pisiform is attached by a stout ligament to the fifth metacarpal base; so we prefer to regard that ligament as part of the tendon of the ulnar wrist flexor, and the pisiform as a sesamoid bone in the tendon. In quadrupedal mammals, the pisiform bone is large and forms a projecting "heel" of the hand, giving Flexor Carpi Ulnaris a powerful lever arm for flexing the wrist in running on all fours. We do not need that lever arm, and our pisiform has been reduced to a pea-sized nubbin as part of the complex of changes that pulled the ulna back away from the wrist bones.

The last of the superficial flexors arising from the medial epicondyle does not cross the wrist joint. (A few of its deeper fibers do not even cross the elbow, since they arise from the ulna's coronoid process.) This muscle lies on the radial edge of the superficial flexor mass; and

Fig. 14-11   Attachment of the two extrinsic flexor tendons to the phalanges of a finger.

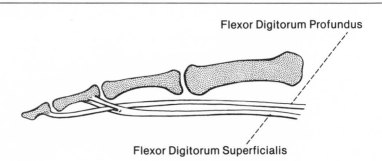

Flexor Digitorum Profundus

Flexor Digitorum Superficialis

Fig. 14-12 Elevator muscles in the forearm. A and B. Schematic comparison between the superficial (epicondylar) flexors (A) and extensors (B). C. Deep extensor muscles. The "outcropping" extensors of the thumb are represented in B by a black arrow. Right forearm, ventral (A) and dorsal (B, C) aspects.

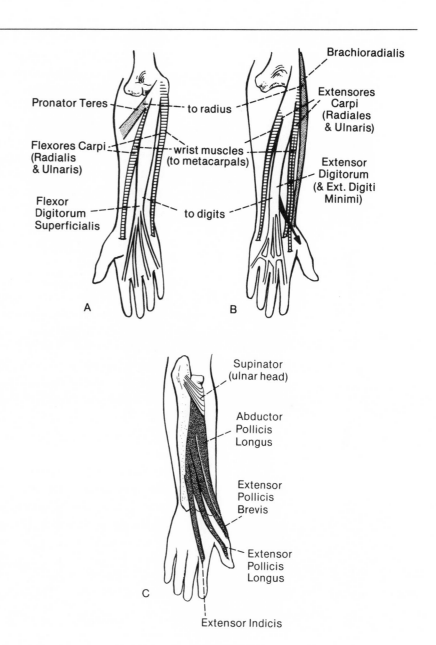

A

Pronator Teres

to radius

Flexores Carpi (Radialis & Ulnaris)

wrist muscles (to metacarpals)

Flexor Digitorum Superficialis

to digits

B

Brachioradialis

Extensores Carpi (Radiales & Ulnaris)

Extensor Digitorum (& Ext. Digiti Minimi)

C

Supinator (ulnar head)

Abductor Pollicis Longus

Extensor Pollicis Brevis

Extensor Pollicis Longus

Extensor Indicis

it inserts high up on the radius, just below the Biceps attachment. When it contracts, it turns the radius medially across the ulna, thus pronating the hand. It is accordingly called **Pronator Teres,** which means "round pronator."

Pronator Teres is so named, not because it is especially round, but to contrast it with the "square pronator"—**Pronator Quadratus**—which is the deepest and most distal of all the depressor muscles in the forearm. It is a flat, rectangular sheet of muscle fibers running across from ulna to radius just above the wrist, where it lies right against the interosseous membrane (Fig. 14-10). Pronator Quadratus is used in pronating with no resistance, as in gesturing or eating. When more powerful pronation is needed—say, in using a screwdriver—Pronator Teres comes into action.

▪ Elevator Muscles

Like the depressor muscles on the ventral side of the forearm, the elevator muscles (Fig. 14-12B and C) on the dorsal side are divisible into two layers—a **deep** layer that arises from the forearm bones and inserts exclusively on the digits, and a **superficial** layer that includes muscles controlling movements of the wrist and the radius as well. The main difference between the dorsal and ventral musculature is that the deep layer on the dorsal (extensor) side is almost wholly concerned with moving the thumb (Table 14-3).

SUPERFICIAL LAYER

The superficial layer of extensors arises from the humerus's lateral, or radial, epicondyle (which is sometimes called the "extensor epicondyle" for that reason, just as the medial one is sometimes called the "flexor epicondyle"). From the lateral epicondyle (and the ridge above it), six elevator muscles fan out and run down past the elbow to insert into the more distal bones of the limb. From the radial side toward the ulnar side of the fan, these are as follows:

1. **Brachioradialis.** As its name implies, this muscle runs from the humerus to the radius. It is thus the equivalent of Pronator Teres on the other side of the limb. But because it is lined up with the radius in all positions, it cannot act to rotate the radius the way Pronator Teres does. Instead, it flexes the elbow. It can do this effectively because it arises up high *above* the lateral epicondyle, from the ridge that ex-

Table 14-3 Elevator muscles in the forearm.

Muscle	Origin	Insertion	Action	Nerve
Superficial layer				
Brachioradialis	Ridge above lateral epicondyle of humerus	Distal radius	Flexes elbow (see Fig. 14-13)	Radial n.
Extensor Carpi Radialis Longus	Lateral epicondyle (and ridge above it)	Base of 2nd metacarpal	Extends (dorsiflexes) and abducts wrist	Radial n.
Extensor Carpi Radialis Brevis	Lateral epicondyle	Base of 3rd metacarpal	Extends (dorsiflexes) and abducts wrist	Radial n.
Extensor Digitorum	Lateral epicondyle	Extensor expansions of digits 2–5 (see Fig. 14-15)	Extends wrist and fingers	Radial n.
Extensor Digiti Minimi	Lateral epicondyle	Extensor expansion of digit 5	Extends little finger	Radial n.
Extensor Carpi Ulnaris	Lateral epicondyle	Base of 5th metacarpal	Extends (dorsiflexes) and adducts wrist	Radial n.
Deep layer				
Abductor Pollicis Longus	Dorsal surface of middle ⅓ of ulna and radius (plus interosseous membrane)	Lateral side of 1st metacarpal and trapezium	Abducts and extends at carpometacarpal joint of thumb	Radial n.
Extensor Pollicis Brevis	Radius below Abductor Poll. Longus origins (plus adjoining interosseous membrane)	Proximal phalanx of thumb	Extends proximal phalanx	Radial n.
Extensor Pollicis Longus	Ulna below Abductor Poll. Longus origins (plus interosseous membrane)	Distal phalanx of thumb	Extends (and laterally rotates) thumb	Radial n.
Extensor Indicis	Ulna below Extensor Poll. Longus origins (plus interosseous membrane)	Extensor expansion of index finger	Extends index finger	Radial n.
Other elevators				
Supinator	Lateral epicondyle and proximal ulna	Lateral edge of proximal ⅓ of radius	Supinates	Radial n.
Anconeus	Lateral epicondyle	Posterior face of proximal ¼ of ulna	Extends elbow	Radial n.

tends back up from the epicondyle onto the humeral shaft. This high origin keeps Brachioradialis far enough away from the axis of elbow flexion to give it fairly good leverage around that axis (Fig. 14-13). Brachioradialis is the only elevator muscle that *flexes* a forelimb joint.

2 and 3. **Extensores Carpi Radiales.** There are *two* wrist extensors on the radial side—a long one and a short one. The long one is longer because it lies more toward the radial side and so arises alongside Brachioradialis—and therefore extends further up on the humerus. Like the radial wrist flexor, it inserts on the base of the second metacarpal. The other radial wrist extensor, arising from the epicondyle, has to settle for the next digit over and inserts on the base of the *third* metacarpal. The names of these two muscles describe them—**Extensor Carpi Radialis Longus** and **Extensor Carpi Radialis Brevis.**

4 and 5. **Extensor Digitorum.** The superficial extensor of the fingers arises from the extensor epicondyle and divides into four tendons—one for every digit except the thumb. The tendons are variably bound together by tendinous bands on the back of the hand (Fig. 14-9). For some reason, the fifth digit receives a second superficial extensor tendon, which is attached to a separate little muscle belly—**Extensor Digiti Minimi.** This special extensor for the little finger is what makes it so easy to "stick out the pinky" independent of the other fingers.

6. **Extensor Carpi Ulnaris.** The wrist extensor on the ulnar side

Fig. 14-13 The "extensor" (elevator) muscle Brachioradialis acts as an elbow flexor.

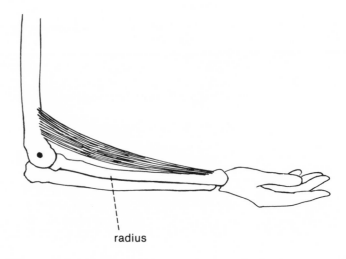

radius

inserts, as might be expected, on the dorsal side of the base of metacarpal 5, opposite the insertion of the ulnar wrist *flexor;* and as might be expected, it extends, or dorsiflexes, the wrist.

Because the wrist joint permits radial and ulnar deviation of the hand as well as flexion and extension, the five wrist muscles can act in various combinations to swing the hand in any direction. If the two ulnar-side wrist muscles (Extensor Carpi Ulnaris and Flexor Carpi Ulnaris) contract together, the result is neither flexion nor extension but adduction (that is, ulnar deviation) of the hand. Similarly, the three radial muscles act together to produce radial deviation.

A more or less detached slip of Triceps Brachii also originates from the lateral epicondyle, from which it runs medially back to insert into the olecranon process and proximal ulna. It is conventionally regarded as a separate muscle, **Anconeus.** It may be fused with Triceps or with the ulnar wrist extensor, and is sometimes absent altogether. When present, it aids Triceps in extending the elbow.

DEEP LAYER

The deep layer of extensor muscles in the forearm, like the deep flexors, arises from the forearm bones and the interosseous membrane. Three of its four muscles attach to the thumb's three bones— one muscle per bone.

The shortest of these three thumb muscles lies on the radial (thumb) edge of the deep extensor mass (Fig. 14-12C). Its tendon passes so far around onto the palmar side of the thumb that it acts as an abductor, not an extensor. It attaches to the metacarpal at the base of the thumb and is called **Abductor Pollicis Longus**—to contrast it with the short (thenar) abductor.

The other two thumb extensors are more dorsal and function as true extensors. They insert on the thumb's two phalanges. The more radial of these two thumb extensors is called **Extensor Pollicis Brevis.** It lies next to Abductor Pollicis Longus, is closely attached to it, and may be fused with it (as it is in most other mammals). It attaches to the next most distal bone—that is, the proximal phalanx. The thumb's third, longest, and most powerful elevator, **Extensor Pollicis Longus,** inserts all the way out on the distal phalanx; hence its name. Because these three deep extensors run across the radial wrist extensors on their way to the thumb, they are sometimes described as the "outcropping" extensors of the thumb.

The fourth and last of the deep finger-extending muscles is a special extensor for the index finger, which gives the second digit the same sort of independent extensibility the fifth digit has. We use this special **Extensor Indicis** in pointing.

SUPINATOR

There is one more elevator muscle in the forearm. It includes both superficial and deep parts and deserves separate treatment. This muscle, the **Supinator** (Fig. 14-14), lies high in the forearm, up near the elbow. It arises partly from the extensor epicondyle and partly from the radial side of the ulna, below the anular ligament. From that double origin, its fibers wrap forward around the lateral side of the radius and insert into its shaft. When they contract, they pull the radius around dorsally and laterally, bringing it into parallel with the ulna and thus supinating it.

Supinator, like Pronator Quadratus in the depressor musculature, is used in rotating the radius without resistance. When more forceful supination is called for, Biceps Brachii is called into play. Although Biceps is mainly an elbow flexor, it also acts as a supinator because it inserts on the ventral side of the radius (Fig. 13-15). When the radius flops across the ulna into the pronated position, the spot where Biceps inserts gets rotated around to the *dorsal* side (Fig. 12-5). This rotation winds the Biceps tendon around the radius. Biceps, in contracting, unwinds itself and spins the radius back to the supinated position.

▪ Extensor Expansions and Lumbricals

Like the flexor tendons, the tendons of the digital extensors have to be tied down at the wrist to keep them from bowstringing outward when the wrist is bent toward them (dorsiflexed). On the back of the wrist, there is no single equivalent of the carpal tunnel. Instead, the extensor tendons lie in bony grooves in the distal radius and ulna. A bracelet-like band of deep fascia, the **extensor retinaculum,** roofs over those grooves and is attached to bone in between them (Fig. 14-9).

Where a single finger receives two extensor tendons (that is, digits 2 and 5, and occasionally others), the two fuse together into a single tendon as they run across the back of the hand. Each of the four resulting tendons then divides into a central band (which attaches to the middle phalanx of its digit) and two lateral bands that run on to reach the distal phalanx (Fig. 14-15).

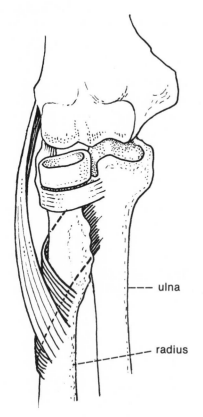

Fig. 14-14   Diagram of the two heads of Supinator. Anterior view. Compare with 14-12.

ulna

radius

Fig. 14-15 Attachment of the extrinsic extensor tendon and associated intrinsic muscles to the phalanges. The digit's dorsal side is toward the top of the figure.

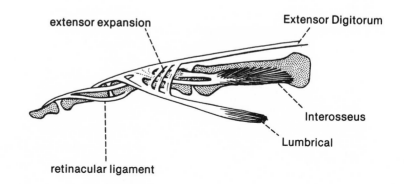

extensor expansion

Extensor Digitorum

Interosseus

Lumbrical

retinacular ligament

The lateral bands of the extensor tendons are joined by small tendons from the hand's intrinsic depressor muscles. Each Interosseus tendon, in addition to attaching to the base of a proximal phalanx, sends tendinous fibers up dorsally toward the lateral bands of its digit. On the radial (thumb) side of each digit, these Interosseus fibers are joined by the tendon of a **Lumbrical** muscle. Each of the hand's four Lumbricals (Fig. 14-6) is a worm-shaped little muscle (L. *lumbricalis,* "wormlike") that connects a deep flexor tendon (Flexor Digitorum Profundus) with the extensor tendon of the same finger (Fig. 14-16). An aponeurotic hood of tendinous fibers—the **extensor expansion** (Fig. 14-15)—covers the back of the proximal phalanx and binds the Lumbrical and Interosseus tendons to each other and to the common extensor tendon. (The thumb has no dorsal Interosseus, no common extensor tendon, and no Lumbricals. Its feeble extensor expansion is composed largely of fibers from Abductor Pollicis Brevis.)

When a Lumbrical muscle contracts, it pulls on its digit's extensor expansion and *extends* the joints between the phalanges. But the Lumbricals' line of pull passes just to the palmar side of the metacarpophalangeal joints' axis of rotation—and so they *flex* those joints when they contract. The resulting posture of the hand, with flexed metacarpophalangeal joints and extended interphalangeal joints (Fig. 14-16), is called the "writing position," because it is the position most of the fingers assume when holding a pen. The Interossei, because of their attachments to the extensor expansion, can help place or hold the hand in this posture, too—but less efficiently and with the added complication of producing adduction or abduction.

Fig. 14-16   A digit in the so-called writing position, showing why a lumbrical muscle (*black*) flexes the metacarpophalangeal (M-P) joint but extends the interphalangeal joints.

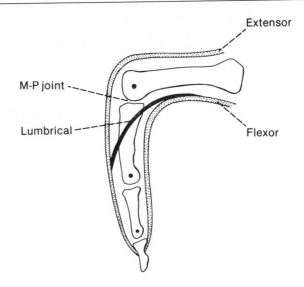

■ Fascial Spaces and Tendon Sheaths

People use their upper limbs almost wholly for handling things, and are often clumsy at it. Our fingers and palms therefore tend to get cut, stabbed, crushed, lacerated, and burned more often than other parts of our bodies. Infections of the hand resulting from such injuries are common. The spread of infection in the hand is confined and directed by the septa that separate the muscle groups and divide the palm into several fascial spaces. The most important of these compartments are the central space in the palm, which contains the long (extrinsic) flexor tendons, and the thenar and hypothenar compartments on either side of it. Infection in one of these spaces cannot readily or quickly spread to the others.

The extrinsic tendons of the fingers have to slide through bony and ligamentous tunnels to get into the palm and the back of the hand. As always where tendons slide across bone, their movement is lubricated by slippery bags of synovial tissue. In the hand, these take the form of hollow tubular bursae called **synovial tendon sheaths.** The sheaths enclose the extrinsic tendons where they slide back and forth under the flexor and extensor retinacula (Fig. 14-9). The flexor tendons in the four fingers are also bound down at the knuckle joints (by fibrous bands that act as retinacula), and separate synovial sheaths surround them there.

A single big synovial sheath surrounds the four fingers' flexor tendons in the carpal tunnel and extends some distance into the palm. Infection within this sheath may produce swelling inside the carpal tunnel, thus compressing the median nerve (which also runs through the tunnel) and producing pain, numbness, and intrinsic-muscle paralysis in the hand. This condition is called "carpal-tunnel syndrome."

■ The Nerves of the Forearm and Hand

Apart from the strictly cutaneous nerves mentioned in the preceding chapter, only three nerves cross the elbow and enter the forearm (Fig. 13-18). The **radial** nerve is the only posterior-division nerve that does so. It supplies *all the elevator musculature* and most of the overlying skin. Its cutaneous distribution usually includes the skin over the back of the hand and over the "outcropping" extensor tendons to the thumb (Fig. 13-18). The *depressor* musculature (and the remaining skin) is innervated by two terminal branches from the anterior divisions of the brachial plexus—the **median** and **ulnar** nerves.

All three nerves are named from their positions at the elbow. The radial nerve winds around the front of the *radial* epicondyle. It thus passes briefly into the depressor compartment before running down the back of the forearm. The ulnar nerve similarly runs behind the *ulnar* epicondyle before passing into the forearm's muscles. (The spot where the ulnar nerve lies behind the medial epicondyle—and can be easily mashed against it by a blow—is commonly called the "funny bone.") The median nerve enters the forearm in a *median* position, between the radial and ulnar nerves, running along the medial edge of Brachialis.

After crossing the elbow, the median and ulnar nerves run along between the superficial (epicondylar) and deep (radioulnar) flexor-muscle layers. Both nerves supply motor fibers to the muscles they touch, in both layers. The ulnar nerve innervates the *ulnar edge* of the two muscle layers—that is, Flexor Carpi Ulnaris in the superficial layer, and the ulnar half or so of the deeper Flexor Digitorum Profundus. *All the rest of the depressor muscles in the forearm are supplied by the median nerve.*

This disproportion is reversed in the hand, where the ulnar nerve innervates almost all the intrinsic muscles. It enters the palm around the radial side of the pisiform. Here it gives off a **deep** branch, which

Fig. 14-17 The ulnar and median nerves in the palm.

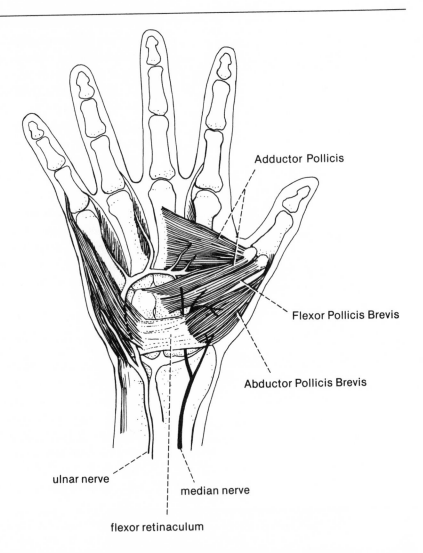

Adductor Pollicis

Flexor Pollicis Brevis

Abductor Pollicis Brevis

ulnar nerve

median nerve

flexor retinaculum

plunges over the distal edge of the flexor retinaculum and dives into the hypothenar muscles. This deep branch of the ulnar nerve then curves over toward the thumb across the ventral surface of all eight Interossei, innervating them. To run across all the Interossei, it has to pierce Adductor Pollicis (Fig. 14-17). It thus divides that muscle into two heads by its passage—and innervates it as it goes by. It also sends motor branches to the hypothenar (little-finger) muscles as it goes through them; and it supplies the Lumbricals of digits 4 and 5.

The only intrinsic hand muscles left for the median nerve to innervate are the three thenar muscles and the other two Lumbricals. It sends branches to those five muscles after it passes through the carpal tunnel in company with the extrinsic flexor tendons.

Both the median and ulnar nerves give off some cutaneous branches before they enter the palm. Those of the ulnar nerve supply the little finger and the adjoining side of the fourth digit; the median nerve's superficial branches supply the skin over the ball of the thumb (Fig. 14-17). The remaining three and one-half digits are innervated by the median nerve *after* it traverses the carpal tunnel. Those digits accordingly suffer pain and numbness in carpal-tunnel syndrome.

Note that the ulnar nerve supplies the two ulnar-side digits (4 and 5) in several ways—with cutaneous innervation (mostly), with motor fibers to their *deep* flexors (but not to their Flexor Superficialis tendons), and with motor fibers to the two Lumbrical muscles attached to those deep flexors.

■ The Arteries of the Arm and Hand

The brachial artery in the arm divides into **radial** and **ulnar** branches (Fig. 13-16) under cover of the bicipital aponeurosis (the fibrous band that joins the Biceps tendon to the forearm's deep fascia). The radial artery runs laterally across the Biceps tendon and simply travels down the *radial* edge of the forearm, on the flexor surface of the septum between elevators and depressors (Fig. 14-18). The ulnar artery runs deeper: it dives under the superficial flexor muscles and passes toward the wrist between the superficial and deep flexors, where it joins and travels with the ulnar nerve. Its branches resemble those of the ulnar nerve, including a deep branch running across the Interossei.

As it enters the forearm, the ulnar artery sends off a **common interosseous** artery. This in turn divides into anterior and posterior branches, which run down opposite sides of the interosseous membrane (Fig. 13-16) and help supply the muscles attached to it. As noted earlier, the anterior interosseous artery is developmentally the continuation of the primary (axial) artery of the limb bud, so it runs in the skeletal plane, directly against the interosseous membrane (Fig. 14-18).

The radial artery is covered by Brachioradialis in most of its course through the forearm. Below that muscle's distal end, the artery lies

Fig. 14-18   Proximal (stump) surface of a diagrammatic section through the right forearm.

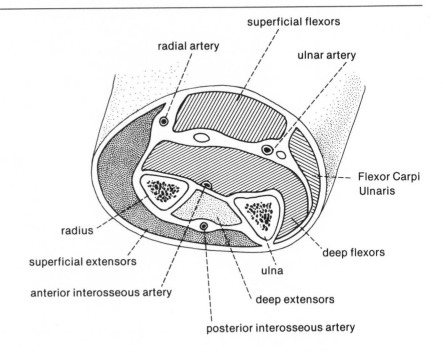

superficial flexors

radial artery

ulnar artery

Flexor Carpi Ulnaris

deep flexors

radius

superficial extensors

ulna

anterior interosseous artery

deep extensors

posterior interosseous artery

directly against the radius, just lateral to the tendon of Flexor Carpi Radialis, and can be distinctly felt there by compressing it with a fingertip. (This is the usual spot for taking a pulse.) The radial artery then wraps around the dorsal side of the thumb's metacarpal and plunges between the two heads of the first Dorsal Interosseous (Fig. 14-5) to reappear in the palm. There it anastomoses with the deep branch of the ulnar artery (Fig. 14-19), forming a **deep palmar arch.** There is also a **superficial palmar arch** of arteries, which is formed by anastomotic superficial branches that the radial and ulnar arteries give off when they reach the wrist. Both arches send off radiating branches, which join and then redivide to send branches to the radial and ulnar sides of each digit.

Fig. 14-19 Arteries and arterial arches of the palm. The deep palmar arch and its branches (*shaded*) accompany the deep branch of the ulnar nerve across the palm. Compare with Fig. 14-17.

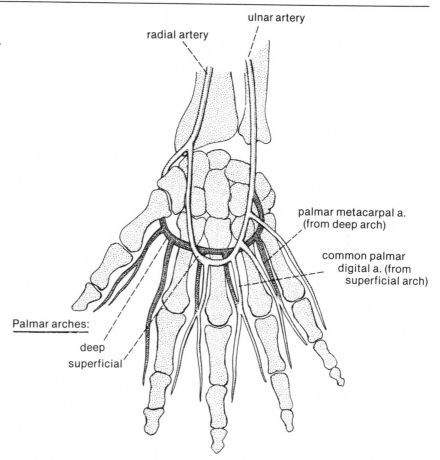

radial artery

ulnar artery

palmar metacarpal a. (from deep arch)

common palmar digital a. (from superficial arch)

Palmar arches:

deep

superficial

15

The Hip
and
the Thigh

■ Limb Posture and Serial Homology

The lobe-finned fishes that first began crawling across dry land from pond to pond must have pushed themselves along on their bellies, holding their fins out sideways and swinging them backward like oars to scoot the body ahead. This is inefficient and involves a lot of wear and tear on the belly. An improved posture for moving around on land (Fig. 15-1) was evolved in early amphibians. In this posture, which is retained in turtles, the limb segment nearest the body—that is, the arm or thigh—sticks straight out laterally. The next segment (forearm or leg) is held vertically, carrying the body's weight down to the ground. The depressor musculature of the limbs acts to keep the belly raised off the ground.

This locomotor posture was a great improvement over the fish condition, but it was still grossly inefficient, especially in big, heavy animals. Too much energy was wasted in heaving the belly up off the ground on limbs that stuck out sideways. Again and again in vertebrate evolution, selection for fast, efficient locomotion on land has resulted in the limbs being rotated around into parallel with the body's midline plane, bringing the feet close together beneath the belly. The early dinosaurs (and their descendants, the birds) managed this by becoming bipedal and swiveling the thigh around so that the knee pointed headward rather than sideways. The early mammals from whom we are descended also rotated their knees forward and pulled them in alongside the body. Because mammals (unlike dinosaurs) remained quadrupedal, they swung the elbow in toward the body as well; but because they swung the elbow around in the opposite direction, the elbow and knee wound up pointing toward each other (Fig. 15-1). This arrangement left the hand and foot facing in opposite directions; hence the hand had to be flopped over into a pronated position to keep the palm facing down toward the ground. (To appreciate this, try crawling on all fours with the hand

Fig. 15-1   Quadrupedal postures in primitive amphibians and reptiles (A) and advanced mammals (B). E, elbow; K, knee.

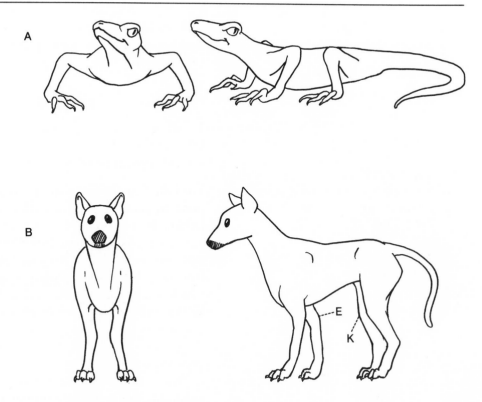

supinated.) This pronation produces the posture seen in a dog or other typical four-footed mammal.

The human locomotor posture is unique. Like dinosaurs and birds, we are bipedal; but unlike those animals, we have risen up on our hind legs by sticking them straight out behind us and throwing our trunk backward until our vertebral column is balanced vertically above our pelvis. Freed from locomotion, the human forearm is held about halfway between full pronation and supination in a relaxed stance. In anatomy textbooks, however, it is always described as fully supinated (because that "anatomical position" keeps the forearm bones neatly parallel and puts the extensors tidily on the dorsal aspect of the forearm). Thus, all the muscles on the *ventral* side of the human upper limb are depressors; but *all the LOWER limb's depressor muscles lie on its DORSAL side.* Mammalian body posture, human uprightness, and anatomical convention all combine to make the back side of our upper limbs correspond to the belly side of our lower limbs (Fig. 15-2). The correspondence is apparent when we recall that the knee and elbow are serially homologous and originally pointed in the same direction—that is, sideways and dorsally, as in a turtle or an early human fetus.

■ The Nerve Supply of the Lower Limbs

The plexus of ventral rami that supply the lower limb is diagrammed in Figure 15-3. Like the brachial plexus, the lower-limb plexus wraps

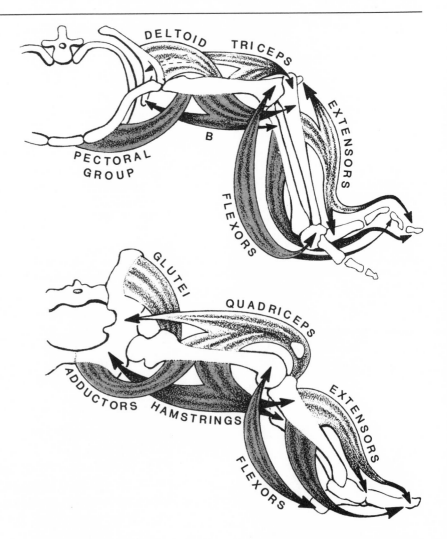

Fig. 15-2 Muscle groups of the fore (upper) and hind (lower) limbs, diagrammed to show serial homologies. B, brachial muscle group.

Fig. 15-3 The nerve plexus of the lower limb. Posterior-division nerves (to elevator musculature) are shaded. O.I., nerve to Obturator Internus; P, parasympathetics (pelvic splanchnic nn.); Pir., nerve to Piriformis; Q.F., nerve to Quadratus Femoris.

✳

Femoral → accompanies external iliac artery → innervates the elevator muscles that extend knee.

Obturator → accompanies obturator artery → innervates the depressor muscles.

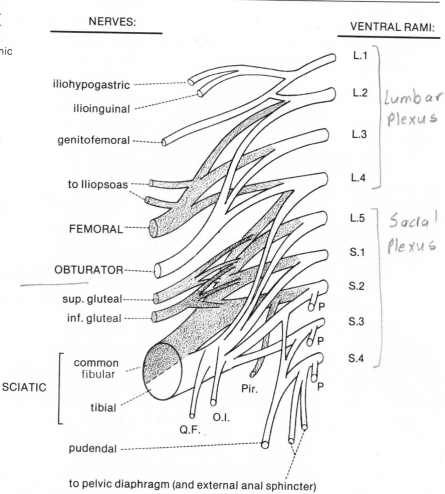

NERVES:

VENTRAL RAMI:

iliohypogastric

ilioinguinal

genitofemoral

to Iliopsoas

FEMORAL

OBTURATOR

sup. gluteal

inf. gluteal

SCIATIC
- common fibular
- tibial

pudendal

Q.F.

O.I.

Pir.

P

to pelvic diaphragm (and external anal sphincter)

L.1

L.2

L.3

L.4

L.5

S.1

S.2

S.3

S.4

Lumbar Plexus

Sacral Plexus

around the old axial artery of the limb bud. But in the lower limb of the human adult, that artery is small and largely replaced by other vessels, and the anterior and posterior divisions of the lower-limb plexus are not neatly held apart by blood vessels the way they are in the brachial plexus.

The plexus of the lower limb has two subdivisions—the **lumbar plexus,** consisting of the upper four lumbar ventral rami, and the **sacral plexus,** consisting of the next five ventral rami (L.5 and S.1–S.4). These two subdivisions are connected by a large branch of the

L.4 ventral ramus that runs down to join the sacral plexus. Each subdivision gives rise to two major nerves: an anterior-division nerve to depressor muscles and a posterior-division one to elevators. (The plexus also gives rise to several lesser nerves, which supply skin or muscles in the hip region.)

The two major branches of the *lumbar* part of the plexus are formed from the ventral rami of L.2–L.4. The anterior divisions of these rami join to form the **obturator** nerve, and the posterior divisions form the **femoral** nerve. Each nerve passes out of the pelvic region in company with an artery. The femoral nerve follows the external iliac artery into the front of the thigh. It innervates the surrounding elevator muscles that extend the knee. The obturator nerve runs out further down, passing through the obturator foramen in company with the obturator artery. It emerges in the midst of the depressor muscles on the medial side of the thigh—which it supplies (Fig. 15-9). Other lumbar-plexus nerves (iliohypogastric, ilioinguinal, genitofemoral) provide mostly cutaneous innervation to the lower body wall and groin region (Fig. 5-7) and do not innervate any limb musculature.

Most of the fibers in the *sacral* part of the lower limb's nerve plexus (including the communicating branch from L.4) feed into a single enormous nerve—the **sciatic** nerve. The sciatic is really two nerves in one: (1) the anterior-division **tibial** nerve that supplies the toe- and ankle-flexing calf muscles on the back of the leg, and (2) the posterior-division **common peroneal** nerve that supplies the corresponding extensors on the front of the leg. The two are bound together where they emerge from the pelvis through the greater sciatic foramen. The resulting composite bundle, the sciatic nerve, runs downward beneath the hamstring muscles on the back of the thigh. It innervates them as it goes by. Five other, much smaller branches of the sacral plexus (superior and inferior gluteal nerves and the nerves to Piriformis, Obturator Internus, and Quadratus Femoris) each supply one or two muscles in the vicinity of the hip joint but do not extend into the more distal parts of the limb.

■ The Muscles of the Hip and Thigh

In our reptilian ancestors, the hipbone and shoulder girdle were both flat, vertical plates of bone with a socket in the middle. Elevator muscles arose from these plates above the socket and depressors arose below it. Things have since gotten more complicated than that in our shoulder region; but the pelvis preserves the simple, primitive arrangement. All the limb muscles that originate from our hipbone *above* the acetabulum are old fin elevators, innervated by posterior-division nerves from the limb plexus. Similarly, all those arising *below* the acetabulum are depressor muscles, innervated by anterior (ventral) divisions of the plexus. Because the hipbone above the acetabulum is formed entirely by the ilium (Fig. 11-1), *all limb muscles attached to the ilium are elevators and all those attached to the ischium and pubis are depressors.* (As we shall see, one muscle—Pectineus—is the sole exception to this rule.)

There are three axes and six possible directions of rotation at the hip joint, identical to those at the shoulder joint: abduction and adduction, flexion and extension, medial and lateral rotation. There are also six muscle groups crossing the hip joint. The six groups correspond roughly to the six movements. But alas, the correspondence is not exact; two muscle groups act to flex the hip, and there is no group of medial rotators. (Medial rotation is handled by the abductor group.) Furthermore, the lateral-rotator "group" is really not a coherent muscle group but a ragbag of phylogenetic odds and ends with diverse innervations and attachments. We will be treating them together just because they happen to lie together in a cluster behind the hip joint—and they all have the same function.

■ The Gluteal Group: Abductors

The four muscles in this group correspond rather closely to the Deltoideus group in the shoulder region. They arise from the outer surface of the ilium and run down laterally across the hip joint to insert into the femur and the overlying deep fascia on the outside of the thigh. Thus they, like Deltoideus, form a sort of hood over the top of the joint and, again like Deltoideus, act as abductors. The two superficial muscles in the group are specialized, but the deeper two—**Gluteus Medius** and **Gluteus Minimus**—are still principally hip abductors. From their broad, fleshy origin from the whole lateral surface of the iliac blade, the fibers of these deep Glutei converge on and insert into a bony prominence—the **greater trochanter**—that sticks up from the top of the femur's shaft (Figs. 15-4 and 15-5). The trochanter provides the deep Glutei with a lever arm; when they pull medially upward on it, the thigh is abducted. The two muscles are

Fig. 15-4 Gluteal musculature, lateral views. A. Deep layer. B. Superficial layer. Dashed line in A indicates outline of Gluteus Minimus: compare Fig. 15-6.

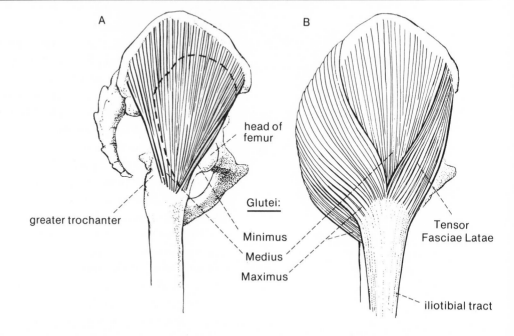

A

B

head of femur

greater trochanter

Glutei:

Minimus

Medius

Maximus

Tensor Fasciae Latae

iliotibial tract

effectively a single mass, separated by their motor nerve, the **superior gluteal** nerve. This nerve emerges through the greater sciatic foramen and breaks up into branches that run forward across the blade of the ilium (Fig. 15-6), thereby splitting the abductor mass into Gluteus Medius and the deeper Minimus.

At its anterior end, the superior gluteal nerve reaches and innervates a small superficial muscle—**Tensor Fasciae Latae** (Fig. 15-4). This muscle arises from the ilium in front (near the anterior superior spine) and inserts, not into bone, but into deep fascia. The thigh's deep fascia is tough and thick, like an elastic stocking around the proximal part of the limb. It receives the special name of **fascia lata** (L. *lata,* "broad"), for which this muscle is named. Tensor Fasciae Latae inserts into a specialized ligamentous band in this fascia, known as the **iliotibial tract** (Fig. 15-4). This tract stretches all the way down the thigh's lateral aspect to insert into the tibia (the shin bone) on the lateral side of the knee. Tensor Fasciae Latae pulls *anteriorly* upward on the tract and therefore acts as a medial rotator of the thigh—as do the anterior fibers of the deeper Glutei, for the

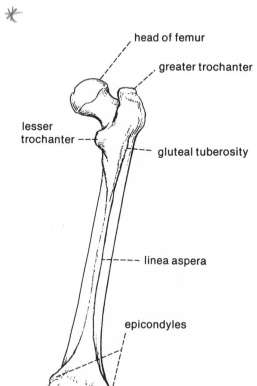

head of femur

greater trochanter

lesser
trochanter

gluteal tuberosity

linea aspera

epicondyles

condyles

Fig. 15-5 The femur. Posterior aspect.

same reason. (Compare the anterior fibers of Deltoideus, which can medially rotate the humerus.)

The most posterior and largest muscle of the gluteal group is **Gluteus Maximus.** Like Tensor Fasciae Latae, it arises from the edge of the iliac crest and inserts into the iliotibial tract—but it does so from behind and so acts as a *lateral* rather than medial rotator. (Compare the *posterior* fibers of Deltoideus; Fig. 13-11.) However, the main job of Gluteus Maximus is to extend the hip. Its fibers pass behind and below the hip joint (Fig. 15-4); so it pulls the thigh backward into an extended position when it contracts. Gluteus Maximus plays no role in normal bipedal striding, but it is crucial in extending the hip against resistance—say, in rising from a squatting position or in climbing a ladder. Its lower fibers (about one-third of the total muscle) insert directly into the femur itself, on a roughened bony crest running downward from the back of the greater trochanter (Figs. 15-4 and 15-6). This crest is called the **gluteal tuberosity** (Fig. 15-5).

Because all the Glutei arise from the ilium, above the acetabulum (as hip abductors must if they are going to abduct), they are elevator muscles and are innervated by posterior-division nerves. The superior gluteal nerve is formed by posterior divisions of ventral rami L.4–L.5 and S.1 (Fig. 15-3). The **inferior gluteal** nerve, which innervates Gluteus Maximus alone, has a similar origin, shifted one segment downward (L.5 and S.1–S.2). Both nerves emerge from the pelvis through the greater sciatic foramen. They are accompanied by similarly named superior and inferior gluteal blood vessels, which run along with the nerves and have similar distributions. These vessels were described earlier as branches of the internal iliac artery and vein (Fig. 11-10).

Gluteus is a bastardized Latin form of the Greek word for buttock, and *gluteus maximus* is often jocularly used as if it were a learned term for the buttocks. This is wrong. The peculiar protuberant buttocks of human beings are not masses of muscle, but humps of tough subcutaneous fascia laden with dense connective tissue. They serve as fat storage bodies at the top of the thigh. The **natal fold** at the bottom of the buttock represents a line along which the superficial fascia is tied down to the fascia lata—which is why the buttock overhangs the skin of the thigh. The buttock only partly overlaps Gluteus Maximus; it extends below its lower edge and does not reach its upper edge. (That upper edge, where Gluteus Maximus is covered only by thin

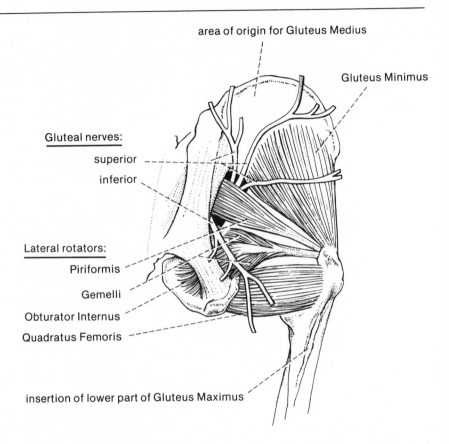

Fig. 15-6   Gluteal region, seen from behind with Gluteus Maximus and Medius removed.

area of origin for Gluteus Medius

Gluteus Minimus

Gluteal nerves:

superior

inferior

Lateral rotators:

Piriformis

Gemelli

Obturator Internus

Quadratus Femoris

insertion of lower part of Gluteus Maximus

and poorly innervated cutaneous tissues, is a favored site for intramuscular injections.) When we sit, our weight is borne by the ischial tuberosities; the overlying soft structures—Gluteus Maximus and most of the buttock fascia—are not squashed underneath us.

It is not clear why we have buttocks. No other mammals have them. Because women have larger buttocks than men, the usual explanatory stories argue either that the buttocks are food-storage organs (like a camel's hump) for pregnancy or sexual stimuli and releasers (like the puffy pink "sexual skin" on the backside of a female chimpanzee in heat). One thing the natal fold does biomechanically is to help keep subcutaneous stored fat localized near the top of the thigh, where it does not have to be accelerated back and forth all the time in walking—as it would if it were distributed further down the limb.

▪ The Lateral-Rotator "Group"

Six small muscles run laterally from the back of the pelvis to the region of the greater trochanter, passing across the back side of the hip joint. They act as lateral rotators of the hip joint (Fig. 15-6). (Gluteus Maximus is a more powerful lateral rotator, but it also extends the hip when it contracts.) The uppermost of these little muscles—**Piriformis** (L., "pear-shaped")—arises from the front of the sacrum and the margins of the greater sciatic foramen. It emerges from the pelvis through that foramen, which it effectively plugs. Phylogenetically, it is a much-reduced vestige of the great caudofemoral elevator muscles that run from a reptile's tail to its femur (and provide propulsion force by pulling the femur backward). Functionally, it is just another lateral rotator in human beings.

The other lateral rotators are all depressor muscles. Here, that fact does not help in learning their innervation, because they (like Piriformis) have separate little motor nerves from the sacral plexus (Tables 15-1 and 15-2); but it may help you to recall that they all originate from the pubis and ischium. There are five of them.

1. **Quadratus Femoris** (L., "square muscle of the femur"). This muscle runs across from the ischial tuberosity to the back of the greater trochanter.

2. **Obturator Internus.** We encountered this muscle when we described the perineum. Its broad, fleshy origin (from the inner surface of the obturator membrane) forms the lateral wall of the ischiorectal fossa (Fig. 11-5). Like the other structures that enter or leave the ischiorectal fossa, the Obturator Internus tendon passes through the *lesser* sciatic foramen, below the sacrospinous ligament (Fig. 15-6). It then winds around the back of the ischium and runs laterally to the greater trochanter. Where it slides back and forth across the ischium, it is provided with a lubricating bursa.

3. and 4. **Superior and Inferior Gemelli.** The tendon of Obturator Internus is provided with two little auxiliary muscle bellies—the Superior and Inferior Gemelli (L., "little twins"). They arise from the margins of the lesser sciatic foramen above and below the Obturator Internus tendon and insert into that tendon.

5. **Obturator Externus.** This muscle (Fig. 15-7) has attachments like those of Obturator Internus, but it originates from the *outer* surface of the obturator membrane; hence its name. Thus its tendon does not

Table 15-1 Elevator muscles of hip and thigh.

Muscle	Origin	Insertion	Action	Nerve
Iliopsoas group (femoral n., lumbar ventral rami)				
Psoas Major	Transverse processes and bodies of vertebrae T.12, to L.5	Lesser trochanter	Flexes hip	Twigs from ventral rami L.2–3 (roots of femoral n.)
Psoas Minor	Vertebral bodies T.12–L.1	Upper edge of pubis	Flexes lumbar vertebrae	L.1 ventral ramus
Iliacus	Inner face of ilium (plus edge of sacrum and the associated ligaments)	Lesser trochanter (with Psoas Major)	Flexes hip	Femoral n.
Gluteal group (gluteal nn.)				
Gluteus Maximus	Posterior end of iliac crest, dorsal surface of sacrum and coccyx, plus associated ligaments	Iliotibial tract and gluteal tuberosity of femur	Extends and laterally rotates at hip joint	Inferior gluteal n.
Tensor Fasciae Latae	Anterior end of iliac crest	Iliotibial tract	Tenses iliotibial tract: medially rotates thigh	Superior gluteal n.
Gluteus Medius	Outer face of ilium	Greater trochanter	Abducts and medially rotates thigh	Superior gluteal n.
Gluteus Minimus	Outer face of ilium (below origin of Gluteus Medius)	Greater trochanter	Abducts and medially rotates thigh	Superior gluteal n.
Quadriceps group (femoral n.)				
Quadriceps Femoris: a. Rectus Femoris	Anterior inferior iliac spine (plus upper rim of acetabulum)	Front of tibia (via the patella)	Extends knee; flexes hip	Femoral n.
b. Vastus Lateralis	Lateral edges of linea aspera (upper half), greater trochanter, and gluteal tuberosity	Front of tibia (via the patella)	Extends knee	Femoral n.
c. Vastus Intermedius	Front of femoral shaft (upper ⅔)	Front of tibia (via the patella)	Extends knee	Femoral n.
d. Vastus Medialis	Medial edge of the whole linea aspera and associated ridges above and below	Front of tibia (via the patella)	Extends knee	Femoral n.
Sartorius	Anterior superior iliac spine	Medial face of upper tibia and deep fascia of leg	Flexes knee and hip	Femoral n.
Other elevators				
Piriformis	Anterior (ventral) face of sacrum (plus adjoining edge of ilium)	Greater trochanter	Laterally rotates thigh	N. to Piriformis

[handwritten annotations: "largest in the group" next to Gluteus Maximus; numbers "2" near Gluteal group, "1" near Tensor Fasciae Latae, circled mark near Psoas Minor]

Table 15-2 Depressor muscles of hip and thigh.

Muscle	Origin	Insertion	Action	Nerve
Lateral rotators ③				
Quadratus Femoris	Ischial tuberosity	Crest below greater trochanter	Laterally rotates femur	N. to Quadratus Femoris
Obturator Internus	Inner face of obturator membrane and surrounding bone	Greater trochanter	Laterally rotates femur	N. to Obturator Internus
Obturator Externus	Outer face of obturator membrane and surrounding bone	Trochanteric fossa (medial to greater trochanter)	Laterally rotates femur	Obturator n.
Gemellus Superior	Spine of ischium	Tendon of Obturator Internus	Laterally rotates femur	N. to Obturator Internus
Gemellus Inferior	Upper edge of ischial tuberosity	Tendon of Obturator Internus	Laterally rotates femur	N. to Quadratus Femoris
Adductors (obturator n.)				
Pectineus	Upper edge of pubis	Upper end of linea aspera (plus crest above leading to lesser trochanter)	Adducts and flexes at hip	Femoral n.: variable additional supply from obturator n.
Adductor Brevis	Pubis in front of obturator foramen	As for Pectineus, but extending a bit lower down	Adduction at hip (and balancing activities in walking)	Obturator n.
Adductor Longus	Front of pubis	Linea aspera (middle third of femur)	Adduction at hip (and balancing activities in walking)	Obturator n.
Adductor Magnus	Lower edge of obturator foramen and ischial tuberosity	Linea aspera and crests above and below it (adductor part); tubercle above medial epicondyle of femur (hamstring part)	Adduction at hip (and balancing activities in walking)	Obturator n. (adductor part); tibial division of sciatic n. (hamstring part)
Gracilis	Lower edge of pubis and ischium	Medial surface of upper tibia	Flexes knee	Obturator n.
Hamstrings (sciatic n.)				
Semitendinosus	Ischial tuberosity	Upper tibia (behind Sartorius and below Gracilis)	Flexes knee; extends hip	Sciatic n. (tibial div.)
Semimembranosus	Ischial tuberosity	~~Ditto, plus surrounding deep fascias~~ Upper tibia	Flexes knee; extends hip	Sciatic n. (tibial div.)
Biceps Femoris	Ischial tuberosity (long head), plus lateral intermuscular septum and linea aspera (short head)	Upper fibula	Flexes knee; long head extends hip	Tibial div. of sciatic n. (long head); plus common peroneal div. of sciatic n. (short head)

Fig. 15-7   Iliopsoas, Pectineus, and Obturator
Externus.

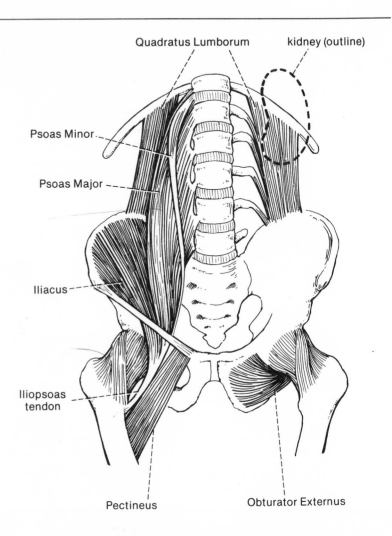

pass through the lesser sciatic foramen but winds around the underside of the hip joint's capsule, on its way to the greater trochanter.

▪ The Iliopsoas Group: Flexors

Another tendon also wraps back underneath the hip joint to insert on
the femur. This second tendon is far larger than that of Obturator
Externus, and it has its own bony epiphysis, which forms a projecting
lump called the **lesser trochanter** on the posterior and medial side of

the upper femur (Fig. 15-5). Two muscle bellies attach to this tendon. One, **Iliacus** (Fig. 15-7), is a fan-shaped muscle arising from the whole inner surface of the iliac blade. The other, **Psoas Major,** is a big spindle-shaped muscle arising from the lumbar vertebrae. Both converge on their tendon as they pass out of the abdomen underneath the inguinal ligament. The two are subdivisions of a single reptilian muscle mass. They can be regarded as one muscle, **Iliopsoas,** which functions as the major flexor of the hip.

Because Iliopsoas arises partly from the ilium, it is an elevator muscle. It is innervated by the same posterior-division nerve that supplies the elevator muscles on the front of the thigh. This is the femoral nerve, which passes *through* the flesh of Psoas Major and across the inner surface of Iliacus on its path from the lumbar plexus to the thigh. The nerves to Iliopsoas come off high up, from the posterior divisions that coalesce to form the femoral nerve (Fig. 15-3). A separate little Psoas slip that inserts on the pelvic rim in front is distinguished as **Psoas Minor.** It receives a motor branch from L.1. The Psoas Minor is an important locomotor muscle in quadrupeds but is vestigial and frequently absent in man.

Where the Iliopsoas tendon slides back and forth around the femoral neck and the hip-joint capsule, it is provided with a bursa, which often communicates with the cavity of the hip joint. Because the kidneys lie against the front surface of Psoas Major in the upper lumbar region, suspected renal inflammation can often be confirmed by pain felt while trying to flex the hip (as the contracting Psoas bulges against the diseased kidney). You may find it helpful to compare the Iliacus part of Iliopsoas with Subscapularis, its equivalent in the upper limb (Fig. 13-13A). Both are elevator muscles; both arise from the *deep* surface of the socket-bearing blade of the limb girdle; and both insert on a "lesser" bump (lesser tubercle, lesser trochanter) on the *depressor* surface of the limb's proximal long bone.

■ The Organization and Muscle Groups of the Thigh

We have described the primary flexors, abductors, and lateral rotators of the hip joint. The remaining three groups—the extensors, the adductors, and a second flexor group—make up the flesh of the thigh. All three groups include muscles that cross the knee and move the knee joint.

Their relationships and organization are most clearly seen in a "ham-steak" cross section through the thigh (Fig. 15-8). The enveloping fascia lata is continuous with three well-marked intermuscular septa that attach to the femur and so divide the thigh into three compartments. (1) The large *anterior* compartment is occupied by the **quadriceps** group of elevator muscles. They cross the front of the hip and knee joints, so they act to flex the hip and extend the knee. (2) The *posterior* compartment contains their opponents, the **hamstrings,** which extend the hip and flex the knee. (3) The *medial* compartment contains the **adductors** of the hip.

The adductors' opponents, the gluteal muscles, are also represented in the thigh—by the iliotibial tract. Our cross section reveals that this tract runs along the lateral boundary between elevators and depressors, which are separated from each other here by a tough **lateral intermuscular septum** attached to both the femur and the iliotibial

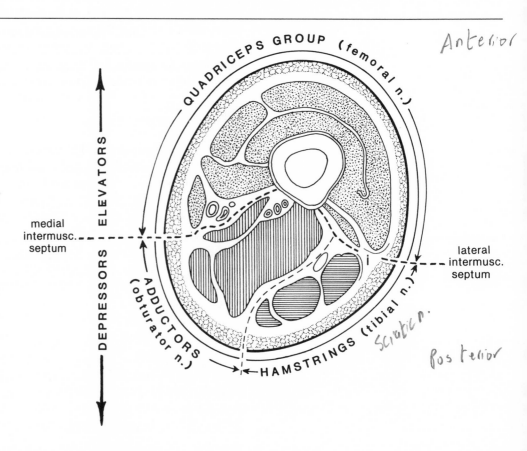

Fig. 15-8 Schematic cross section through the right thigh, showing muscle groups and the septa between them. The anterior side of the thigh is toward the top of the drawing. i, iliotibial tract.

tract. Gluteus Maximus and Tensor Fasciae Latae, inserting into the tract, pull on the femur via this lateral septum.

Each of the thigh's three compartments is supplied by a different motor nerve—the femoral nerve to the anterior compartment, the obturator nerve to the medial compartment, and the sciatic nerve (tibial division) to the posterior compartment. This picture is complicated slightly by the fact that each of the septa between the compartments has one composite muscle associated with it. These composite muscles—Pectineus, Adductor Magnus, Biceps Femoris— lie at the boundaries between muscle groups. Each composite muscle incorporates fibers from two adjoining groups and is therefore supplied by two nerves. We shall describe them in more detail as we come to them.

Most of the femoral shaft is covered by the origins of the knee extensors (Quadriceps group) in the anterior compartment. Only a narrow strip down the back of the shaft is left bare for attachments of other muscle groups. To increase the space available for muscle attachments to the femur, this strip develops after birth into a bony ridge, the **linea aspera** (L., "rough line"; Fig. 15-5). The adult femur is therefore a bit pear-shaped, not circular, in cross section (Fig. 15-8).

▪ The Quadriceps Group

The quadriceps group (Fig. 15-9) consists of two muscles. **Quadriceps Femoris** is by far the larger and more important of the two. It arises by a long head from the ilium and by three short heads from the shaft of the femur (L. *quadriceps,* "four heads"). All four heads insert into the front of the larger of the two leg bones—the **tibia** (shin bone) on the medial side of the leg. They share a single powerful tendon of insertion, which contains a huge sesamoid bone—the **patella,** or kneecap. Quadriceps extends the knee when it contracts. Its three short heads are the Vasti—**Vastus Lateralis, Vastus Medialis,** and **Vastus Intermedius.** The Vastus Intermedius (Fig. 15-11) has a fleshy origin from the upper two-thirds or so of the whole front surface of the femoral shaft; the medial and lateral Vasti arise by aponeuroses from the corresponding (medial and lateral) edges of the linea aspera. The fourth and longest head of Quadriceps is called **Rectus Femoris.** It arises from the ilium (anterior inferior iliac spine) and crosses in front of the hip joint as it runs straight down (L. *rectus,* "straight") toward the kneecap. It therefore flexes the hip in addition to extend-

Fig. 15-9 Muscles of the quadriceps (A) and adductor (B) groups, with their respective motor nerves. The deepest muscle in each group (Vastus Intermedius, Adductor Magnus) is shown elsewhere (Figs. 15-10 and 15-11).

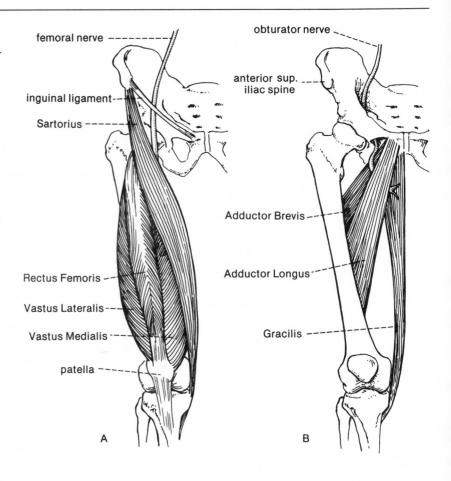

ing the knee. The whole Quadriceps Femoris is equivalent and rather similar to the elbow extensor, Triceps Brachii.

The other muscle in the quadriceps group is the **Sartorius** (Fig. 15-9). This extremely long, straplike muscle arises just above Rectus Femoris, from the anterior *superior* iliac spine (the palpable bump where the inguinal ligament's lateral end is attached). From there, Sartorius winds medially down around the front of the thigh toward the tibia. It follows the medial boundary between elevators (Quadriceps) in front and the adjoining depressors (the adductor group) in back. Like Quadriceps, the Sartorius inserts into the tibia. But it attaches to the side of the tibia, behind the axis of knee rotation, so it acts as a knee *flexor*. Looking at its course and attachments, you would expect it to flex the knee and hip joints and to rotate the thigh laterally—thus putting the limb into position for sitting cross-legged on the floor ("tailor-sitting"). It got its name (L. *sartor,* "tailor") from that line of reasoning. In fact, its functions are debated.

■ The Adductor Group

The adductors of the thigh lie in the medial compartment. They are depressor muscles, innervated by the obturator nerve. They originate from the margin of the obturator foramen (through which their motor nerve emerges from the pelvis) and insert via aponeuroses into the linea aspera, between the attachments of the medial and lateral Vasti. The most anterior of the three, **Adductor Longus** (Fig. 15-9) arises high up from the front of the pubis. The next, **Adductor Brevis,** arises from a point further back and lower down on the rim of the obturator foramen and inserts a bit further up the femur. It is therefore shorter than Adductor Longus—hence its name. The third Adductor, **Adductor Magnus** (Fig. 15-10), arises furthest back, from the ischial border of the obturator foramen (just in front of the ischial tuberosity). (It is "magnus" because it spreads out in a big fan from its origins, inserting into almost the whole of the linea aspera.) The three Adductors are stacked up from front to back like a three-layered sandwich; Adductor Longus is the only one easily seen from in front when the skin is removed (Fig. 15-9).

Besides the three Adductors, the adductor group contains one-and-a-half other muscles. The half muscle is **Pectineus** (Fig. 15-7). This is one of the three composite muscles in the thigh. It inserts like an Adductor (into the linea aspera) and functions as an adductor (of the hip joint). It occasionally receives some motor innervation from the obturator nerve that supplies the adductor group. But it is not wholly an adductor. It lies on the boundary between Iliopsoas and the adductor group, and it receives most of its innervation—all of it, in the majority of cases—from the **femoral** nerve that supplies Iliopsoas. Its origin, from the upper edge of the pubis, is similarly intermediate between the Adductor and Iliopsoas attachments. Arising from the pubis but innervated by the femoral nerve, Pectineus is the sole exception to the rule that elevator muscles never attach to the pubis or ischium.

The remaining adductor-group muscle is **Gracilis** (Fig. 15-9). It

Fig. 15-10 Hamstrings (A) and the underlying Adductor Magnus (B), viewed from behind.

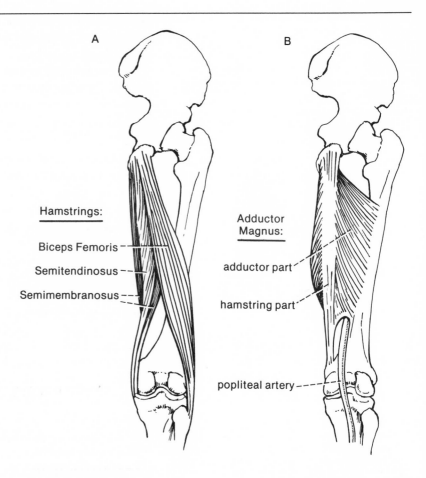

Hamstrings:

Biceps Femoris

Semitendinosus

Semimembranosus

Adductor Magnus:

adductor part

hamstring part

popliteal artery

arises from the pubis and runs down past the knee to insert into the upper part of the tibia, just behind the Sartorius attachment. Gracilis is the only adductor-group muscle that crosses the knee joint. Besides adducting the thigh, it also flexes the knee.

▪ The Hamstrings

The hamstring muscles arise from the ischial tuberosity and insert into the upper ends of the two leg bones (Fig. 15-10). Two of the three hamstrings (**Semimembranosus** and **Semitendinosus**) attach to the tibia. The third hamstring, **Biceps Femoris**, attaches to the much smaller *fibula,* on the lateral side of the leg. All three extend the hip and flex the knee. They are depressor muscles, innervated by the sciatic nerve (tibial division), which passes deep to them on its way down the thigh.

We would need to say no more about the hamstrings, were it not for the fact that two bundles of hamstring musculature have fused secondarily with muscles outside the group. In most mammals, the hamstring group includes an accessory semimembranosus. This fourth hamstring does not quite manage to cross the knee joint; it inserts just above the knee, on the medial side of the distal femur. In man, this accessory muscle has fused with the Adductor Magnus. The definitive Adductor Magnus (Fig. 15-10) therefore includes a hamstring part, which has a separate insertion and (like a hamstring) gets its motor supply from the tibial division of the sciatic nerve.

On the other side of the knee, Biceps Femoris inserts into the fibula. Its tendon of insertion receives a bundle of elevator-muscle fibers, which arise from the linea aspera medial to the femoral attachment of Vastus Lateralis. This elevator bundle is referred to as the **short head of Biceps Femoris.** Like the other hamstrings, the short head of Biceps is innervated by the sciatic nerve; but unlike them, it is supplied by the sciatic's *elevator*-muscle division, the **common peroneal** nerve. Therefore, Biceps Femoris, like Pectineus and Adductor Magnus, is a composite muscle with a dual innervation. You can remember both its attachment and secondary (peroneal) innervation by associating it with the fibula, because *peroneal* means *fibular* (L. *fibula* = Gk. *perone*, "safety pin").

■ The Vessels of the Thigh

The major blood vessels of the lower extremity—the **external iliac artery and vein**—pass from the pelvis into the thigh in front, below the inguinal ligament (Fig. 15-11). This places them on the boundary between elevators and depressors in front, and they simply run down through the thigh between the two groups, along the medial intermuscular septum (Fig. 15-8). They are covered over along most of this course by Sartorius, which also follows the elevator-depressor boundary down toward the knee. The fascial space in which the thigh's big blood vessels run is therefore sometimes known as the **subsartorial canal.** (The proper term, **adductor canal,** is less informative.)

The external iliac vessels change names twice before they reach the

Fig. 15-11 Arteries of the thigh. Anterior (A) and posterior (B) aspects. The three superficial heads of Quadriceps have been removed in the anterior view.

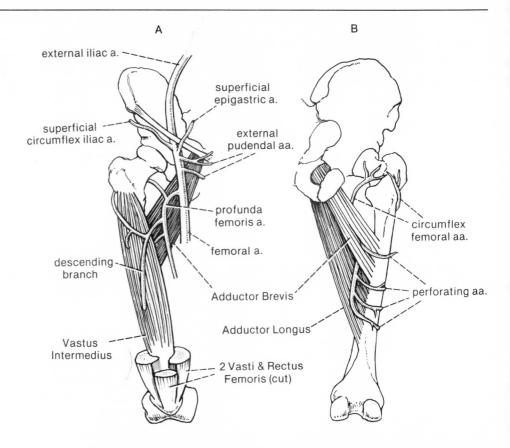

knee joint. When they enter the thigh, they are rechristened the **femoral** artery and vein. At the distal end of the subsartorial canal, they pass backward around the medial side of the femur to enter the depressor musculature behind the knee. They do this by passing between the adductor and hamstring groups—that is, between the two parts of Adductor Magnus, of which one is a true adductor-group muscle and the other a hamstring in adductor's clothing (Fig. 15-10). The gap in Adductor Magnus through which the vessels pass is called the **tendinous hiatus.** As they pass through it, they change names again, becoming the **popliteal** artery and vein.

Up in the abdomen, the external iliac vessels lie on the inner surface of Iliacus, from which they are separated by the transversalis fascia (here called iliac fascia) that lines the inner surface of the body wall. When they enter the thigh and become the femoral vessels, they are surrounded by a tubular prolongation of this fascia. The tube is called the **femoral sheath.** In addition to the femoral artery and vein, it also encloses the lymphatic vessels following the vein. Under sufficient intraabdominal pressure, a loop of intestine can sometimes rupture out into this sheath underneath the inguinal ligament, thereby producing a **femoral hernia.**

The femoral artery follows a tidy course through the thigh, running along the boundary between elevators and depressors. Its branches do not. As it enters the thigh, it gives off a radiating spray of small arteries to the lower body-wall structures (Fig. 15-11A)—a **superficial epigastric** artery running upward toward the navel, a **superficial circumflex iliac** artery running laterally alongside the inguinal ligament, and a couple of **external pudendal** arteries running medially to the scrotum or labia. The femoral artery's largest branch is the **profunda femoris** artery. The profunda femoris follows a course parallel to that of the femoral artery, but on a deeper plane, running backward into the adductor musculature through the gap between Pectineus and Adductor Longus. High up, the profunda femoris gives off a **lateral circumflex femoral** artery. This artery ramifies on the surface of Vastus Intermedius and supplies the Quadriceps. Its branches join with a similar **medial circumflex femoral** branch of the profunda femoris to produce an anastomotic arterial network around the upper femur. As the profunda femoris artery continues downward, it sends **perforating** arteries back through little tendinous arches in Adductor Magnus's aponeurosis. These perforating arteries wrap laterally across the linea aspera, piercing and supplying the muscles attached to it (Fig. 15-11B).

The obturator and gluteal vessels are much smaller than the femoral vessels and supply restricted areas—the adductor and hamstring origins, and the gluteal region, respectively. Developmentally, the inferior gluteal artery was the axial artery of the lower limb, and the popliteal artery was originally just its continuation below the knee. The two are connected in the adult by a tiny vestige of the old axial artery, which follows the sciatic nerve down through the hamstring muscles. As a rare anomaly, this **sciatic** artery may persist as a major vessel; when it does, the femoral artery is correspondingly reduced.

Like those of the upper extremity, the superficial veins of the lower limb are big and important. The largest is the **great saphenous** vein, which roughly follows the medial elevator-depressor boundary up the limb and pierces the femoral sheath to end in the femoral vein. The **small saphenous** vein does not follow a muscle-group boundary; it just runs straight up the back of the calf and ends in the popliteal vein behind the knee. A dorsal venous arch on the back of the foot drains at either end into the two saphenous veins, which also receive all the other superficial veins of the leg and thigh. (Note that in anatomical terminology, the "leg" begins at the knee and does not include the thigh.)

In the upper extremity, blood can pass freely from the deep veins to the superficial ones, which provide an alternative channel for venous return during prolonged contraction of the limb muscles. In the lower limb, the reverse tends to be the case; the vessels connecting the deep and superficial veins contain valves that prevent blood from flowing toward the limb's surface. If these valves become incompetent, blood flows from the deep veins into the superficial ones, which often become distended and varicose as a result.

The Leg
and the Foot

16

■ Differentiation of Limb Functions

In monkeys, apes, and lemurs, our closest living animal relatives and fellow members of the order Primates, the hand and foot are similar in appearance and function; both are grasping organs, used in hanging on to tree branches. But even in these animals, there is an important difference between the fore and hind limbs. The limb at the head end of the body is the one that first touches new things as the animal moves along. The hand is therefore used far more than the foot as a tactile "feeler" for exploration. In monkeys and apes, the hand becomes important as a manipulatory organ for grabbing, carrying, and disassembling objects of all sorts. In ourselves, this differentiation of the limbs is complete; the foot never grasps, and the hand never walks. Although the anatomy of the human foot still betrays the fact that it was once very much like the hand, our feet and legs have lost a lot of their primitive flexibility.

The differences between the two limbs can be better appreciated if we imagine the steps we might take to convert a human hand into a human foot.

1. *Tie the thumb to the second digit.* In the hand, all the metacarpal heads are bound together by deep transverse ligaments—except that of the thumb. Our thumb is therefore free to swing away from the four fingers and oppose them in grasping. The elongated "thumb" of the human foot—the big toe, or **hallux**—is tied tightly to the side of the second toe by a deep transverse ligament and is permanently adducted. Grasping is no longer possible, and the hallux's joints and muscles have been modified accordingly.

2. *Shrink the phalanges and elongate the metacarpals.* The phalanges of the toes are extremely short, but the foot's "metacarpals"—properly called **metatarsals**—are long and stout. They form a sheaf of sturdy, parallel bones with a fringe of stubby toes projecting

299

The free movement of the thumb permits grasping.

from their distal ends. The toes aid in balancing and stabilizing, but they normally do not bear any weight in standing or walking. Half the body's weight in a standing person is borne by the metatarsal heads, with the other half being carried by the heels of the feet.

3. *Enlarge the triquetrum and attach all the superficial flexor muscles to it.* The triquetrum, the proximal carpal on the ulnar edge of the wrist, is the serial homolog of the foot's heel bone, or **calcaneus.** In quadrupedal mammals, both these bones bear projecting lever arms. Flexor muscles attach to these bony processes, which give the muscles better leverage for flexing the wrist and ankle in running on all fours. In quadrupeds, the triquetrum's lever arm is the attached pisiform bone, which juts back across the wrist and serves as a "heel" for the ulnar wrist flexor. Our own pisiform is greatly reduced, but it still forms a prominent bony lump known as the heel of the hand— which we find useful in kneading bread dough and delivering karate blows.

The corresponding lever arm in the foot is the bony heel of the calcaneus. Early in mammalian evolution, *all* the superficial flexor muscles on the back of the calf shifted their insertions over onto this bony lever. As part of this new mammalian arrangement, the calcaneus moved medially to line up with the pull of the superficial flexor muscles straight down the back of the calf. This medial shift and enlargement of an originally fibular "wrist" bone has produced many changes in the intrinsic and extrinsic flexor muscles of the toes—much like the changes that would result if you inflated the pisiform to the size of a golf ball and shoved it over thumbward into the carpal tunnel.

4. *Shorten the palmar aponeurosis.* The **plantar aponeurosis** (L. *planta,* "sole") underlying the skin of the sole is the equivalent of the hand's palmar aponeurosis. It stretches from heel to metatarsal heads. It is shorter than the foot's bony elements would be if laid out end to end; so the foot skeleton is kinked upward in the middle, producing a *longitudinal arch* of the foot. This arch is kept from collapsing principally by the tautness of the plantar aponeurosis, which ties the front and back ends of the arch together (Fig. 16-1) and keeps them from moving away from each other. The aponeurosis, and the longitudinal arch it helps preserve, ensures that body weight is borne only at the two ends of the arch—the heel and the ball of the foot.

Fig. 16-1 Foot bones and collateral ligaments of the ankle. Medial (A) and lateral (B) aspects of right foot. The two-headed black arrow in B represents the plantar aponeurosis. The center of the deltoid ligament is represented by a dashed line only, to expose the underlying head of the talus (the stippled bone) supported by the "spring" ligament.

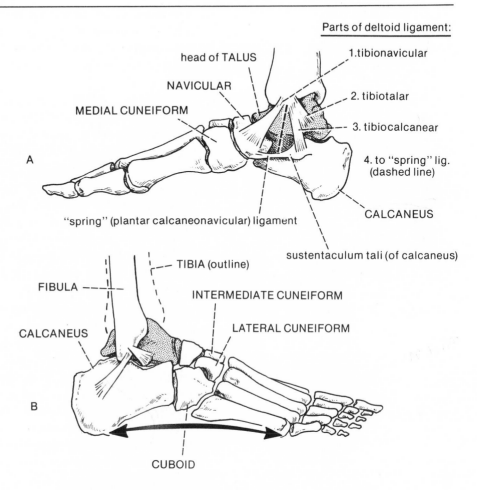

Parts of deltoid ligament:

head of TALUS

NAVICULAR

MEDIAL CUNEIFORM

1. tibionavicular

2. tibiotalar

3. tibiocalcanear

4. to "spring" lig. (dashed line)

CALCANEUS

"spring" (plantar calcaneonavicular) ligament

sustentaculum tali (of calcaneus)

TIBIA (outline)

FIBULA

INTERMEDIATE CUNEIFORM

LATERAL CUNEIFORM

CALCANEUS

CUBOID

▪ Movements of the Foot

The two leg bones (tibia and fibula) are permanently fixed in parallel to each other and can be regarded as a single bone for most purposes. The metatarsals can wiggle a little bit but are also more or less fixed in parallel. The toes have fingerlike movements (flexion–extension, abduction–adduction), but these movements are restricted and are not crucial for foot function. (If they were, we could not walk wearing stiff shoes, and we would have to clothe our feet in something more like gloves.) Most of the foot's movements occur among the ankle bones (tarsals) that separate the leg bones from the five metatarsals.

The musculature in the leg is thus mainly devoted to ankle movements, flopping a more or less rigid foot around at the end of the rigid leg skeleton.

There are seven tarsal bones, but the tibia and fibula only touch one of them. This is the **talus,** which sits atop the arch of the foot like a keystone (Fig. 16-1). It articulates with four other bones, two above and two below. Its upper articular surface, shaped something like the curved surface of a spool, fits into a reciprocal socket formed by the two leg bones. The tibia and fibula press against the flat medial and lateral ends of the spool. Because the upper surface of the spool rests wholly against the tibia, body weight is carried downward to the talus through the tibia alone; the fibula bears no weight. (At its upper end, it does not even touch the femur.)

The other two bones that articulate with the talus lie below it and receive the weight that the tibia imposes on the talus. The calcaneus, which lies directly underneath the talus, carries most of the weight and transmits it downward—to its own heel in back, and to the lateral two metatarsals in front. It passes weight to those metatarsals (4 and 5) via the intervening **cuboid** bone (Fig. 16-1). The rest of the body's weight is transmitted from the talus (via its downward-slanting, rounded **head**) to the bowl-shaped **navicular** bone—and from the navicular to the medial three metatarsals (digits 1–3) through three cuboidlike elements called *cuneiforms,* one per metatarsal. Note that in both upper and lower limbs, digits 4 and 5 share a single "wrist" bone at the base of their metapodials—the hamate in the hand, the cuboid in the foot.

Most of the foot's movements occur at the joints between the talus and the neighboring bones above and below it. The upper joint—between the talus and the leg bones—is a simple hinge, capable only of flexion and extension. Like other hinge joints, it has collateral ligaments on each side that help restrict its movements to a single axis of rotation. These ligaments are attached to conspicuous bony bumps, the **malleoli,** at the bottom ends of the two leg bones (Fig. 16-4). (You can feel these malleoli on either side of your own ankle.) The collateral ligaments run from the malleoli down to the calcaneus. The one from the fibular malleolus is a round cord; the one on the tibial side has a more broadly spread-out attachment, including bundles running to the talus and navicular. Its radiating fibers fanning out from the tibial malleolus give it a triangular delta shape, so it is called the **deltoid** ligament (Fig. 16-1).

The talus's lower articulations (with the underlying calcaneus and the navicular) share a single fore-and-aft axis (Fig. 16-2), around which the rest of the foot rotates as a unit on the immobile talus. The foot swings from side to side around this axis, turning the sole of the foot in toward the other foot or outward and away from it. Turning the sole inward is called **inversion**; the reverse movement is **eversion.**

Both kinds of ankle movement—flexion–extension at the top of the talus and inversion–eversion below the talus—are needed in normal walking. If you walked all the time on hard, flat floors with your feet close together, extension and flexion would be the only movements needed. But when you stand with your feet far apart, you have to invert them to keep the soles on the ground; and when you walk on an uneven surface, your feet are continually everting and inverting to adjust to the irregularities of the terrain. Sometimes we make the wrong adjustment; and the ankle buckles under our weight, thereby resulting in a *sprain*—that is, a wrenching or tearing of the joint's ligaments.

Fig. 16-2 Inversion and eversion take place chiefly at the joints between the talus (here removed) and the rest of the foot. The rod represents the principal axis of rotation in these movements.

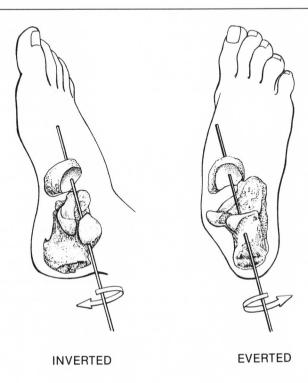

INVERTED   EVERTED

The muscles in the leg that move the foot and toes can be divided into three groups—a thick depressor mass at the back of the leg and two smaller elevator groups arising from the anterolateral aspect of the leg bones. The antero*medial* aspect of the leg is occupied by a long, exposed surface of the tibia—the so-called shin—that lies just below the skin. Here, the tibia itself separates elevators from depressors. The other two boundaries between the three muscle groups are formed by stout intermuscular septa (Fig. 16-3).

■ The Depressor Muscles of the Leg

Although the depressor muscles that form the flesh at the back of the calf all share a single innervation and a similar arrangement, it is convenient to divide them into a superficial layer and a deeper layer (Table 16-1). The superficial layer comprises the muscle bellies that attach to the heel. The deeper muscles have tendons that continue on into the sole of the foot.

Fig. 16-3 Diagrammatic cross section of the right leg; cut surface as seen from above.

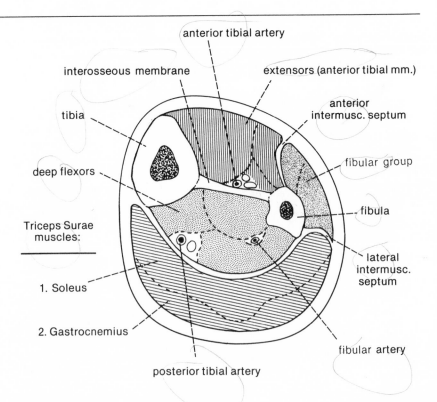

Table 16-1   Depressor muscles in the leg.

Muscle	Origin	Insertion	Action	Nerve
Superficial layer (Triceps Surae)				
Gastrocnemius	By two heads, from the back of the femur above the two condyles	Bony heel of the calcaneus, via the achilles tendon	Flexes ankle (and knee)	Tibial n.
Plantaris	Ridge above lateral condyle	Bony heel of the calcaneus, via the achilles tendon	Flexes ankle (and knee)	Tibial n.
Soleus	Tibia and fibula, above the origins of the deep flexors (Fig. 16-4)	Bony heel of the calcaneus, via the achilles tendon	Flexes ankle	Tibial n.
Deep layer				
Flexor Hallucis Longus	Lower ⅔ of fibula and attached septa	Distal phalanx of big toe (plus slip to Flexor Digitorum Longus)	Flexes hallux (and variable number of other toes) and ankle	Tibial n.
Flexor Digitorum Longus	Posterior surface of middle ⅓ of tibia	Distal phalanges of toes 2–5	Flexes toes and ankle	Tibial n.
Tibialis Posterior	Tibia and interosseous membrane, deep to and in between origins of Soleus and the two toe flexors	Tuberosity of navicular; sustentaculum tali (of calcaneus); two medial cuneiforms and metatarsal bases of toes 2–4; variable slips to cuboid and lateral cuneiform (Fig. 16-7)	Inverts foot; weak plantarflexor of ankle and intertarsal joints	Tibial n.
Other depressors				
Popliteus	Lateral condyle of femur (plus joint capsule and lateral meniscus of knee)	Tibia above the Soleus origins	Rotates tibia medially	Tibial n.

SUPERFICIAL LAYER: TRICEPS SURAE

The three superficial depressor muscles arise from the tibia, fibula, and lower end of the femur and insert together into the bony heel of the calcaneus via the powerful **achilles tendon**. Contracting, these muscles volarflex the ankle, swinging the front end of the foot down toward the ground. If the foot is already touching the ground, this movement lifts the body, as in rising on tiptoe. These muscles are the major propulsive muscles in *Homo sapiens*.

The most superficial of these three muscles is the two-headed **Gastrocnemius** (Fig. 16-4). Its two heads arise just above the two big bony **condyles** (Gk., "knuckles") protruding backward from the distal end of the femur. Both of its heads converge on a common tendon that feeds into the achilles tendon. Its name (Gk., "belly of the knee") comes from the prominent bulge that Gastrocnemius produces near the top of the calf in a well-muscled person. The deeper, one-joint muscle **Soleus** (L., "flatfish") is less conspicuous but larger and more powerful. It has an arch-shaped origin from the tibia and the fibula—and from the interosseous membrane that stretches between them like the interosseous membrane in the forearm. Soleus and Gastrocnemius considered together as one muscle make up the **Triceps Surae** (L., "three-headed [muscle] of the calf"). The third superficial depressor muscle is the trivial little **Plantaris**. It arises from the femur above the lateral condyle and usually intersects into the achilles tendon. A hind-limb equivalent of Palmaris Longus, Plantaris is an important propulsive muscle in reptiles, but vestigial in man.

DEEPER LAYER: EXTRINSIC TOE FLEXORS

This group also contains three muscles. Like the equivalent deep layer of finger flexors in the forearm, this muscle layer includes two digital flexors—one for the first toe and one for the other four. They are respectively named **Flexor Hallucis Longus** and **Flexor Digitorum Longus**. Oddly enough, they arise from the "wrong" sides of the leg. The hallux (big toe) is on the *tibial* edge of the foot, but its flexor arises from the *fibula*; Flexor Digitorum Longus, the flexor for the four lateral toes, arises medially from the *tibia*. It is not clear what the functional value is of having the tendons cross like this. (In primitive mammals, both muscles sent tendons to all five toes, and the hallux flexor in *Homo* still usually gives off little tendinous slips to toes 2 and 3.) The two tendons cross each other as they enter the sole. The Flexor Digitorum Longus tendon then divides into its four tendons of insertion; and all five extrinsic-flexor tendons continue onto the five distal phalanges—exactly like their equivalents in the hand.

Between the two digital flexors, a third muscle of this deeper layer—**Tibialis Posterior**—arises from the leg bones and interosseous membrane (Fig. 16-4). It lies a bit deeper than the two toe flexors, which overlap it. Tibialis Posterior does not send tendons to the toes; it just fans out to insert into all the tarsal bones (except the talus; Fig. 16-7).

Fig. 16-4 Depressor musculature of the leg, shown in successively deeper layers (A, B, C). In C, Flexor Digitorum Longus is pulled medially to expose Tibialis Posterior. Posterior view of right leg.

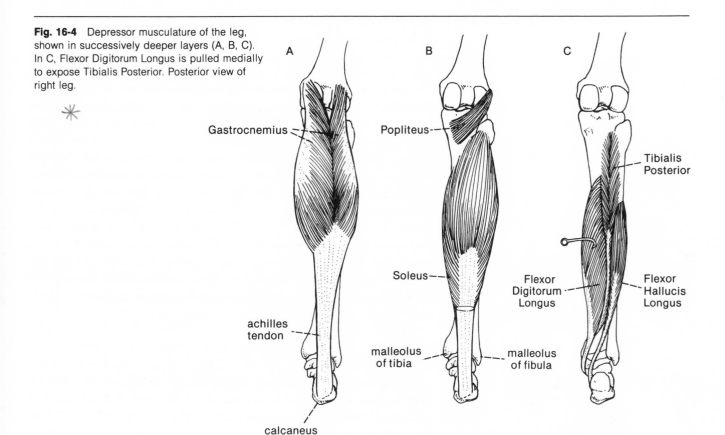

A

B

C

Gastrocnemius

Popliteus

Tibialis Posterior

Soleus

achilles tendon

Flexor Digitorum Longus

Flexor Hallucis Longus

malleolus of tibia

malleolus of fibula

calcaneus

The tendons of Tibialis Posterior and the toe flexors pass into the sole in a bundle that runs just behind the tibial malleolus. (They are held in place there by a fibrous **flexor retinaculum,** which runs from the malleolus back to the bony heel and prevents bowstringing of the tendons.) Because the axis of ankle flexion and extension passes through the two malleoli and these tendons pass behind that axis, all three muscles can act as ankle flexors. But they do so with much less leverage and power than the Triceps Surae muscles, and their main jobs involve movements at more distal joints in the foot. The two long toe flexors flex all the joints of the toes. Tibialis Posterior acts chiefly on the joints between the tarsal bones, inverting the foot and producing some slight flexion between the proximal and distal tarsals.

One additional muscle that is often regarded as a fourth member of this group is **Popliteus.** It runs medially from the femur's lateral condyle (just above the top of the fibula) down across the back of the knee joint to insert high up on the tibia (Fig. 16-4). In primitive reptiles, Popliteus served as a sort of hind-limb Pronator Teres, twisting the tibia around to keep the sole touching the ground as the limb was thrust backward during crawling. Our own tibia still has a little of this rotatory mobility left, as you will discover if you sit with your knee flexed and feel the sharp front edge of your tibia (your "shinbone") while swiveling your foot back and forth to point the toes inward and outward. Popliteus is one of several muscles that can rotate the tibia medially. It is not clear what function this serves. Most anatomy textbooks claim that the rotation Popliteus produces is needed in walking, to "unlock" the extended knee when the foot leaves the ground. This seems unlikely. Electromyography shows no consistent Popliteus action during walking. Furthermore, the extended knee is not really locked in place; an unexpected shove in the backs of the knees will cause a standing person to collapse, without any muscles rotating the tibia beforehand.

■ The Elevator Muscles of the Leg

Although none of the elevator muscles in the leg cross the knee joint, they otherwise correspond in a general way to the superficial extensor layer in the forearm. They are divided into two groups (Fig. 16-5) that have different innervations (Table 16-2) and are separated by the anterior intermuscular septum (Fig. 16-3).

Fibularis Group   These two muscles lie behind the anterior septum. As their name implies they arise from the fibula, on the lateral side of the leg. The shorter and deeper of the two—**Fibularis** (or **Peroneus**) **Brevis**—ends on the lateral side of the foot by inserting into a prominent bump on the base of the little toe's metatarsal. The longer and more superficial **Fibularis** (or **Peroneus**) **Longus** follows the same course down to the ankle; but instead of running forward from there to the fifth metatarsal, it hooks medially around the side of the calcaneus and runs all the way across the sole (in a bony groove on the underside of the cuboid) to insert into the base of the *first* metatarsal (Fig. 16-7). In other primates, this insertion enables Fibularis Longus to adduct the thumblike big toe in gripping tree branches. In *Homo,* the foot's grasping ability has been lost, and both Fibulares act mainly

Fig. 16-5 Elevator musculature of the leg.

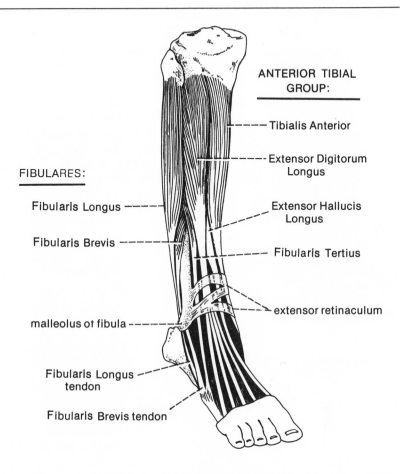

FIBULARES:

Fibularis Longus

Fibularis Brevis

malleolus of fibula

Fibularis Longus
tendon

Fibularis Brevis tendon

ANTERIOR TIBIAL
GROUP:

Tibialis Anterior

Extensor Digitorum
Longus

Extensor Hallucis
Longus

Fibularis Tertius

extensor retinaculum

as evertors of the foot. Their tendons pass behind the fibular malleolus, so they also plantarflex the ankle. Like the toe-flexor tendons that wind behind the other malleolus, they are tied down by retinacula at the ankle and enclosed in synovial tendon sheaths to protect them from rubbing against bone and ligament. A separate synovial sheath encloses the distal end of the Fibularis Longus tendon where it runs across the sole of the foot.

Anterior Tibial Group Four elevator muscles lie in the leg's anterior compartment (in front of the anterior septum). The largest is **Tibialis Anterior.** It arises from the front of the tibia and has the same insertion as Fibularis Longus—into the base of the first metatarsal (and

Table 16-2 Elevator muscles in the leg.

Muscle	Origin	Insertion	Action	Nerve
Fibularis group (superficial fibular nerve)				
Fibularis Longus	Upper ⅔ of lateral face of fibula	Base of 1st metatarsal (plus a slip to the medial cuneiform)	Everts foot (and plantarflexes ankle)	Superficial branch of common fibular n.
Fibularis Brevis	Lower ⅔ of lateral face of fibula (anterior to Fibularis Longus origins)	Tubercle on lateral side of base of 5th metatarsal	Everts foot (and plantarflexes ankle)	Superficial branch of common fibular n.
Anterior tibial group (deep fibular nerve)				
Tibialis Anterior	Upper ½ of tibia (lateral to subcutaneous "shinbone" part of tibia)	Base of 1st metatarsal (plus medial cuneiform)	Dorsiflexes ankle and inverts foot	Deep branch of common fibular n.
Extensor Hallucis Longus	Middle ¾ of fibular shaft, plus interosseous membrane	Distal phalanx of big toe	Extends big toe; dorsiflexes ankle	Deep branch of common fibular n.
Extensor Digitorum Longus	Upper ¾ of fibular shaft, plus interosseous membrane	Distal phalanges of toes 2–5	Extends toes and dorsiflexes ankle	Deep branch of common fibular n.
Peroneus Tertius	Lower ⅓ of fibula, plus attached fascias	Base of 5th metatarsal	Dorsiflexes ankle and everts foot	Deep branch of common fibular n.

into the adjoining medial cuneiform bone). Tibialis Anterior pulls upward on the first metatarsal, so it *inverts* the foot and dorsiflexes the ankle—actions precisely opposite to those produced by Fibularis Longus.

Recollect the forearm for a moment. The superficial extensors of the hand comprise a wrist extensor on either side (the radial one is double) and a mass of digital extensors lying in between. The same setup is found in the leg: the extensor of the toes, **Extensor Digitorum Longus,** is flanked by the "wrist" muscles that move the ankle (Tibialis Anterior and the Fibulares). From each edge of Extensor Digitorum Longus, a small muscle has split off and become independent. The first of these two Extensor Digitorum Longus spin-offs is merely a separate belly for the extensor tendon to the big toe. It is known (reasonably enough) as **Extensor Hallucis Longus.** The second, on the opposite (fibular) side of Extensor Digitorum Longus, is a slender muscle that inserts next to Fibularis Brevis on the fifth metatarsal. Like Fibularis Brevis, this extensor slip pulls upward on the lateral side of the foot and everts it. It is accordingly called **Fibularis Tertius,** the "third Fibularis." Despite its name, it belongs with the other anterior tibial muscles (and not the Fibulares) by virtue of its developmental history, position, and innervation (Table 16-2). Another difference between the true Fibulares and the anterior tibial muscles (including "Fibularis" Tertius) is that the tendons of the true Peronei pass behind the fibular malleolus at the ankle and so act as ankle *flexors*. The anterior tibial tendons all lie in front of the line connecting the two malleoli; so they *extend* or dorsiflex the ankle when they contract.

■ The Sole of the Foot

The major differences between the foot and the hand result mostly from the medial shift of the calcaneus. That shift left the heel parked squarely in the midline of the limb. As the extrinsic flexor tendons approach this obstacle, they have to duck around it and enter the sole on the medial side of the calcaneus, instead of running through a midline carpal tunnel. This arrangement means that the tendons of Flexor Digitorum Longus (Fig. 16-6) have to run obliquely across the sole to reach the four lateral toes and are not lined up with their digits. Their obliquity may be compensated for by a little muscle called **Flexor Accessorius,** which has no equivalent in the hand. A Y-shaped muscle, it arises by two heads from the calcaneus and runs forward to insert directly into the radiating fan of Flexor Digitorum Longus tendons. It *looks* like it ought to help straighten out the oblique direction of the long flexor's pull, but nobody really knows whether it does.

In the hand, the long flexor tendons entering the palm are flanked by the thenar and hypothenar muscles. Similar clusters of intrinsic muscles attach to the two marginal toes. The most superficial muscles in both of the foot's marginal-digit clusters attach to the sides of the calcaneus's projecting heel, so the foot's extrinsic flexor tendons have to pass deep to the superficial "thenar" muscle (Fig. 16-6) as they enter the medial side of the sole. You would get a similar effect in the hand if you shifted the origin of Abductor Pollicis Brevis over to the pisiform bone.

Because our metatarsals and toes are much less mobile than our metacarpals and fingers, the "thenar" and "hypothenar" clusters in

Fig. 16-6 Muscles of the sole. A. Superficial layer. B. Extrinsic flexor tendons and the muscles (Lumbricals, Flexor Accessorius) attached to them. Dashed lines in B indicate the extrinsic flexor tendons and the medial head of Flexor Accessorius, seen through the Abductor Hallucis (*white*).

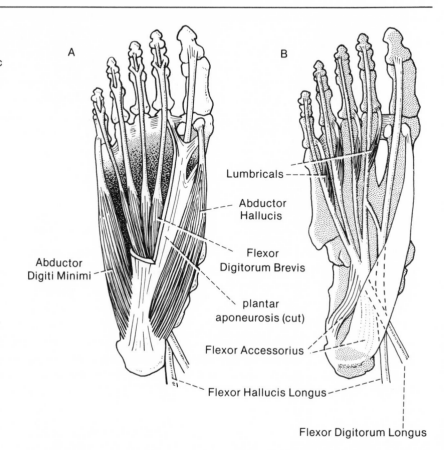

A

B

Lumbricals

Abductor Hallucis

Flexor Digitorum Brevis

plantar aponeurosis (cut)

Abductor Digiti Minimi

Flexor Accessorius

Flexor Hallucis Longus

Flexor Digitorum Longus

the human foot (Table 16-3) are simplified and have different functions from their counterparts in the hand. Neither cluster in the foot normally includes an Opponens muscle; only the Abductor and Flexor Brevis are retained. The two *Abductors* (**Abductor Hallucis** and **Abductor Digiti Minimi**) are not important as abductors; they are named by analogy with their equivalents in the hand. Their main function seems to be to help out the plantar aponeurosis in maintaining the foot's longitudinal arch when stress on that arch is increased—say, in running or in standing on tiptoes.

The short *flexors* of the two marginal digits—**Flexor Hallucis Brevis** and **Flexor Digiti Minimi Brevis**—arise more distally and deeply in the sole, deep to the extrinsic flexor tendons and Flexor Accessorius (Fig. 16-7). As in the hand, they insert on the bases of

Table 16-3 Intrinsic depressor muscles in the foot.

Muscle	Origin	Insertion	Action	Nerve
"Thenar" muscles				
Abductor Hallucis	Flexor retinaculum, medial face of heel process, and plantar aponeurosis	Medial side of big toe's proximal phalanx and medial sesamoid	Flexes and abducts big toe; helps in arch support	Medial plantar n.
Flexor Hallucis Brevis	Bifurcated tendon, from (a) the cuboid and (b) the Tibialis Posterior tendon (cf. Fig. 16-7)	Proximal phalanx of big toe, via two sesamoids underlying head of 1st metatarsal	Flexes hallux	Medial plantar n.
"Hypothenar" muscles				
Abductor Digiti Minimi	Lateral face of bony heel; plantar aponeurosis	Lateral side of 5th toe's proximal phalanx	Flexes (and weakly abducts) 5th toe: helps in arch support	Lateral plantar n.
Flexor Digiti Minimi Brevis	Base of 5th metatarsal	Base of proximal phalanx of 5th toe	Flexes 5th toe	Lateral plantar n.
Superficial digital-flexor layer				
Flexor Digitorum Brevis	Plantar aponeurosis and bony heel	Via four perforated tendons (like those of the superficial *finger* flexor) to toes 2–5	Flexes toes	Medial plantar n.
Muscles attached to long flexor tendons				
Lumbricals	As in the hand	As in the hand	Uncertain	Lateral plantar n., except the 1st Lumbrical (medial plantar n.)
Flexor Accessorius (Quadratus Plantae)	Bifurcated tendon, from (a) medial and (b) inferior surface of heel process of calcaneus	Slips to tendons of Flexor Digitorum Longus (Fig. 16-6)	Uncertain	Lateral plantar n.
Other depressors				
Adductor Hallucis	Transverse head from the heads of metatarsals 3–5 and attached ligaments; oblique head from bases of metatarsals 2–4 and sheath of Peroneus Longus tendon (Fig. 16-7)	Lateral sesamoid at base of hallux	Uncertain	Lateral plantar n.
Interossei	(See Fig. 16-8 for origins, insertions, and actions of Interossei)			Lateral plantar n.

Fig. 16-7 Deep muscles and tendons of the sole. Light stipple indicates tarsal bones; dark stipple, metatarsals.

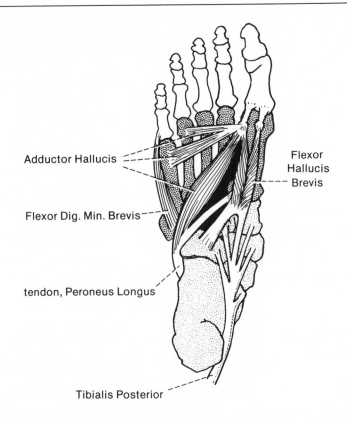

Adductor Hallucis

Flexor Hallucis Brevis

Flexor Dig. Min. Brevis

tendon, Peroneus Longus

Tibialis Posterior

their digits' proximal phalanges. Nobody really knows what function they serve. Flexor Hallucis Brevis forks into two tendons of insertion, which attach to the phalanx via two little **sesamoid bones** lying under the first metatarsal head. (Other intrinsic muscles of the hallux may also have attachments to these sesamoids.) The sesamoids of the hallux probably serve to keep the body's weight from squashing the big toe's long flexor tendon under the first metatarsal head. The sesamoids transmit the weight from that metatarsal down to the underlying skin (the "ball" of the foot) and form a little bony arch underneath which the tendon can slide back and forth freely. (As might be expected, the tendon is surrounded there by a lubricating synovial sheath.) The Flexor Hallucis Brevis may act as a sort of active ligament for adjusting the position of these two sesamoids.

In primitive quadrupedal mammals, all the Interossei of the hands and feet had similar little sesamoids in their tendons, which kept weight off the flexor tendons to the other toes as well. Our own Interossei generally lack such sesamoid bones. The Interossei of the human foot, like those of the hand, can be divided into an abducting dorsal series and an adducting ventral (plantar) series. They all arise from metacarpals and pass into the toes on the corresponding (dorsal or ventral) sides of the deep transverse ligaments that connect adjacent metatarsal heads. The only interesting difference between the Interossei of hand and foot is that the foot's axis, around which abduction and adduction occur, lies through the second digit rather than through the third. The second toe, like the hand's third digit, thus has two Dorsal and no ventral Interossei—and so on and so forth (Fig. 16-8). Note that there is not a separate ventral Interosseus for the first toe as there is for the thumb.

The Lumbricals of the foot (Fig. 16-6) and the Adductor of the hallux (Fig. 16-7) are arranged more or less like their counterparts in the hand. The two heads of Adductor Hallucis are more widely separated than those of the thumb adductor. It is not of much use as an adductor because the hallux is permanently adducted. Its functions (if any) are unclear.

▪ What Happened to Flexor Digitorum Superficialis?

In our reptilian ancestors, the superficial flexor of the four fingers was an intrinsic hand muscle arising from the palmar aponeurosis. During our evolution, this muscle shifted origins back through the carpal tunnel and took over most of the superficial flexor musculature in the forearm, becoming Flexor Digitorum Superficialis (Chapter 14). But in the leg, the superficial flexor muscles were not available for a similar takeover by the intrinsic toe-flexor, for they had become the Triceps Surae, shifting their insertion from the old plantar aponeurosis to the new mammalian heel. The superficial flexor of the toes stayed put underneath the plantar aponeurosis. It is still an intrinsic muscle of the foot in ourselves, just as it is in a lizard. The belly of this muscle—**Flexor Digitorum Brevis** (Fig. 16-6)—still arises from the deep surface of the plantar aponeurosis (and from the heel of the calcaneus as well). It splits into four tendons, which enter digits 2–5 and wrap around the sides of each deep flexor tendon to attach to the middle phalanx of each toe—just like the four forked tendons of Flexor Digitorum Superficialis in the hand. Because the fleshy belly of Flexor Digitorum Brevis fills in the space between the "thenar" and

Fig. 16-8 Interosseus muscles of the foot. Dorsal views. A. Plantar Interossei. B. Dorsal Interossei.

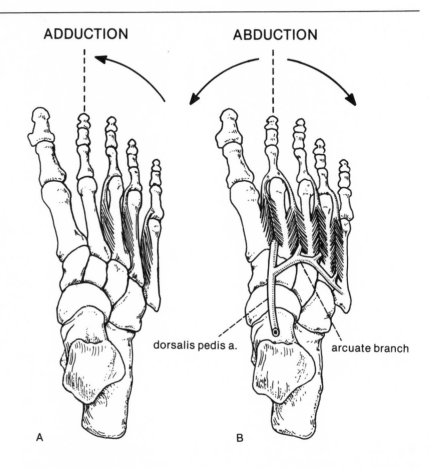

ADDUCTION

ABDUCTION

dorsalis pedis a.

arcuate branch

A

B

"hypothenar" muscles in the sole, the sole does not have a central cup or hollow like that of the hand.

■ The Dorsal Muscles of the Foot

The final group of foot muscles has no obvious equivalent in the hand. This is a fan of short *intrinsic* toe extensors—**Extensor Hallucis Brevis** and **Extensor Digitorum Brevis**—lying deep to the *extrinsic* extensor tendons on the back of the foot (Fig. 16-9). These short extensors arise laterally from the calcaneus and send little tendons down to feed into the extrinsic extensor tendons. Again, the marginal digits are exceptional: the little toe usually does not receive a short extensor tendon, and the one to the big toe (Extensor Hallucis Brevis) attaches directly to the proximal phalanx.

Fig. 16-9 Intrinsic extensors of the toes.

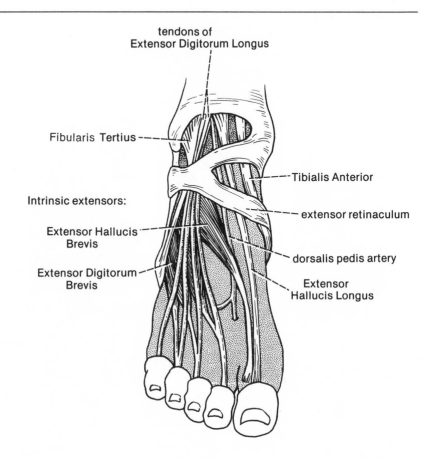

tendons of
Extensor Digitorum Longus

Fibularis Tertius

Tibialis Anterior

Intrinsic extensors:

extensor retinaculum

Extensor Hallucis
Brevis

dorsalis pedis artery

Extensor Digitorum
Brevis

Extensor
Hallucis Longus

These short toe extensors look as though they ought to be a hind-limb equivalent of the forearm's deep, "outcropping" extensor layer that has slipped down below the ankle. They probably are not—but thinking of them that way may help you remember the deep position and differing insertions of the two intrinsic elevator muscles on the back of the foot (Table 16-4), which parallel those of the deep extensors Extensor Indicis and Extensor Pollicis Brevis in the forearm.

■ The Innervation of the Leg and Foot

The sciatic nerve innervates all the muscles below the knee, sending its elevator-muscle branch (common fibular n.) into the elevators and its depressor-muscle branch (tibial n.) into the depressors. Little

Table 16-4   Intrinsic elevator muscles in the foot.

Muscle	Origin	Insertion	Action	Nerve
Extensor Hallucis Brevis	Upper and lateral face of calcaneus and attached ligaments	Proximal phalanx of big toe	Extends hallux (metacarpophalangeal joint)	Deep branch of common fibular n.
Extensor Digitorum Brevis	Upper and lateral face of calcaneus and attached ligaments	Dorsal extensor expansions of toes 2–4	Extends toes	Deep branch of common fibular n.

more need be said. The picture is complicated only slightly by the fact that each of the sciatic nerve's divisions has two major branches.

The tibial and common fibular nerves gradually separate from each other as they run down the back of the thigh deep to the hamstrings. They separate before they reach the popliteal fossa (the hollow at the back of the knee). The common fibular nerve follows the tendon of Biceps Femoris to the head of the fibula and hooks around the side of that bone—which is why it is called the fibular nerve. As it does so, it divides into a superficial branch, which supplies the fibular compartment (Fibularis Longus and Brevis), and a deep branch, which runs down along the interosseous membrane and supplies all the extensors in the anterior compartment (including Fibularis Tertius and the short extensors down in the foot).

The tibial division of the sciatic nerve courses downward through the calf between the superficial (Triceps Surae) and deep flexor layers (Fig. 16-3). It follows the toe-flexor tendons around behind the tibial malleolus at the ankle, where it divides into **medial** and **lateral plantar** branches. These two are *equivalent to the median and ulnar nerves respectively and have almost precisely equivalent distributions*. The medial plantar nerve innervates the "thenar" muscles of the big toe; the lateral plantar nerve innervates the "hypothenar" muscles, the first-digit Adductor, and all the Interossei (via a deep branch that runs across their plantar surface, just like the deep branch of the ulnar nerve). The medial plantar nerve supplies cutaneous innervation to three-and-a-half digits, just as the median nerve does; it even mimics the median nerve in innervating Flexor Digitorum Brevis, the hind-limb equivalent of the superficial flexor of the fingers.

The single difference worth noting between the nerves of sole and palm is that the medial plantar nerve innervates only the second-digit

Lumbrical. It does not (as the median nerve does) supply that of the third digit—which has been taken over by the lateral plantar nerve. The lateral plantar nerve innervates not only most of the Lumbricals but also the other muscle that attaches to the long flexor tendons: the peculiar little Flexor Accessorius, which has no equivalent in the hand. The lateral plantar nerve runs across (and sends motor fibers into) this muscle's plantar surface on its way to the "hypothenar" muscles of the little toe.

■ The Arteries of the Leg and Foot

The femoral artery passes through the gap between the hamstring and adductor parts of Adductor Magnus and enters the popliteal fossa as the **popliteal** artery (Figs. 15-10 and 16-10). This artery divides into two branches, one to the front of the leg and one to the back of the leg. The posterior one is the **posterior tibial** artery, which simply follows the tibial nerve down into the sole. Shortly after crossing Popliteus, the posterior tibial artery gives off a large branch to the fibular side of the calf. This branch, the fibular (or peroneal) artery, runs down the back of the fibula and supplies all the depressor muscles arising from that bone (Soleus, Tibialis Posterior, Flexor Hallucis Longus)—and also the two Fibulares that arise from it more laterally.

The remaining leg muscles, the elevators in the anterior compartment, get their blood via the popliteal artery's anterior branch, the **anterior tibial artery.** This vessel branches off the popliteal artery behind the knee, immediately ducks forward between the two leg bones, and continues downward on the front surface of the interosseous membrane (Fig. 16-3). It gives off branches to the anterior tibial muscles and ends on the dorsal surface of the foot as the **dorsalis pedis** artery (Figs. 16-8 and 16-9).

All this is very much like the arrangement in the forearm, where there are also two parallel arteries (radial and ulnar) following the depressor surface of the limb bones and a third, smaller artery that runs on the elevator side of the interosseous membrane (posterior interosseous artery). The main difference is that the lower limb's ulnar-artery equivalent—the fibular artery—does not continue into the "palm" of the foot. Instead, it collides (so to speak) with the enlarged calcaneus and ends in a network of tiny branches on the bony heel. The posterior tibial artery (the "radial" artery of the leg) is left with the task of supplying blood to the entire sole. It does this by

Fig. 16-10 Popliteal artery and its branches. Back of knee and sole of foot are shown separately, connected by the posterior tibial artery (*white dashes*).

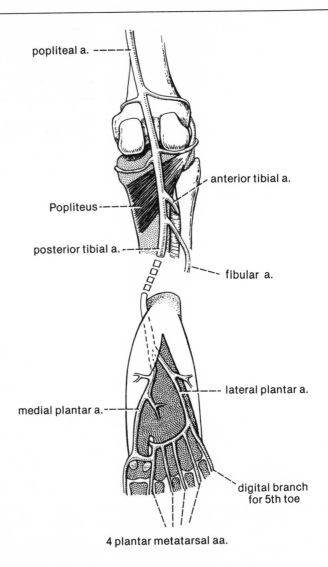

popliteal a. ------

anterior tibial a.

Popliteus -----

posterior tibial a. ------

fibular a.

lateral plantar a.

medial plantar a. ------

digital branch for 5th toe

4 plantar metatarsal aa.

dividing into **medial** and **lateral plantar** branches (Fig. 16-10), which have the same course (and much the same distribution) as the similarly named nerves. The *lateral* plantar artery, which does the job of the ulnar artery in the hand, imitates the ulnar artery satisfactorily by sending a branch curving across the Interossei to form a deep **plantar arch.** The *medial* plantar artery, however, does not do a very good imitation of the terminal end of the *radial* artery. It does not send a superficial branch over to anastomose with the lateral plantar artery, so there is no *superficial* plantar arch; and it does not wrap around to the dorsal side the way the radial artery does. Here the dorsalis pedis artery has to take over its job, sending a branch in between the two heads of the first Dorsal Interosseus to complete the (deep) plantar arch. An **arcuate** branch of the dorsalis pedis artery (Fig. 16-8) curves laterally across the backs of the metatarsals. Its branches run on to the toes—and down through the Dorsal Interossei, making further anastomoses with the plantar arch in the sole.

17

Upright Posture and Locomotion

▪ Advantages of Upright Posture

People (and some of their close extinct relatives) are the only mammals to date that have given up the use of the forelimbs in locomotion. Some flightless birds (for example, ostriches, kiwis, and dodos) and certain extinct reptiles (for example, *Tyrannosaurus*) developed similar specializations, but their forelimbs tended to become atrophic and useless. We have retained our large forelimbs and put them to use in handling, carrying, and making things. *instead of locomotion.*

Human bipedalism has two major advantages. The first and most obvious is that it facilitates the construction and use of tools, a habit that has guided our evolutionary history for the last two million years and has enabled us to become almost disastrously successful. The second, which is less obvious, is that upright posture and locomotion are extremely efficient in themselves. Although our upright stance is unstable, it does not take much muscular effort. A man or woman can go on standing in one spot for many hours; a dog or cat has to sit or lie down rather frequently to relieve the postural strain on its limb muscles. Similarly, our striding gait is slow, but it can be kept up longer than the pacing or trotting gaits of typical quadrupeds. Men in good condition can run a hundred miles in twenty-four hours. Within historical times, some human groups used to hunt horses and deer by chasing them for days until the animals fell exhausted. With their huge brains, their quiet and tireless locomotion, and their flexible forelimbs grasping deadly weapons, human beings make very efficient predators.

▪ Disadvantages of Upright Posture

Bipedal locomotion has its disadvantages. For one thing, it is relatively slow. (If you doubt this, trying chasing a cat sometime.) It also involves a 90° change in the direction of gravitational pull on all the parts of the body. This change produces a lot of new stresses that the old anatomical structures are not built to take. The body of a quadrupedal mammal is built like a suspension bridge; the cablelike vertebral column is slung between the columnar limbs, and from this "cable" the body wall and viscera dangle on their mesenteries and ligaments like the roadway hanging from a bridge's cables. Obviously, standing a suspension bridge on one end causes problems. The chief problems (and their adaptive "solutions") are tallied below.

1. In the bipedal posture, the heart and the surrounding sac of fibrous pericardium no longer are suspended from the structures in the posterior mediastinum but slump downward against the diaphragm. The problem of supporting the human heart has been solved by attaching the fibrous pericardium to the diaphragmatic fascia. The diaphragm itself supports our heart, and the heart rides up and down with it.

2. The loops of abdominal intestine dangling from the dorsal mesentery also slump tailward when we stand erect. We have had to evolve new supports for the mobile parts of the gut. This has been accomplished by hanging some of the intestinal weight from the posterior abdominal wall through secondary mesenteric adhesions (for example, those of the colon). This arrangement reduces the strain on the lower body-wall muscles and helps to prevent the intestinal twisting and obstruction that might otherwise result.

3. Our pelvic viscera tend to fall through the lower pelvic opening. This tendency has been countered by tucking the reduced tail between the legs and pasting some of the old tail muscles to the hindgut to form a pelvic diaphragm.

4. Our upright posture greatly increases the pressure on our lower abdominal wall. A simple experiment will show why. Fill a milk carton with water and punch two small holes in it, one near the top and one near the bottom. Water dribbles out of the upper hole but gushes in a stream from the lower one—because the greater weight of overlying water increases the pressure at the bottom hole. Similar distribution of pressure in the human abdomen tends to force loops of gut out at the lower end, into the inguinal canal and the femoral sheath. We have an exceptionally strong inguinal ligament that helps guard both openings—but hernias are still a common problem.

5. Upright posture forces the venous blood draining from our hind

limbs, abdomen, and pelvis to flow uphill over a much longer course than it would have if we were quadrupeds. The resulting strain on the veins often produces pathological dilatations of the vessel walls—varicose veins in the legs, hemorrhoids around the anus, and so on.

6. Compressed by the downward thrust of the body's weight, the human vertebral column tends to break down. Ligaments tear; weak vertebral arches pull loose; intervertebral disks rupture and allow vertebral bodies to grind together around their edges, thus resulting in nerve compression, osteophytic growth, and abnormal curvatures of the column. Most of these pathological conditions, however, result from abnormal strain or involve congenital abnormalities of some sort. Our vertebral adaptations are adequate to bear the stresses of normal upright posture and locomotion.

■ Human Postural Adaptations

The adaptations of our viscera to upright posture and locomotion are not uniquely human characteristics. We share them with chimpanzees, orangutans, and the other living apes. People and apes also share several peculiarities of forelimb anatomy. Unlike typical quadrupedal mammals, people and apes have an articular disk between the ulna and the radius, a short olecranon process that allows the elbow to be extended fully, a loose glenohumeral joint capsule, and a scapula that sticks out sideways rather than ventrally (Fig. 13-7). These specializations give people and apes exceptionally limber forelimbs. They allow living apes to hang and swing along easily underneath branches and to reach out in any direction when moving from one tree to another. This kind of clambering and dangling locomotion is typical of big animals that live in trees. Being heavy, such animals have to be careful in moving from branch to branch, and they find it easier to hang below branches than to balance on top of them. Their locomotor adaptations are very different from those of smaller monkeys, which run atop branches on all fours in a more primitive quadrupedal fashion.

Because hanging underneath branches by one's hands places the vertebral column in a vertical position, it produces the same strains on the viscera that we suffer in standing on our hind legs. The peculiar features of visceral anatomy that we share with the apes thus probably evolved as adaptations to hanging rather than to standing. Those features, together with our apelike upper extremities, testify to our descent from a large, cautious arboreal primate resembling a modern orangutan or chimpanzee.

Arm-swinging in the trees and bipedal walking on the ground put similar strains on the *viscera;* but our bipedalism produces different strains on the *skeleton.* The most obvious difference is that the vertebral column is compressed rather than stretched in standing upright.

In a standing person, the weight of the body is transmitted downward through the chain of vertebral bodies to the pelvis. From there, it is passed through the hip joints to the lower limbs and the ground. The upright human body is kept balanced around this jointed pile of bones by continual little muscular tugs and tensions in various directions as the pile sways gently in and out of equilibrium. The whole performance is a complicated balancing act, resembling that of a circus juggler carrying a stack of cups and saucers on his head. It is nevertheless surprisingly efficient, requiring very little muscular exertion. The fatigue that results from long standing is mainly vascular; venous blood tends to pool in the lower parts of the legs unless it is driven upward through its valved channels by occasional contractions of the limb muscles.

To understand the mechanisms involved in maintaining an upright posture, we need to understand how weight is distributed in a standing human being (Fig. 17-1). The center of gravity in an upright human body is usually located just in front of the second sacral vertebra. A plumb line dropped through this point would pass ventral to the whole vertebral column; just behind a line connecting the two hip joints; in front of a line connecting the two knee joints; and in front of the ankles. A standing person thus tends to collapse in different directions at different joints. There is a tendency for the vertebral column to flex and buckle ventrally, for the trunk to topple backward on the thighs, for the knees to fold the wrong way, and for the entire body to pitch forward on its face through rotation at the ankle joint. These tendencies must be resisted by ligaments or by the contraction of muscles.

■ What Keeps the Vertebral Column from Buckling?

Because the line of gravity passes in front of the vertebral bodies, most of the intervertebral joints tend to flex in the upright posture. This tendency is resisted by a continual low level of activity in the epaxial muscles whenever we stand or sit upright. The resulting pos-

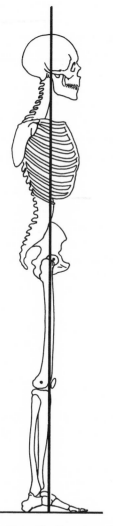

Fig. 17-1 The line of gravity.

tural strain on these muscles has been kept to a minimum by the evolution of two dorsal concavities in the vertebral column (Fig. 2-2). The **lumbar curve** swings the thorax backward over the front end of the sacrum, drawing the line of gravity in close to the vertebral column. Likewise, the **cervical curve** throws the weight of the head backward, thus reducing the postural work that the epaxial neck muscles have to do. Nevertheless, epaxial muscles in the lumbar region (Erector Spinae) and neck (Semispinalis) are always slightly active in upright postures.

The sacrum is the least vertical part of the human vertebral column; it lies at an angle of about 45°, halfway between vertical and horizontal. There are two possible reasons for this sacral slope. First, the cranially facing tilt of the sacrum's dorsal surface presents a broader bony surface for the origin of the epaxial muscles that maintain the lumbar curve. Second, if the sacrum rotated into a vertical position, the tail end of it would swing forward and block the birth canal. As might be expected from this second rationale, human females have even less vertical sacra than males have; the sacrum is almost horizontal in many women. This orientation maximizes the front-to-back diameter of the pelvic opening, thereby making it easier to get a baby out through it.

Because the sacrum does not participate in the lumbar curve, there is a fairly sharp bend in the column between vertebrae L.5 and S.1 (Fig. 2-2). The fifth lumbar vertebra therefore has a tendency to slide forward off the sacrum. This is resisted by **iliolumbar** ligaments (Fig. 11-3) that stretch from the crest of the ilium to the fifth lumbar transverse processes. In about one out of every twenty people, through a poorly understood combination of traumatic and congenital factors, the arch and body of vertebra L.5 become detached from one another. The body may then slide forward while the arch stays behind, held in place by the iliolumbar ligaments.

The oblique orientation of the sacrum also means that the body's weight tends to rotate the sacrum forward. This rotation is resisted by the sacroiliac, sacrospinous, and sacrotuberous ligaments (Chapter 11).

■ The Hip Joint

The line of gravity in a standing man or woman passes just behind an imaginary line drawn through the two hip sockets, so the trunk has a tendency to topple over backward at the hip. This tendency is resisted by ligamentous thickenings in the hip joint's fibrous capsule. The most important of these is the strong, triangular **iliofemoral** ligament (Fig. 17-2) that runs across the front of the joint. A standing man can lean or topple backward at the hip only a few degrees, whereupon his iliofemoral ligament becomes taut. The joint is then secured against further extension without any muscular effort.

The twisted arrangement of the capsular ligaments in our hip joint (Fig. 17-2) reflects both ontogeny and phylogeny. In a mammal standing on all fours, the hip is held in a flexed position and the capsular ligaments run straight across laterally, from the rim of the hip socket to the margin of the femoral "ball." When the thigh of a dog or a horse swings backward in running, the capsule winds around the neck of the femoral head and becomes tighter. In full extension, the capsule is wound taut, checking movement. The human fetus devel-

Fig. 17-2 Capsule of the hip joint. Anterior view.

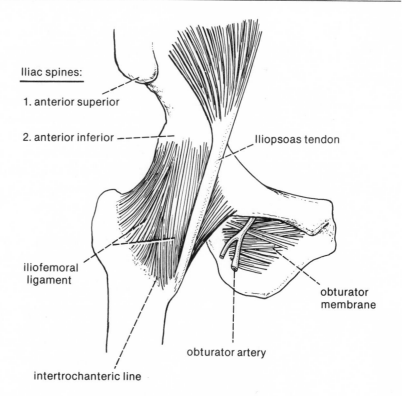

Iliac spines:

1. anterior superior

2. anterior inferior

Iliopsoas tendon

iliofemoral ligament

obturator membrane

obturator artery

intertrochanteric line

ops with its thigh in a doglike, flexed position; and the capsular fibers of our hip joint grow straight across from hipbone to femur, like those of a quadruped. But after birth, when we start to walk on our hind limbs, we fling them straight out behind us, thus twisting the capsular fibers and drawing the capsule almost completely taut. The capsule has developed local thickenings to take advantage of this tautness. Our specialized iliofemoral ligaments allow us to lean backward and rest (so to speak) on the twisted hip-joint capsule when we stand upright. The attachments of those powerful ligaments are marked by bony protuberances—the ilium's **anterior inferior spine** and the **intertrochanteric line** that runs across the front of the femur between the two trochanters—found only in human beings.

The human hip socket is deep, surrounding more than half of the femoral "ball." The lower anterior quadrant of the hip socket carries no weight in standing, however; and this part of the socket is not ossified. In a skeleton, the socket appears to have a bite out of its edge at this point. In a living person, the "bite" (or acetabular notch) is bridged by the **transverse acetabular** ligament (Fig. 17-3). This ligament completes the margin of the acetabulum and helps to provide attachment for a circular fibrocartilaginous lip—the **acetabular labrum**—that projects from the acetabulum's margin and makes the hip socket effectively even deeper.

Our deep hip socket strengthens the joint against dislocation. Unless there is some congenital weakness such as an unusually loose joint capsule, it generally takes something on the order of an auto accident to wrench the femoral head out of the acetabulum. The shoulder joint, with its lax capsule and shallow socket, is far more mobile—and much more vulnerable to tearing and dislocation.

■ The Knee Joint

The line of gravity passes in front of the knee in a standing human being; so this joint tends to hyperextend and collapse. As in the hip, this tendency is prevented by ligamentous mechanisms, which require no muscular exertion.

The femur ends distally in two large knuckles—the **medial** and **lateral condyles** (Gk., "knuckle")—which articulate with matching depressions in the top of the tibia. Seen from the side (Fig. 17-4), the femoral condyles are ovoid in shape, longer from front to back than from top to bottom. From the outer side of each condyle, a stout

Fig. 17-3   Hip socket. A. Lateral view. B. Schematic vertical section through socket and greater trochanter. Black arrow in B indicates gap (acetabular foramen) through which branches of the obturator vessels enter the joint to supply the articular tissues.

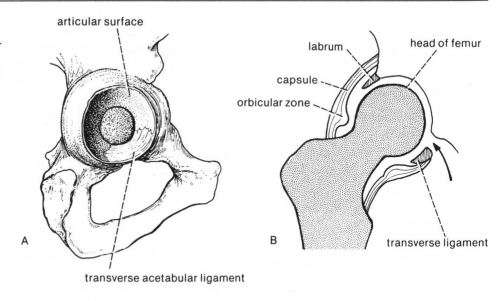

Fig. 17-4   Collateral ligaments of the knee joint. A. Medial aspect. B and C. Lateral aspects. The ligaments are eccentrically attached to the femur and are accordingly taut in extension (A and B) and slack in flexion (C).

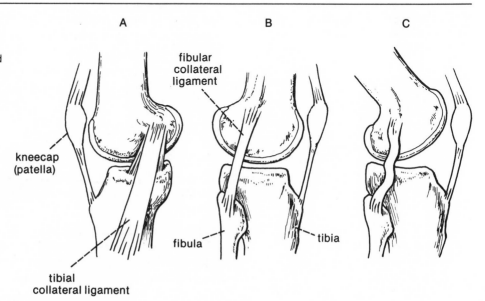

ligament runs down to attach to the leg bone below—to the tibia on the medial side and to the top of the fibula on the lateral side. These **tibial** and **fibular collateral** ligaments lie behind the knee joint's axis of rotation. Because the femoral condyles are ovoid, the position and attachments of the collateral ligaments cause them to grow taut as the knee moves into full extension (Fig. 17-4). They thus keep the knee from hyperextending in the standing position and resist the body's tendency to topple forward at the knee. Like the collateral ligaments of other hinge joints, they also prevent abduction, adduction, and other unwanted movements.

The knee is the most complicated joint in the body. It develops as three separate joint cavities—two **tibiocondylar cavities** (one between each femoral condyle and the tibia) and a **subpatellar cavity** in front between the femur and kneecap. The fibrous capsules of the two tibiocondylar joints are thin and insubstantial, and they soon get resorbed where the patella slides across them. The tibiocondylar joint cavities thus come to open directly into the subpatellar cavity in front. A separate perforation also generally develops in the septum between the two tibiocondylar cavities (Fig. 17-5).

Fig. 17-5 Diagrammatic vertical section through the knee. Lateral view. The cruciate ligaments (A) are embedded in a septum of softer tissues (B) separating the two condyles.

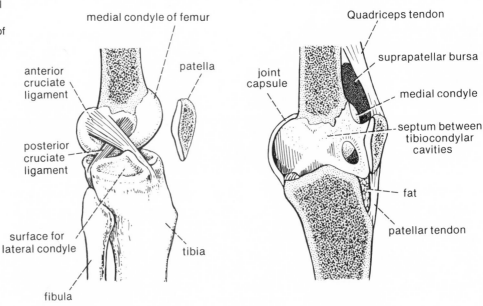

A

B

That septum also contains two strong **cruciate** ligaments, which run slantwise down from the notch between the condyles to attach to the tibia (Fig. 17-5). They cross each other like the limbs of the letter X—hence their name (L. *cruciatus,* "crossed"). The cruciate ligaments keep the femur from sliding backward or forward off the top of the tibia.

From the inner surface of each tibiocondylar joint's fibrous capsule, a fibrocartilaginous ring grows inward, forming a C-shaped articular disk or **meniscus** (Fig. 17-6) that intervenes between the condyle and the tibia. The outer edge of each meniscus is closely attached to the top of the tibia by a thickening of the joint capsule called the **coronary** ligament. The menisci (especially the medial one) thus cannot move much on the tibia, and so they do not have the usual articular-disk function of allowing different types of motion against their opposite sides. When they are removed surgically, there is no loss of knee function. The main purpose of the menisci seems to be filling in the

Fig. 17-6 Tibia and menisci, seen from superior (A) and lateral (B) aspects.

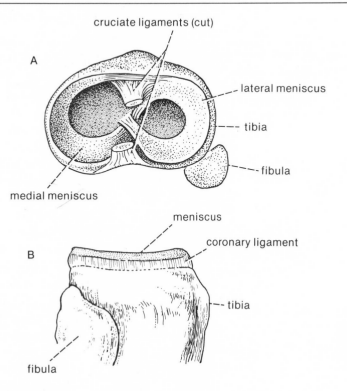

ever-changing gaps between the ovoid condyles and the flat top of the tibia. They apparently help to keep body weight and synovial fluid spread more evenly over the joint surfaces as the knee flexes and extends.

Because the femoral condyles are so large and protuberant, most of the numerous muscle tendons converging on the knee wind up sliding back and forth over bony surfaces as they move; so they have to be provided with lubricating bursae. The large number of these bursae (at a minimum, there are three for the Quadriceps tendon and the associated patella, one for each of the three hamstring tendons, one for each head of Gastrocnemius, and one for the Popliteus tendon) and their variable connections with the knee's joint cavity help to make the knee the most complicated joint in the body. People who spend a lot of time kneeling are apt to develop inflammation ("housemaid's knee") in one or more of these bursae—or in the knee joint itself, via the bursae around the kneecap that communicate with the subpatellar part of the joint cavity.

■ Foot and Ankle Stability

The line of gravity (Fig. 17-1) passes in front of the ankle. When you stand up, there is thus a natural tendency for you to pitch forward onto your nose. This tendency is resisted by muscular effort.

When we stand upright, our heel-raising muscles (Gastrocnemius and Soleus) contract a trifle whenever we start to topple forward. Their contraction raises the heel slightly. This shifts the support point abruptly forward to the balls of the feet—which lie *in front* of the line of gravity. The body then begins to topple *backward* around the new support point, the heel-raising muscles relax again, and the cycle repeats. A gentle back-and-forth sway of this sort goes on continually in a standing person; it becomes more evident when postural reflexes are slowed by fatigue or drunkenness.

The necessary swift transfer of weight to the ball of the foot when the heel rises is made possible by another human peculiarity, the longitudinal arch of the foot. When we stand up without moving around, this arch is maintained effortlessly, by ligaments running in various directions from the calcaneus. Four of these are particularly strong and important (Fig. 17-7):

1. The plantar aponeurosis, which is the major ligamentous defense against fallen arches.

Fig. 17-7 Supporting ligaments of the sole. A. Plantar aponeurosis. The attachments of the aponeurosis ensure that it grows taut when we rise on our toes (*arrow*) and extend the metatarsophalangeal joints. B. Plantar ligaments. The black arrows indicate the passage of the Fibularis Longus tendon across the sole.

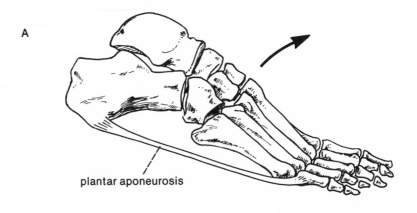

A

plantar aponeurosis

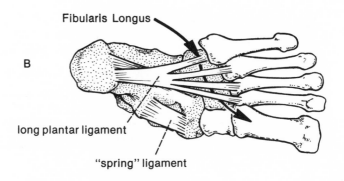

Fibularis Longus

B

long plantar ligament

"spring" ligament

2. The **plantar calcaneonavicular,** or "spring" ligament. This short but thick band of fibrocartilage runs medially forward underneath the ball-like head of the talus, from the calcaneus's talus-supporting shelf (the **sustentaculum tali**) in back to the navicular in front (Fig. 16-1). As long as this ligament is tight, the head of the talus is kept away from the ground, thereby ensuring that body weight transmitted through the talus will be borne by the heel and ball of the foot, not by the sole under the talus itself.

3,4. The **long plantar** and **short plantar** ligaments running directly forward from the underside of the calcaneus to attach to the metatarsals and cuboid.

When we stand on tiptoes, run, or lift the heel in walking, the arch is put under more strain, and its supporting ligaments get some active assistance from intrinsic and extrinsic muscles of the foot. The most important of these seem to be the (intrinsic) Abductors of the marginal digits, which run from the heel to the region of the metatarsal heads and thus provide a muscular parallel to the plantar aponeurosis. Under extraordinary loads, practically all the muscles of the foot and leg become active—and some of this activity probably contributes to maintaining the longitudinal arch.

A surprisingly large number of people—fifteen percent or so of the population—have "fallen arches," or **flatfoot.** This does not prevent them from walking, but it tends to make them walk abnormally. In a flatfooted person, the ligaments supporting the arch have been stretched, allowing the head of the talus to drop toward the sole. If it drops far enough, a lot of the body's weight gets carried to the ground through the arch's "keystone," the talus. The downward slump of the talus results in a partial eversion of the foot, so flatfooted people often have a distinctive ducklike waddle, with feet turned outward and knees turned inward. When the flatfoot is lifted during swing phase (see below), it tends to be picked straight up as a unit, without transferring much weight to the front of the foot. This is inefficient and tiring and produces muscle fatigue and pain if kept up for a long time. The abnormal standing posture, caused by the shift in the tarsals' positions, commonly results in widespread joint pain and even backache.

▪ Bipedal Locomotion and Its Antecedents

When a typical four-footed mammal like a dog or a cat runs, its limbs swing back and forth in arcs parallel to the midline plane of the body. The animal does not need to stick its limbs out sideways, and this movement—abduction—is accordingly very limited. (You can demonstrate this by experimenting with a tolerant dog.) In the human (or ape) shoulder, abduction is enhanced by the shape of the thorax. The human thorax is wider from side to side than it is deep from back to front. (In a typical quadruped, the reverse is true.) As a result, the human shoulder socket faces laterally instead of ventrally, thus facilitating abduction and increasing the range of forelimb movements. This reshaping of the thorax is another one of the apelike features we seem to have inherited from arm-swinging ancestors, but it later turned out to be useful for bipedalism; it has the effect of moving the vertebral column ventrally in toward the line of gravity in the upright posture (Fig. 13-7).

The human lower limb, like the limbs of a typical quadruped, has more limited abduction and merely swings back and forth in a fore-and-aft arc during walking or running. But in human-style bipedal locomotion, the hind limb is used as a propulsive *strut,* rather than (as in quadrupeds) as a propulsive *lever.*

A quadrupedal mammal's hind limb generates propulsive thrust when it is placed on the ground and retracted backward, thus shoving the animal forward. This is the **stance phase** of the limb's repeating cycle of movements (Fig. 17-8). Most of the propulsive "push" consists of a tailward thrust, produced throughout stance phase by the hamstrings and heel-raising muscles. At the end of the stance phase, the hip is fully extended and the knee is straightened out somewhat by Quadriceps. The straightening limb becomes a rigid thrust member along which the animal's heel-raising muscles and toe flexors exert a final push. The foot is then raised from the ground and the femur swung forward again (the **swing phase** of the locomotor cycle). When the foot is brought all the way forward and lowered to the ground, the stance phase begins once more, and the cycle repeats. The performance is mechanically something like propelling a canoe with a paddle.

Normal human walking is more like pushing a boat along with a pole. Our stance phase corresponds to a prolongation of the last part of the quadruped's stance phase, when the limb is straightened out behind the pelvis for a final shove backward. In human beings, the hip stays almost wholly extended throughout the walking cycle, and the knee joint is held in extension whenever the foot is on the ground. (In effect, we have flung our hind limbs straight out behind us and stood upright on them.) The backward "push" that moves us forward is produced not by drawing the limb backward like a canoe paddle but by lifting the heel at the end of the stance phase—and thus exerting a thrust *along* the rigid "pole" formed by the stiffly extended lower limb. The most important hind-limb propulsive muscles in a quadruped are the hamstrings; for us, the plantarflexors of the ankle (Triceps Surae) are more important.

Figure 17-8 details some of the muscle actions in our striding gait, beginning with the start of the swing phase. As the foot leaves the ground, Iliopsoas contracts to start the thigh swinging forward. The calf lags behind the thigh, and this lag automatically and passively flexes the knee. The extensors of the ankle and toes contract during swing phase to keep the toes from dragging on the ground as the foot

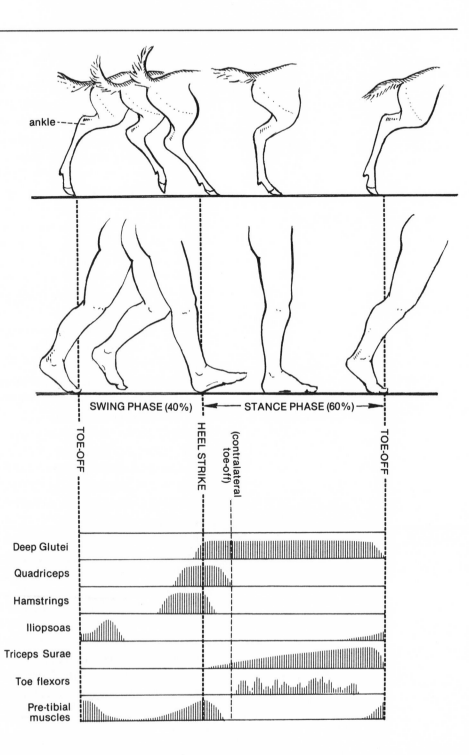

Fig. 17-8 Limb movement in quadrupedal and bipedal locomotion. The graphs at the bottom show muscle activity during the human locomotor cycle.

swings forward. (Injury to the common fibular nerve, which supplies these extensor muscles, produces a characteristic toe-dragging limp.)

At the end of the swing phase, there is a brief burst of activity in our hamstrings, which brings the forward swing of the thigh to a halt. The leg is kept swinging forward into extension by a surge of Quadriceps contraction, which keeps the knee extended as the heel touches down. The knee stays more or less locked in extension throughout the stance phase. (There is a little flexion of the human knee during the first half of the stance phase, but far less than in a quadruped; see Fig. 17-8.)

In a quadruped, the hamstrings would go on contracting through most of the limb's stance phase, pulling the femur backward and causing the foot to thrust backward against the ground. Our stance phase is mostly passive. Our heel-raising muscles (Triceps Surae) contract during stance, reaching a climax just before the foot is lifted; this flexes the ankle and produces the propulsive thrust along the stiffened "pole." The toe flexors, Fibulares, and adductors of the thigh contract unpredictably to keep the body more or less balanced over the foot while the other foot is lifted off the ground. This balancing act is abetted by the hip abductors (Gluteus Medius and Minimus), which resist adduction and thus prevent the pelvis from dropping toward the unsupported side (Fig. 17-9). If you walk along with your fingers dug into the top of your thigh between the iliac crest and the greater trochanter (the bony bump on the side of your thigh near the top), you can feel Gluteus Medius rhythmically contracting during stance to maintain balance. At the end of the stance phase, the heel is raised, and weight is carried almost entirely by the ball of the big toe. The two sesamoids flanking the tendon of the Flexor Hallucis Longus prevent this pressure from hurting the tendon.

Human running is a less efficient procedure than a striding walk. The lower limb of a running man or woman goes through a more quadrupedlike cycle of movements, with the hip and knee continually flexed. As in a quadruped, a running person's hamstrings help to provide propulsive thrust. The forelimbs, which do most of the propulsive work in a dog, stay off the ground even in running in human beings—which greatly handicaps us in trying to catch up with or run away from more typical mammals. Nevertheless, our forelimbs have an active role to play in running. When we run we swing each forelimb vigorously back and forth in synchrony with the hind limb

Fig. 17-9 The deeper Glutei (Medius and Minimus) tilt the trunk toward the supporting foot when the foot of the opposite side is lifted. In walking, they contract to keep the pelvis from dropping on the unsupported side.

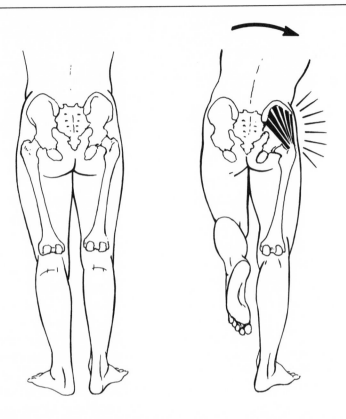

on the *opposite* side. In a horse, this pattern of limb movement would be called a trot. The function of this two-footed "trotting" in us bipeds seems to be to damp out the oscillations produced by the pelvis's swiveling to-and-fro around a vertical axis (as we swing each hip socket forward during swing phase). You will understand why this damping action is useful if you try running as fast as you can with your arms folded across your chest.

THE HEAD AND THE NECK

PART V

18

The Specializations of the Head

The head of a vertebrate consists mainly of the expanded front ends of the neural tube (the brain) and the gut tube (the pharynx). They have the same relationship in both the head and the typical body segment: the brain is dorsal to the pharynx.

There is not much else about the head that could be called typical. The rear half of the vertebrate head does consist of fused segments; *but* but they have been so greatly altered and specialized that *their* serial homologies are hard to make out. The front half of the head is even stranger. The notochord, which seems to be involved in producing the segmentation of the embryo, never grows out into this anterior, **prechordal** part of the head, so *has* no truly segmental structures ever develop there. The eyes, nose, and other prechordal organs are utterly unlike anything we see in the typical body segment. The whole prechordal part of the head seems to be a mainly ectodermal elaboration that the early vertebrates tacked onto the front end of an otherwise *Branchiostoma*-like body.

All the components of a vertebrate's head, including the parts that are still faintly segmented, are specialized for doing jobs that the typical body segment cannot do: sensing the environment in special ways, procuring food, and absorbing oxygen from the surrounding air or water. Although the eyes of human beings are still more or less like those of primitive fish, all the other parts of our head have been massively reworked again and again by evolution as our ancestors developed jaws, came out onto dry land, became warm-blooded, took to suckling their young, and repeatedly changed their food preferences over the course of the past 500 million years. These changes have still further scrambled the vestiges of the original segmental pattern. The chief peculiarities of the head's components are summarized in the paragraphs that follow.

Gut   At its head end, the gut tube has several openings onto the body surface. The largest appears in the midline, forming the **mouth;**

but lesser openings appear above and behind the mouth on either side. Two **nostrils** form as pits in the ectoderm above the mouth opening. In air-breathing vertebrates, these pits open into the roof of the mouth, producing a pair of nasal passages separated by a midline partition.

Behind the eye, six more pockets of ectoderm form on each side and invaginate until they meet corresponding outpouchings of the gut lining. In a fish, these ectodermal clefts and endodermal pouches open into each other, thereby forming **gill slits.** The side walls of the pharynx are reduced to a series of **gill arches,** columns of tissue in between the slits.

In a human embryo, the clefts and pouches never open up to form actual slits—and, of course, no gills are developed. The gill arches are accordingly rechristened **pharyngeal** arches in human embryology. Most of the clefts and pouches separating them eventually disappear. Various glands develop from the pouches' endodermal lining, however; and the air-filled channels of the ear represent the most anterior "gill slit," with an eardrum stretched across it and a crinkly, cartilaginous funnel surrounding its outer opening.

Special Sense Organs   The nose, eye, and ear have no equivalents in a typical body segment. They all begin as pits in the ectoderm of the embryonic head. The nasal passages, described above, contain the end organs of smell: specialized patches of ectodermal cells that turn into neurons and send axons back into the developing brain. A second invagination further back on each side is pinched off from the embryonic "skin" and buried under the body surface to become the **lens** of the eye. The light-sensitive **retina** forms from a cup-shaped outgrowth of the brain that wraps around the lens. The inner ear starts out like the lens, but the invaginating pit retains its central cavity and turns into a fluid-filled sac lying alongside the embryonic hindbrain. In the adult, this sac becomes a system of tubules—the **membranous labyrinth**—buried in bone at the base of the skull. It contains the receptor organs of balance and hearing.

Dorsal Nerve Cord   The head end of the dorsal nerve cord develops three bulges, or **primary vesicles** (Fig. 18-1), originally associated with the three special sense organs. The first bulge—the **forebrain**—forms behind the nasal passages and receives the **olfactory** nerves growing back from the nose. Clusters of nerve cells in the forebrain

Fig. 18-1 The three primary vesicles of the brain and their relationship to the nerves of special sense in a six-week embryo.

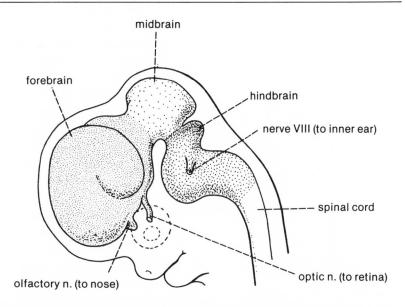

are still the primary centers for processing olfactory sensations. The retinal cells also develop from the forebrain, but they originally sent their axons back to visual centers in the second primary vesicle—the **midbrain.** In human beings, newer visual centers in the forebrain have taken over most of the job of processing visual information; however, the old midbrain centers play an important role in coordinating eye movements. The senses of hearing and balance still have their primary centers in the **hindbrain** vesicle that forms between the fluid-filled sacs of the embryonic ear.

A great elaboration of the forebrain vesicle to form a **cerebral cortex** is characteristic of mammals and is carried to an almost grotesque extreme in *Homo sapiens.* The cerebral cortex can be thought of as a huge mass of internuncial neurons, into which all sensory data are channeled and integrated into a detailed "picture" of the world. This internal map facilitates more complex motor responses than are possible with simple reflex arcs like those found in the spinal cord. It also probably permits us to be conscious of the world—and therefore of ourselves.

Somites Clear, indisputable somites still form alongside the notochord at the rear of the head, behind the developing ear sacs. The sclerotomes of these **occipital somites** help form the floor of the braincase; their myotomes develop into the muscles of the tongue. More anterior somites are hard to make out in most vertebrates. Some vertebrates' eye muscles unmistakably develop from three hollow blocks of mesoderm lying behind the eye, and these have generally been regarded as three vestigial somites. Until recently, most authorities have concluded that all the other somites of the head disappeared early in vertebrate evolution and that the striated muscles of the pharyngeal arches correspond to the smooth muscles surrounding the rest of the gut.

New discoveries have thrown all this into doubt. Scanning electron micrographs of bird embryos show that the eye-muscle somites are just part of a long series of paired mesodermal bumps alongside the front end of the notochord. All these bumps, which have been christened **somitomeres,** appear to be vestigial somites. Unlike proper somites, they do not develop a vertebral component (sclerotome) or a dermis-forming layer (dermatome). They just give rise to striated muscles—including all those of the pharyngeal arches. The gill-arch muscles thus seem to correspond to the myotomes, not to the gut musculature of the typical body segment. However, they are innervated differently from the eye and tongue muscles that develop from the head's more clearly recognizable somites.

Neural Crest   In the typical body segment, bone, connective tissue, and smooth muscle are all derived from mesoderm. This pattern also holds in the occipital region, where true somites still develop; but in the rest of the head, all these types of tissue form chiefly from ectoderm—especially that of the neural crest. Neural-crest ectoderm has been described as "the mesoderm of the head." In the head, it not only gives rise to pigment cells and to sensory and autonomic ganglia (as in the typical body segment; Fig. 1-11) but also forms the dermis and the underlying dermal bones of the face and most of the cartilage of the nonoccipital part of the head. Even the smooth muscle coat of the aortic arches develops from ectodermal cells of the neural crest.

Arteries   Two major arterial channels on each side traverse the neck to supply the head. The **common carotid** arteries develop from the ventral aorta, and their continuations into the third aortic arches and paired dorsal aortae (Fig. 6-4) become the internal carotid arteries that supply the forebrain and midbrain. The hindbrain is supplied by the brain's other major arterial channels, the **vertebral arteries.** These branches of the subclavian arteries develop as longitudinal anastomoses that connect (and eventually replace) the intersegmental arteries on each side of the neck.

In a human adult, almost all the blood passing through the vertebral and internal carotid arteries goes to supply the brain. Branches of these arteries also supply the special sense organs—nose, eye, and ear. Early in prenatal life, the internal carotid also supplies blood to the rest of the head; but this job is soon taken over by a new vessel, the external carotid artery, which grows out from the base of the third aortic arch and captures most of the internal carotid's branches. This takeover recapitulates the evolutionary history of these two arteries in our mammalian ancestors.

■ The Twelve Cranial Nerves

The peripheral nervous system of the lower chordate *Branchiostoma* has a delightful simplicity. Ventral roots carry motor impulses into the myotomes; separate dorsal roots carry sensory information back into the dorsal nerve cord. The only complication involves the strip of striated muscle running down the underside of the pharynx, which gets its motor innervation via *dorsal* roots.

Early vertebrates added new muscles of two sorts: striated muscles in the gill arches, and smooth muscles in the walls of the viscera. The motor nerves to smooth muscles and gill muscles, like the pharyngeal motor nerves of *Branchiostoma,* seem to have emerged originally through the dorsal roots. But in our spinal nerves, the autonomic fibers supplying smooth muscle leave the spinal cord via ventral roots. Our dorsal roots are wholly sensory, our ventral roots are wholly motor, and the two roots merge to form a mixed spinal nerve in each segment.

The nerves that come out of our brain (Table 18-1) preserve a more ancient vertebrate pattern, in which the dorsal roots remain separate and contain the autonomics and gill-arch motor fibers (Fig. 18-2). Ten of our twelve cranial nerves can be grouped into two classes:

1. **Primitive ventral roots.** Like the ventral roots of *Branchiostoma,* these are strictly motor nerves to myotomes. They supply the specialized myotomes that develop into the muscles of the tongue and eyeball.
2. **Primitive dorsal roots.** These include all the sensory fibers di-

Table 18-1   Cranial nerves and their constituents.

Nerves	Motor innervation			Sensory innervation			
	Voluntary motor		Autonomic motor (para-sympathetic)	Body surface (somatic)		Gut tube (visceral)	
	To somites	To branchial mm.		General (touch)	Special	General (touch)	Special
Atypical sensory nerves							
I. Olfactory					Smell		
II. Optic					Sight		
Primitive ventral roots (to somites)							
III. Oculomotor	Eye mm.		Ciliary and pupillary mm.				
IV. Trochlear	Superior Oblique m.						
VI. Abducent	Lateral Rectus m.						
XII. Hypoglossal	Tongue mm.						
Primitive dorsal roots (gill-arch nn.)							
V. Trigeminal (Arch I)		Arch I mm.		Face		Arch I and II	
VII. Facial (Arch II)		Arch II mm.	Lacrimal and salivary glands (sublingual and submandibular)[a]	Tiny patch of skin near ear hole			Taste, front ⅔ of tongue
VIII. Vestibulocochlear (from n. VII)					Hearing, Balance		
IX. Glossopharyngeal (Arch III)		Arch III mm.	Parotid salivary gland[a]	Perhaps small area of skin near ear hole		Arch III territory and middle ear	Taste, rear ⅓ of tongue
X. Vagus (Arches IV to VI)		Mm. of arches IV to VI; upper esophagus	Most of gut and its glands; heart, etc.	Small area of skin near ear hole		Arch IV territory and rest of gut down to L. colic flexure	A few taste buds at rear of tongue
XI. Accessory (Arches IV to VI)		Mm. of arches IV to VI; upper esophagus (cranial root), plus Sternocleido-mastoid and Trapezius mm. (spinal root)		—[b]			

a. Severing either nerve VII or nerve IX results in decreased secretion in all three major salivary glands. The two nerves probably swap preganglionic parasympathetic fibers at several places (for example, between the greater and lesser petrosal nerves), but the details are uncertain.

b. Nerve XI's spinal root often has connections with the dorsal (sensory) root of spinal nerve C.1, and may distribute C.1 sensory fibers to the meninges and atlantooccipital joint as it runs up into the braincase.

Fig. 18-2 Spinal and cranial nerve components. Schematic sections of the dorsal nerve cord. A. The primitive arrangement preserved in the cranial nerves, with separate dorsal and ventral roots. B. A typical (mixed) spinal nerve.

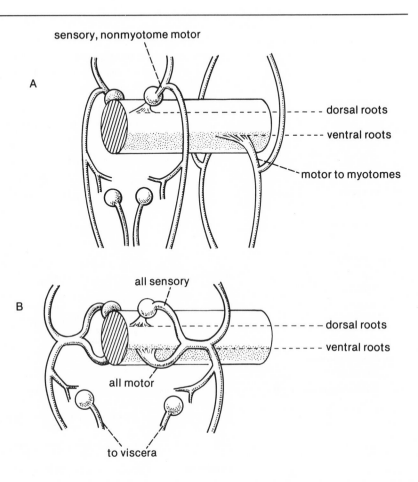

rectly entering the brain and also contain the motor nerves to the gill-arch muscles. Almost all the autonomic (parasympathetic) fibers leaving the brain also emerge via these primitive dorsal roots.

All the primitive dorsal and ventral roots emerge from the midbrain or from even more posterior parts of the central nervous system. The remaining two cranial nerves, which convey the special sensations of smell and sight, emerge more anteriorly, from the forebrain. They are accordingly numbered as cranial nerves I and II. Like everything else in the most anterior, prechordal part of the head, they are simply weird and do not fit into any general pattern.

The **olfactory nerve,** cranial nerve I, is the only sensory nerve whose neurons are not derived from neural crest. Instead, they are derived from the ectodermal cells that invaginated to form the air passages of the nose. In an adult, the bodies of the olfactory nerve cells lie in the mucous membrane in the roof of the nasal passages. They send non-myelinated axons back through a series of tiny holes in the overlying braincase. These axons synapse in the forebrain. The whole complex of these axons on each side is called the olfactory "nerve," although it does not form a single bundle like other named nerves.

The other atypical cranial nerve is the **optic** nerve, cranial nerve II. Like the olfactory nerve, it is not really a nerve in the usual sense of the word. It is simply the narrow stalk of the forebrain outgrowth that enfolds the lens of the developing eye and turns into the retina. Unlike a true sensory nerve, this outgrowth contains many internuncial neurons, which form layers in the retina. Nerve impulses triggered by light falling on the retina's receptor cells pass through many synapses and get extensively reprocessed in the retina itself before they ever enter the braincase. The eye, in effect, is a lobe of the brain that sticks out of the skull; and the optic nerve is merely a tract of white matter connecting that lobe to the rest of the central nervous system.

■ Primitive Ventral Roots

Like all other ventral roots in any vertebrate body, the primitive ventral roots emerging from our brain are strictly motor nerves. There are two clusters of them: one in front that supplies the eyeball muscles and one in back that innervates the tongue muscles. The front group consists of cranial nerves III (**oculomotor**), IV (**trochlear**), and VI (**abducent**). They supply the small muscles that attach to the outside of the eyeball and turn it this way and that. Nerve III supplies most of these muscles and is considerably larger than the other two. The rear group of primitive ventral roots forms the last cranial nerve, nerve XII (**hypoglossal**). It is really a composite bundle of four (or maybe five) primitive ventral roots, which supply the myotomes of the occipital somites. In mammals, these myotomes migrate forward beneath the floor of the mouth and develop into the muscles of the tongue.

■ Primitive Dorsal Roots: The Gill-Arch Nerves

The remaining six cranial nerves are primitive dorsal roots. Like the dorsal roots of our spinal nerves, the primitive dorsal roots carry all the general sensory information—touch, pain, heat, and so on—back from the tissues they innervate. They have sensory "dorsal-root" ganglia, just as do the dorsal roots in a typical body segment. But they are also the motor nerves to the gill arches.

In advanced vertebrates, each of the first three arches has its own primitive dorsal root; a fourth dorsal-root nerve innervates all the rest of the arches. These four gill-arch nerves (cranial nerves V, VII, IX, and X) provide four types of innervation to the territories they cover (Table 18-1):

1. **General sensory** fibers, for tactile sensations. These can be divided into *visceral sensory* nerves to the gut lining and *somatic sensory* nerves to everything else.
2. **Special visceral sensory** fibers to the tongue and palate, for the receptor organs of the taste sense.
3. **Parasympathetic motor** fibers to smooth muscles and glands.
4. **Branchial-motor** fibers to the gill-arch muscles. Anatomy texts usually call these "special visceral motor" nerves, as though they were a sort of parasympathetic fiber that did not bother to synapse with a second neuron. This label reflects the old theory that the striated gill-arch muscles are serial homologs of the smooth muscles surrounding the rest of the gut, rather than of the myotomes (as we assume here).

These four components are differently emphasized in the four gill-arch nerves. A couple of them lack one or two components altogether. Furthermore, the second and fourth gill-arch nerves each have one component that is so functionally specialized and so anatomically distinct that it is reckoned as a separate cranial nerve (nerve VIII separate from VII, and nerve XI from X). These four cranial nerves are thus conventionally counted as six.

The **trigeminal** nerve (V) is the nerve of the first arch and the largest of the twelve cranial nerves. It consists mostly of general sensory fibers, which innervate the whole surface of the face back to the ear holes (Fig. 18-3) and the anterior end of the gut lining—and practically everything in between as well. Its branchial-motor component is

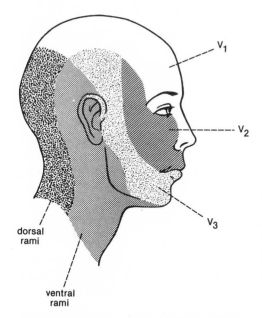

Fig. 18-3 Cutaneous innervation of the head. The face and most of the scalp are innervated by the three branches of the trigeminal nerve (V_1, V_2, V_3).

also important; the first-arch muscles it supplies include the large **masticatory** muscles that we use in chewing. However, the trigeminal does not contain any taste fibers or parasympathetics.

The **facial** nerve (VII) is the nerve of the second arch. It lacks general visceral sensory fibers but provides taste fibers to the anterior two-thirds of the tongue. (The trigeminal and facial nerve join forces to innervate this part of the tongue, furnishing it with touch and taste fibers respectively.) Across the face, the facial nerve overlaps with the trigeminal in a different way; it supplies purely motor fibers to the little second-arch muscles that move the skin of the face in mammals.

The third arch is innervated by nerve IX, the **glossopharyngeal** nerve. It takes its name from its sensory distribution to the pharynx and the posterior third of the tongue, which it supplies with taste fibers as well as with general sensation. In human beings, the third-arch musculature has almost disappeared; only one little muscle of the pharynx (Stylopharyngeus) remains for nerve IX to innervate.

The **vagus** nerve (X) is familiar to us from the typical body segment, because it provides sensory and parasympathetic motor innervation to most of the rest of the gut, from the root of the tongue all the way down to the left colic flexure. It also supplies the striated muscles derived from arches 4, 5, and 6 (including the muscles of the larynx) and brings taste sensation back from a few taste buds on the back of the tongue.

All four primitive dorsal roots provide sensory innervation to the skin, but this somatic (nonvisceral) sensory component is significant only in the trigeminal nerve (Fig. 18-3). The other three gill-arch nerves supply only tiny patches of skin in and around the ear hole. They also differ from the trigeminal in containing autonomic—specifically, parasympathetic—motor fibers.

The facial nerve (VII) actually plays an important role in innervating the skin of the head, but the "skin" it innervates has sunk into the head to become the inner ear. In fish, the body surface carries ciliated sensory receptors that detect vibrations in water. These make up the so-called **lateral-line** system and are innervated by nerves VII, IX, and X (arches 2 through 6). In the early vertebrates, some of these receptors in the ectoderm overlying the second arch invaginated to form a sealed-off acceleration-sensing organ—the **semicircular canals.** After our ancestors crawled out onto dry land, the lateral-line system was lost (except perhaps for those patches of skin around the ear that are still innervated by the three rear gill-arch nerves). The buried semicircular canals were retained intact, however. They eventually developed a new vibration-sensing outgrowth—the **cochlea**—through which sound waves in the air around the head could be indirectly detected.

The branch of the facial nerve that innervates the inner-ear sac is now reckoned as a separate cranial nerve, the **vestibulocochlear** nerve (VIII). Its evolutionary connection with the nerve of the second arch is apparent in its embryology. It can also be seen in its exit from our brain stem (Fig. 18-4), where it is usually bound up as a single bundle with the sensory root of nerve VII. (The ambiguous position of nerve VII's sensory root—starting out with VIII, but crossing over immediately to join the rest of VII—has won it a separate name, the **nervus intermedius.** Luckily, nobody thought to number *it* as a separate cranial nerve.)

As Figure 18-4 shows, the primitive dorsal roots arise more or less in line with each other from the ventral surface of the brain: V in front, followed by VII, VIII, IX, and X arising progressively further back. The primitive ventral roots arise along a similar, more ventrally

Fig. 18-4 Ventral surface of the adult human brain, showing the roots of the cranial nerves.

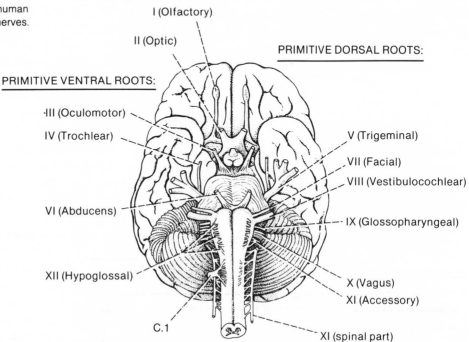

I (Olfactory)

II (Optic)

PRIMITIVE DORSAL ROOTS:

PRIMITIVE VENTRAL ROOTS:

III (Oculomotor)

IV (Trochlear)

V (Trigeminal)

VII (Facial)

VIII (Vestibulocochlear)

VI (Abducens)

IX (Glossopharyngeal)

XII (Hypoglossal)

X (Vagus)

XI (Accessory)

C.1

XI (spinal part)

positioned line drawn through the origins of nerves III, VI, and XII. The one major exception is the trochlear nerve (IV), which seems to emerge through the roof of the brain stem. In fact, the cell bodies of its motor axons are clustered in the ventral part of the brain stem, in line with those of the other primitive ventral roots. The peculiar course of the trochlear nerve's axons was fixed early in vertebrate evolution when the eye muscle that they innervate (the Superior Oblique) lay dorsal to the tiny brain and the trochlear nerve had to run up dorsally to reach it.

■ The Cervical Segments and the Accessory Nerve

The ventral roots of the cervical spinal nerves do not have any autonomic component; they contain only motor fibers to myotomes. They thus resemble the ventral-root cranial nerves that supply the eye and tongue muscles—and, as might be expected, they are lined up with the primitive ventral rootlets emerging from the brain stem (Fig. 18-4).

The *dorsal* roots of the cervical nerves are of the usual, purely sensory sort seen in a typical body segment. Of the four components found in dorsal-root *cranial* nerves, they lack three (taste, parasympathetic, and branchial motor). In fact, some branchial motor fibers do emerge from the cervical part of the spinal cord. But instead of following the cervical dorsal roots, these fibers take an intermediate course, coming out of the cord *laterally* between the dorsal and ventral roots (Fig. 18-4). All these gill-arch motor fibers from the upper neck segments are gathered together into a bundle called the **spinal root of the accessory** nerve. The most anterior rootlets of this series arise inside the skull, from the very tail end of the brain stem, and form the so-called **cranial root of the accessory** nerve. The spinal root runs up into the skull alongside the spinal cord and joins the cranial root. The resulting bundle is counted as a separate cranial nerve, the **accessory** nerve (XI).

Both roots of the accessory contain only branchial motor fibers to the muscles of arches 4, 5, and 6. Both join the vagus and leave the skull together with it. The *spinal* root immediately splits off from the vagus and runs right back down into the neck to innervate the Trapezius and the associated Sternocleidomastoideus, which are derived from the gill-lifting muscles of the posterior arches (Fig. 21-1 and Chapter 13). The *cranial* root of the accessory sticks with the vagus and is distributed with it to branchial muscles of the pharynx and larynx. Things would be a great deal simpler if the cranial root of the accessory nerve were just counted as part of the vagus; we could then say that the vagus nerve supplies all the voluntary and involuntary muscles surrounding the gut tube from the back of the pharynx all the way down to the left colic flexure, and leave it at that.

▪ Relay in Cranial Nerves

The cranial nerves start out in an embryo as fairly discrete entities, innervating the well-defined territories we have been describing—nerve I to the organs of smell, nerve II to the retina, nerves III, IV, and VI to the eyeball muscles, nerve V to the first pharyngeal arch, and so on. But as development proceeds, some of the cranial nerves send out branches that join branches of other cranial nerves and are distributed along with them. The simplest case is the vagal distribution of the cranial root of the accessory nerve, described above. Relay of this sort becomes more complicated where it involves the cranial parasympathetic outflow.

Most of this parasympathetic outflow emerges via the vagus nerve. The vagal parasympathetics enter the thorax and abdomen, where they synapse on little ganglion cells buried in the walls of their target organs. Three other cranial nerves also contain parasympathetic fibers. Two of these are gill-arch nerves (primitive dorsal roots) like the vagus—nerve VII (arch 2) and nerve IX (arch 3). The third is a primitive *ventral* root, nerve III (oculomotor). Parasympathetic impulses in the gill-arch nerves VII and IX cause tears and saliva to flow; those in the oculomotor nerve help focus the eye and adjust the size of the pupil.

None of these other cranial parasympathetic fibers run all the way to their target organs the way the vagal parasympathetics do. Instead, they synapse in discrete clumps of ganglion cells located some distance from the target organs. There are four pairs of these parasympathetic ganglia in the head. They dangle underneath major branches of the trigeminal nerve (V)—the only gill-arch nerve that does not contain any parasympathetic outflow of its own. From these ganglia, postsynaptic parasympathetic fibers proceed on to their target organs by traveling with branches of the trigeminal. The resulting motor pathways can be absurdly complicated (Chapter 21). We will describe them as we come to them in the chapters that follow.

The Brain
and the Skull

19

■ The Brain—General Organization

The internal structure of the brain constitutes most of the subject matter of neuroanatomy and is outside the scope of this book. Nevertheless, a few facts about the brain may help you to understand the anatomy of the skull.

The brain develops from three local thickenings in the dorsal nerve cord (Fig. 18-1) associated with the three special sense organs (eye, nose, and ear). In early developmental and evolutionary stages, the brain is just another regional specialization of the spinal cord, like the thickenings associated with the nerve plexuses of the limbs. The embryonic brain starts out with an internal structure much like that of the spinal cord: a hollow tube, with white matter (axons) on the outer surface and gray matter (cell bodies) on the inner surface. Subsequent changes blur the brain's resemblance to the spinal cord. The central canal is elaborated into a series of connected chambers called **ventricles,** the columns of cell bodies are split up into more or less discrete clusters called **nuclei,** and the bundles of axons are divided and rearranged into **fiber tracts** that connect one mass of cell bodies to another.

The midbrain stays relatively simple and tubular in mammals, but the forebrain and hindbrain blow up like balloons, thereby producing spherical masses of tissue that swell out over the top of the more primitive brain stem. Each of these dorsal bubbles has a wrinkled outer coating, or **cortex,** of gray matter and an internal filling of white matter that provides the "wiring" for the cortical cells (see Fig. 19-11). The wrinkling up and folding of the cortex affords more gray coating per ounce of white stuffing than we would get if the cortex were smooth.

The forebrain vesicle gives rise to two dorsal bubbles—the left and right **cerebral hemispheres** (Fig. 19-1). The neurons in the cerebral gray matter are connected (1) to lower forebrain sensory centers, by a

The brain has a cortex of gray matter and an internal filling of white matter.

Fig. 19-1 Dorsal outgrowths of the mammalian brain. A. Early developmental stage. B. Human adult.

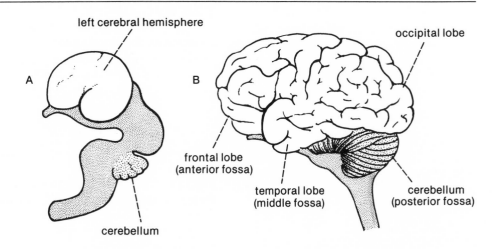

fan of fibers called the **corona radiata;** (2) to spinal motor neurons, by **corticospinal tracts;** (3) to other cortical cells in the same hemisphere, by **association fibers;** and (4) to cells in the opposite hemisphere, by **cerebral commissures.** The most important of our commissures is a great bridge of white matter called the **corpus callosum,** found only in placental mammals (Fig. 19-11). Certain kinds of severe epilepsy have been treated by severing the corpus callosum. The apparent result is that each hemisphere becomes capable of learning and responding separately; so the patient has something like two minds in the same body.

A single dorsal bubble—the **cerebellum** (Fig. 19-1)—develops from the hindbrain vesicle. Through it, proprioceptive input (the "muscle sense" that enables you to tell, for example, where your left foot is without looking at it) and vestibular input (from the acceleration-sensing apparatus of the inner ear) are integrated with other sensory information to help coordinate habitual voluntary movements such as walking. Injury or disease of the cerebellum can produce staggering, dizziness, palsy, speech defects, and so on.

The **brain stem** comprises the older, basal parts of the brain, where the cranial nerves emerge. Most of them (Fig. 18-4) are connected to the hindbrain, which contains the primitive motor and sensory centers for the branchial-arch nerves (including the nerve to the inner ear) and the tongue muscles. The primitive visual centers in the midbrain receive some of the fibers from the retina; here, too, arise most of the nerves to the muscles of the eyeball. (The hindmost eye-muscle nerve, cranial nerve VI, emerges from the front end of the hindbrain). Only the two atypical sensory ("weird") nerves—I (olfactory) and II (optic)—enter the forebrain directly.

After they enter the skull, the optic nerves of each side come together and swap about half their fibers at the so-called **optic chiasm** (Gk., "crossing," from the letter *chi*). The resulting mixed bundles— the optic **tracts**—continue backward into the basal part of the forebrain, which is known as the **thalamus.** Just behind the chiasm, from the most ventral part of the forebrain (the **hypothalamus**), a glandular body called the **hypophysis cerebri,** or pituitary gland, projects downward into a pit in the base of the skull. The hypophysis has a double developmental origin. The front part of it develops as a globular outpocketing from the roof of the mouth (Fig. 9-4). Its rear part is a lobe of the brain that has become a neurosecretory organ like the suprarenal gland. The two parts secrete different but equally important hormones into the bloodstream, thereby controlling such diverse functions as body growth, the contraction of the uterus in childbirth, and the production of milk and urine.

▪ The Bones and Foramina of the Cranial Base

While reading the following paragraphs, you might find it helpful to study an actual human skull. The bones that make up our skull can be grouped into three series.

1. The skull-base bones, which lie underneath the brain stem and are preformed in cartilage.
2. The membrane or dermal bones (Chapter 1), which form the sides and roof of the skull and make up the skeleton of the face.
3. The cartilage-replacement elements that form in the branchial arches.

Some of the bones of the skull base correspond to vertebral bodies, but the membrane bones and gill-arch bones do not have any equivalents in the typical body segment. Because the skull-base bones are more complicated than the other bones of the skull and have important relationships to the nerves and blood vessels passing in and out of the braincase, we will describe them in more detail.

The mass of cartilage that condenses beneath the embryonic brain is called the **chondrocranium,** and the bones that replace this cartilage are together referred to as the **basicranium.** Initially, two sets of cartilaginous lumps form below the brain in the embryo: a series of paired elements near the midline and a more lateral series that form capsules around the three pairs of special sense organs (nose, eye, and ear). All these elements fuse to form the cartilaginous chondrocranium, and ossification centers appear and spread in the cartilage later on. The bones that replace the chondrocranium represent the primitive vertebrate braincase, and so all the nerves and vessels passing to and from the brain traverse holes in or between these bones. The adult's basicranium comprises all or part of five bones: (1) the **ethmoid** bone, which surrounds the olfactory apparatus and olfactory nerves; (2) the **sphenoid** bone, which surrounds the optic nerves and contains the hypophysis's bony cradle, the **hypophyseal fossa** (Fig. 20-1B); (3) and (4) the left and right **temporal** bones, which surround the labyrinth of the inner ear on each side; and (5) the **occipital** bone, which surrounds the spinal cord as it passes into the skull.

ETHMOID BONE

The ethmoid (Fig. 19-2) is the only basicranial bone that is entirely preformed in cartilage; the others incorporate some dermal (membrane-bone) elements as well. The ethmoid encapsulates the receptors of smell. It roofs them over with a horizontal **cribriform plate** riddled with holes for the olfactory nerves (L. *cribriformis,* "sievelike"), and it walls them in on either side with a **lateral mass** full of **ethmoid air cells.** The left and right cribriform plates are separated below by the ethmoid's **perpendicular plate,** which forms the top of the midline septum between the two nasal passages. A smaller midline crest—the **crista galli** (L., "cock's comb")—sticks up between the cribriform plates inside the braincase. A fold of dura mater (the **falx cerebri**) that dips down between the two cerebral hemispheres attaches to this little crest. The pocket on each side between the ethmoid's air-filled lateral masses and its perpendicular plate is lined with olfactory receptor cells, from which the fibers of the olfactory nerves stream up through the cribriform plate to enter the brain. Viewed from behind, the ethmoid has roughly the shape of a face-down capital E—for "ethmoid," of course.

Seen from inside the braincase, the ethmoid is almost completely surrounded by the **frontal** bone, one of the dermal bones that form the skull's roof and walls. The front ends of the cerebral hemispheres lie on top of the ethmoid here and are surrounded by the frontal bone.

Fig. 19-2 The ethmoid bone (diagrammatic). A. The isolated ethmoid. B. Schematic section through the ethmoid in the complete skull. Anterior view.

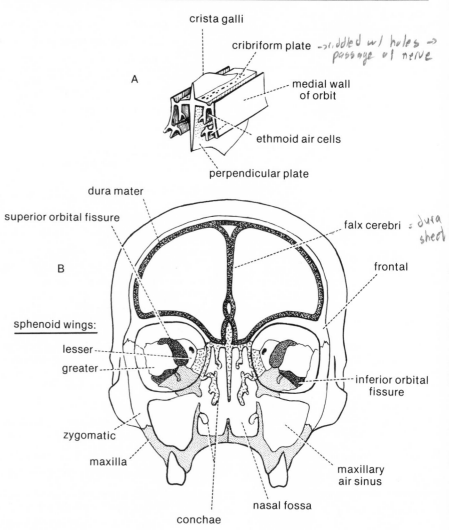

crista galli

cribriform plate —*riddled w/ holes → passage of nerve*

medial wall of orbit

ethmoid air cells

perpendicular plate

A

dura mater

superior orbital fissure

falx cerebri = *dura sheet*

frontal

B

sphenoid wings:

lesser

greater

inferior orbital fissure

zygomatic

maxilla

maxillary air sinus

nasal fossa

conchae

They are called the **frontal lobes** of the brain, and their bony cradle is the **anterior cranial fossa** (Figs. 19-1 and 19-3).

SPHENOID BONE

The sphenoid bone, unlike the ethmoid, is formed from both cartilaginous and dermal elements. Viewed from behind (Fig. 19-4), the sphenoid looks vaguely like some sort of flying creature with spread

Fig. 19-3 The interior surface of the skull base. View from above with the top of the braincase removed.

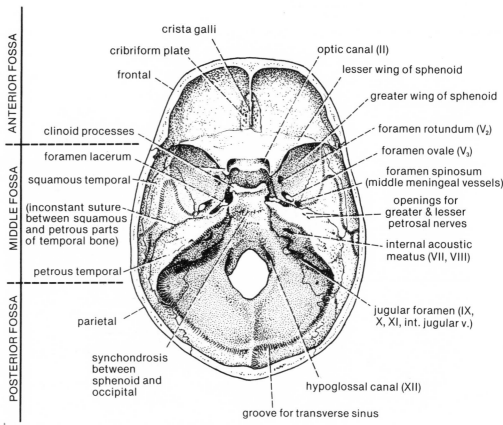

ANTERIOR FOSSA

MIDDLE FOSSA

POSTERIOR FOSSA

crista galli

cribriform plate

frontal

clinoid processes

foramen lacerum

squamous temporal

(inconstant suture between squamous and petrous parts of temporal bone)

petrous temporal

parietal

synchondrosis between sphenoid and occipital

groove for transverse sinus

optic canal (II)

lesser wing of sphenoid

greater wing of sphenoid

foramen rotundum (V₂)

foramen ovale (V₃)

foramen spinosum (middle meningeal vessels)

openings for greater & lesser petrosal nerves

internal acoustic meatus (VII, VIII)

jugular foramen (IX, X, XI, int. jugular v.)

hypoglossal canal (XII)

Below → 2 pterygoid plates
Above → 4 clinoid processes
→ hypophyseal fossa

wings and dangling talons. The dangling talons—the **pterygoid plates**—are its dermal elements. They project down from the cranial base behind the bony palate (Fig. 19-5), and various muscles that move the lower jaw and soft palate arise from them.

The sphenoid **body** is the bone's central mass in the midline. It bears the hypophyseal fossa on its upper surface. Four **clinoid processes** projecting from the sphenoid surround the fossa (Fig. 19-3) and support its roof of dura mater. The two posterior clinoid processes are conjoined by a bony bar called the **dorsum sellae** (Fig. 19-4), which marks the point where the notochord ends in the embryo.

Two bony flaps, known as **wings,** stick out on each side from the prechordal part of the sphenoid body. These wings start out as independent cartilage-replacement bones. The lower flap, or **greater wing,**

Fig. 19-4 The sphenoid bone (*stippled*). Front half of the skull, viewed looking forward and slightly downward from behind.

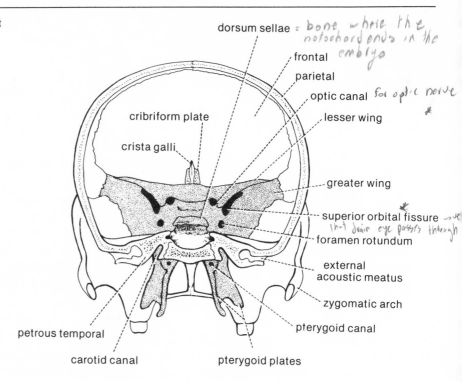

dorsum sellae = *bone where the notochord ends in the embryo*

frontal

parietal

optic canal *for optic nerve*

lesser wing

cribriform plate

crista galli

greater wing

superior orbital fissure → *that drain eye passes through*

foramen rotundum

external acoustic meatus

zygomatic arch

pterygoid canal

petrous temporal

carotid canal

pterygoid plates

is an old bone of the first branchial arch, serving here to patch a hole in the side wall of the mammalian braincase. The **lesser wing** above it was originally one of the paired sense-organ capsules—for the eye, as the ethmoid is for the nose. It develops from a cartilaginous ring that forms around the embryo's optic nerve, and it later co-ossifies with the sphenoid's body. (Associating the eye with the lesser wing and the first arch with the greater wing should help you remember that the eye socket's contents and the first-arch derivatives are all innervated via nerves that traverse holes in the sphenoid [see Fig. 19-6].)

Because the lesser wing of the sphenoid forms as a ring around the optic nerve, of course the optic nerves of the adult leave the braincase through holes in the lesser wing. These **optic canals** (Figs. 19-3 and 19-4) also transmit the **ophthalmic** branch of the internal carotid artery, which carries blood out of the braincase to the contents of the bony eye socket. The veins draining the eye socket go back into the braincase—not through the optic canals, but through the cleft between the greater and lesser wings. This large cleft—the **superior**

Fig. 19-5   The skull, viewed from the side (A) and from beneath (B).

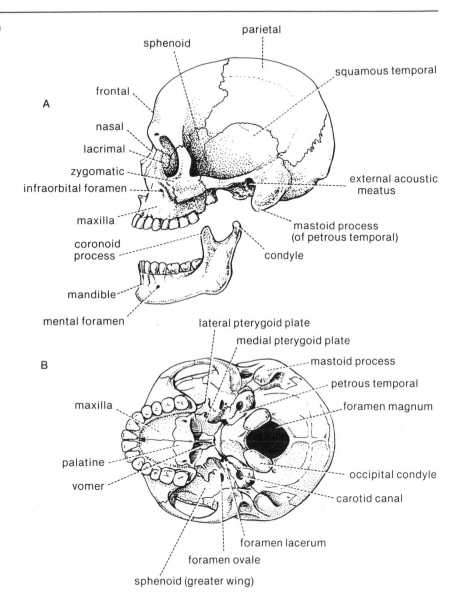

A

parietal
sphenoid
squamous temporal
frontal
nasal
lacrimal
zygomatic
infraorbital foramen
maxilla
coronoid process
mandible
mental foramen
external acoustic meatus
mastoid process (of petrous temporal)
condyle

B

lateral pterygoid plate
medial pterygoid plate
mastoid process
petrous temporal
maxilla
foramen magnum
palatine
occipital condyle
vomer
carotid canal
foramen lacerum
foramen ovale
sphenoid (greater wing)

orbital fissure (Figs. 19-2 and 19-4)—also transmits the other nerves that supply the orbit's contents (Fig. 19-6): the motor nerves (III, IV, and VI) to the eye muscles and the **ophthalmic** division of the trigeminal nerve (V).

The trigeminal nerve takes its name from the fact that it splits into

Fig. 19-6 Cranial nerve foramina. A. Foramina for atypical sensory nerves and primitive ventral roots, seen looking down on the floor of the braincase. B. Foramina for primitive dorsal roots. C. Base of skull seen from underneath, showing exit points for nerves VII (stylomastoid foramen) and XII (hypoglossal canal).

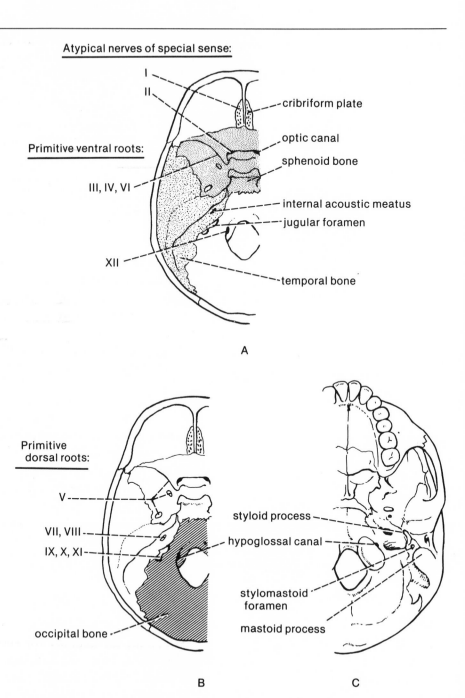

Atypical nerves of special sense:

I
II
cribriform plate
optic canal
sphenoid bone

Primitive ventral roots:

III, IV, VI

internal acoustic meatus
jugular foramen

XII

temporal bone

A

Primitive dorsal roots:

V
VII, VIII
IX, X, XI

occipital bone

B

styloid process
hypoglossal canal

stylomastoid foramen
mastoid process

C

All divisions run through separate holes in the sphenoid bone.

three major divisions, which are identified by subscripts: V_1, V_2, V_3. The ophthalmic nerve (V_1) is the general sensory nerve of the eye and orbit. If you get punched in the eye, the stars you see are optic-nerve hallucinations; but the pain you feel comes to you by courtesy of V_1.

The other two divisions of the trigeminal leave the skull through separate holes, also in the sphenoid bone (Fig. 19-4). The **maxillary** division (V_2), which is the sensory nerve of the upper jaw and the overlying skin (Fig. 18-3), exits through a round foramen located just below the superior orbital fissure. From this **foramen rotundum,** nerve V_2 emerges into a deep cleft between the sphenoid and the inflated back face of the upper jaw. This cleft is called the **pterygopalatine fossa** (Fig. 21-14). (If you can, get a human skull, pass a probe through the foramen rotundum, and check this for yourself; it is hard to visualize without actually seeing it.)

Behind and lateral to the foramen rotundum, the **mandibular** division (V_3) of the trigeminal leaves the braincase through a larger, oval hole—the **foramen ovale** (Fig. 19-3). The mandibular nerve sends sensory fibers to the *lower* jaw—and to the neighboring skin and gut lining, including the front two-thirds of the tongue. *It also carries all the motor fibers that supply the muscles of the first branchial arch.*

Seen from the inside of the braincase, the sphenoid's lesser wings form the sharp back edge of the anterior cranial fossa. The *greater* wings contribute to the floor of the **middle cranial fossa,** where the brain's temporal lobes lie (Figs. 19-1 and 19-3). The line separating the two fossae runs through the sphenoid's body in the midline. Like the anterior fossa, the middle fossa is roofed and walled by dermal bones (parietals and the squamous parts of the temporal bones).

TEMPORAL BONE

The core of the temporal bone is its **petrous** part (Fig. 19-4), which surrounds the ear apparatus. It is the third and last of the bony sense-organ capsules. It starts out as a mass of cartilage that condenses around the inner ear's labyrinth. The first pharyngeal pouch grows out of the pharynx underneath this cartilage and expands to form the middle-ear cavity. The cavity's connection with the pharynx narrows to become the **auditory** (or eustachian) **tube.** After the cartilage is replaced by bone, the bone and the middle-ear cavity get intimately entangled with each other. First, the petrous temporal sends out bony shelves that enclose the cavity in a hard protective shell. Then branching outgrowths from the cavity penetrate these shelves, inflating them

[Handwritten margin notes:]

Temporal bone:
- petrous part (that includes the mastoid processes).
- squamous part - flat bone
- tympanic part - bony ring around the eardrum
- styloid processes

In the petrous part:
1. internal acoustic meatus — entrance for → facial nerve VII / vestibulocochlear VIII
2. stylomastoid foramen → exit for VII
3. carotid canal → exit for carotid artery
4. foramen lacerum → not a real foramen because in real life it is filled with cartilage.

---

into masses of small air cells separated by thin osseous walls—a sort of bony foam. The largest cluster of these air cells invades the back end of the petrous temporal, expanding it into a projecting air-filled lump called the **mastoid process** (Gk., "breast-shaped"). You can feel your own mastoid process as a hard bump directly behind the point where your external ear sticks out from your head (Fig. 19-5).

An adult's temporal bone incorporates three other bones that fuse with the petrous temporal after birth:

1. The **squamous** part is a large thin sheet of dermal bone that forms the lateral wall of the braincase above the ear hole. It also spreads medially in front of the ear to form the socket of the jaw joint (Figs. 19-3 and 19-5).

2. The **tympanic** part of the temporal bone forms as a ring of dermal bone around the eardrum. After birth, it expands laterally and becomes a bony tube surrounding the ear hole (the **external acoustic meatus**) that leads in to the eardrum from outside (Fig. 19-4).

3. The **styloid process,** projecting down from the underside of the skull (Figs. 19-6 and 21-10), is derived from cartilages of the second gill arch. It fuses with the petrous temporal, in front of and medial to the mastoid process. Several muscles and ligaments derived from the old gill-arch apparatus attach to it.

Even without these three add-ons, the petrous temporal all by itself would be the most complicated bone in the body, because so many nerves, veins, and arteries pass into, around, or through it. The facial (VII) and vestibulocochlear (VIII) nerves enter it on its inner surface, alongside the back end of the brain stem, through the so-called **internal acoustic meatus** (Fig. 19-3). (Note that this internal "meatus" is a nerve foramen; it has nothing in common with the *external* acoustic meatus [Fig. 19-4], through which nothing ordinarily passes except sound waves and earwax.) Nerve VIII ends on the organs of the inner ear, so it never emerges from the petrous temporal bone. Its companion nerve, VII, follows a winding course through the bone and comes out via the **stylomastoid foramen,** between the mastoid and styloid processes (Fig. 19-6). The internal carotid artery also traverses a sinuous channel—the **carotid canal**—through the petrous temporal bone. The artery curves upward along the medial side of the middle-ear cavity (Figs. 19-4 and 21-12) and enters the braincase through a hole at the front end of the petrous temporal. It then runs forward, lateral to the hypophyseal fossa, leaving a **carotid groove** on the body of the sphenoid.

The anterior tip of the human petrous temporal usually does not get replaced by bone, so a dollop of cartilage persists here in the adult. When a skull is cleaned for study, this cartilage is removed, thus leaving a jagged hole called the **foramen lacerum** (L., "jagged hole"; Figs. 19-3 and 19-5). This is not a real foramen, and should not be confused with the carotid canal.

The glossopharyngeal (IX), vagus (X), and accessory (XI) nerves— that is, the motor nerves to the last four pharyngeal arches—leave the skull through a hole between the petrous temporal and the basicranial bone behind it, the occipital (Fig. 19-6). This hole also transmits the internal jugular vein that drains blood from the brain. It is accordingly called the **jugular foramen.**

OCCIPITAL BONE

There are two major parts to the occipital bone. Its *squamous* part is a large dermal bone that forms the projecting back end of the head. The *basilar* part of the occipital is a cartilage-replacement bone, representing the pasted-together vertebral elements of the occipital somites. It forms as four separate bones that fuse together into a vertebralike ring around the spinal cord and then merge with the squamous part above. The hole enclosed by the occipital "vertebra" is the **foramen magnum** (Fig. 19-5). Through it, the spinal cord enters the braincase, along with the vertebral arteries and the spinal root of the accessory nerve (XI). The basilar part of the occipital is also pierced on each side by the hypoglossal nerve (XII), which innervates the occipital myotomes that become the muscles of the tongue.

The petrous temporal has a sharp upper edge where it is exposed on the inside of the braincase (Fig. 19-3). This edge marks the boundary between the middle cranial fossa (for the brain's temporal lobes) and the **posterior cranial fossa,** where the cerebellum lies. The floor of the posterior fossa is formed by the occipital bone, with a little help from the two petrous temporals in front. The fossa's back, walls, and roof are formed by dermal bones—the two **parietals** (L. *paries,* "wall"), which cover most of the back half of the cerebrum, and the squamous (or dermal) part of the occipital.

■ The Membrane Bones of the Skull

The cartilage-replacement bones of the skull base are ancient associates of the brain, and each is pierced by some of the cranial nerves streaming out from the brain stem. The dermal or membrane bones*:flat bones* that form the roof of our braincase originally had nothing to do with the brain at all.

In the first land-dwelling vertebrates, the basicranium was all the braincase there was (Fig. 19-7A). It did not cover the dorsal surface of the brain, but merely cradled it from underneath. Far above the top of the tiny brain, just below the skin, a **head shield** or skull roof of membrane bone enclosed and protected all the soft tissues of the head—including the jaw muscles. These muscles originated from the *inner* surface of the head shield and ran down between the head shield and brain to attach to the lower jaw. The head of an amphibian or a primitive reptile like a turtle is thus mostly full of muscle.

In the reptiles that evolved into mammals, part of the head shield on each side was reduced to a sheet of tough fascia (Fig. 19-7B). Other lines of reptiles developed similar defects elsewhere in the head shield, so there must have been some advantage to doing this—but nobody knows for sure what it was. For whatever reason, the new "hole" in our ancestors' skull roof expanded, thereby leaving the brain unprotected on either side. The defect was filled in by new, deeper-lying bony walls that grew down from the skull roof, between

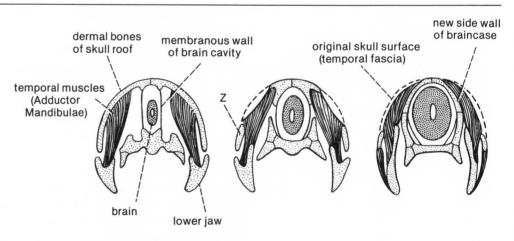

Fig. 19-7 Evolution of the skull roof. Schematic cross sections through the heads of a typical primitive reptile (A), mammal-like reptile (B), and mammal (C). Z, zygomatic arch.

dermal bones of skull roof

membranous wall of brain cavity

new side wall of braincase

original skull surface (temporal fascia)

temporal muscles (Adductor Mandibulae)

Z

brain

lower jaw

A　　　　　B　　　　　C

the jaw muscles and the dura mater. In the early mammals (Fig. 19-7C), these new side walls extended all the way down to the basicranium and formed a complete tube of bone around the brain—the condition seen in a human skull. The chewing muscles lie *outside* this new skull roof. The original edges of the head shield remain sticking out to either side like jug handles. From these handles—the **zygomatic arches**—the **masseter** component of the mammalian jaw muscles stretches downward to the lower jawbone (Fig. 21-13).

The bones of the face also are dermal bones, derived from the snout part of the old head shield. In fish, they protect the eyes and nose and provide a tooth-bearing covering for the primitive upper and lower jaws. Their homologs in our skull—the **frontal, zygomatic, nasal, vomer, lacrimal, palatine,** and **maxillary** bones, and the **mandible** (Fig. 19-5)—still serve similar functions.

■ The Gill-Arch Bones of the Skull

The rest of the bones in our skull are derived from the gill arches. Inside each gill arch of a fish, there forms a chain of small cartilage-replacement bones linked by synovial joints. The branchial muscles bind these bones to each other and to the skull, and flex the joints between them.

Primitive vertebrates, like living lampreys and hagfishes, had no jaws. The first jaws were formed from two bones of the first, or **mandibular,** gill arch (Fig. 19-8B). One of these first-arch bones grew forward under the braincase to form a primitive upper jaw on each side; the other swung forward below the mouth to become the lower jaw. The synovial hinge between upper and lower jaw elements persisted as the jaw joint. This joint was held in place by a bone of the second, or **hyoid,** arch that moved up to prop the back of the upper jaw against the braincase (Fig. 19-8C). The muscles of the first arch became jaw adductors, pulling the two first-arch bones together when they contracted. The resulting setup, retained in sharks, delivers a very satisfactory bite (from the shark's viewpoint, at any rate).

In our fishy ancestors, the primitive upper and lower jaws became sheathed in, and eventually replaced by, dermal bones bearing **teeth.** Teeth apparently evolved from fish scales. (Many sharks have tiny teeth all over their skin in addition to the big ones set in their jaws.) Like the skin itself, our teeth have a living inner layer and a dead outer layer. The tooth's living core, made of a sort of dense bone

Fig. 19-8 How jaws evolved. Primitive verte-brates (A) lacked jaws and probably had more than six gill arches. After the first two or three arches were lost, the bones of the mandibular arch became the primitive upper and lower jaws (B), and second-arch elements eventually moved forward to prop the upper jaw against the base of the skull (C). H, hyomandibular (mammalian stapes); S, spiracle (first gill slit).

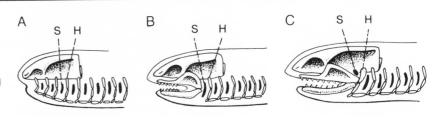

called **dentin,** extends into a socket in the maxilla or mandible. A layer of hard **cementum** encases the tooth's embedded **root.** The cementum is bound to the bone of the socket by fibrous tissue that allows the tooth to wiggle a bit in the socket, giving us a delicate sense of the pressures on each tooth when we chew. The exposed **crown** of the tooth is protected by a white shell of **enamel.** This extremely hard coating is deposited by specialized neural-crest cells, which surround the developing crown within the jaw and get stripped off when the tooth erupts into the mouth.

The tooth has a central hollow—the **pulp cavity**—containing nerves and blood vessels. Nerve fibers and other cellular processes radiate from the pulp cavity into microscopic canals in the surrounding dentin, enabling the dentin to feel pain when it is damaged. Cells in the pulp cavity can repair such damage to a limited extent by laying down new dentin. But the enamel can neither feel pain nor repair itself when damaged. Tooth decay is therefore painless until it eats through the enamel into the dentin core of the tooth, whereupon it become both painful and dangerous. Unchecked infections of the teeth may spread to other organs and even kill. Primitive people, like other mammals, ate mostly tough or abrasive foods that kept the teeth scoured clean and helped prevent tooth decay. The soft, sweet, sticky diets that civilized folk relish nowadays make dental bills a necessary part of life.

The gill-arch bones that formed the primitive vertebrate jaws were gradually replaced by the tooth-bearing dermal bones surrounding them. In even the most primitive reptiles, the jaw muscles attached directly to the mandible, and the primitive lower jaw was reduced to a nubbin in back. This nubbin articulated with a similar remnant of the old upper jaw to form the jaw joint. In the reptiles that evolved into mammals, a new jaw joint developed between the mandible and the squamous part of the temporal bone. The little first-arch remnants were not needed any longer as part of the chewing machinery, and they lost their connection to the jaws. But they did not simply disappear; they moved into the middle ear and became two of the three tiny bones that link the eardrum to the fluid-filled inner ear (Chapter 21).

As already mentioned, another bone derived from the old first-arch skeleton was called into service to help fill in the side wall of the new mammalian braincase. This vagrant first-arch bone became the greater wing of the sphenoid in our own skulls.

▪ The Arteries of the Brain

The brain is ordinarily the blood-thirstiest organ in the human body, accounting for about 22 percent of the body's consumption of oxygen when at rest. There are no reserves of food or oxygen in the brain, so even a brief interruption of blood flow to our brain produces unconsciousness. Widespread cell death sets in if the flow is interrupted for more than a few minutes. Accordingly, the brain receives a copious blood supply via four major arteries: the two vertebral arteries and the two internal carotids. The primary branches of all four anastomose with each other and with their fellows of the opposite side and form an arterial circle at the base of the brain. This circular anastomosis—the **circulus arteriosus cerebri** (the circle of Willis)—forms a vascular ring around the optic chiasm and the stalk of the hypophysis.

The typical, symmetrical arrangement of the circulus arteriosus is shown in Figure 19-9. After entering the skull through the foramen magnum, the two vertebral arteries merge to form a midline **basilar** artery. The basilar artery runs forward below the brain stem, sending off branches to the hindbrain (including the cerebellum above). It ends by dividing into a pair of **posterior cerebral** arteries, which supply the rear ends of the cerebral hemispheres. The rest of the brain gets its blood via the internal carotids. Each internal carotid divides alongside the hypophysis into **anterior** and **middle cerebral** branches. The anterior cerebral artery supplies the medial surface of each hemisphere, where it presses against the other hemisphere. The middle cerebral artery takes care of the remainder. Three **communicating** arteries complete the arterial circle, linking the two anterior cerebral arteries and connecting the middle and posterior cerebrals on each side. However, the textbook setup shown in the figure is found in only about 40 percent of us; most people lack one of the communicating arteries or have some other harmless anomaly.

Beyond the arterial circle, there are few important anastomoses between cerebral arteries. The superficial arteries running over the

Fig. 19-9   The cerebral arterial circle and its branches, seen looking downward from inside the skull with the brain removed. The diaphragma sellae, which is the dura mater that roofs over the hypophyseal fossa, has been removed on the right side to expose the internal carotid in the cavernous sinus.

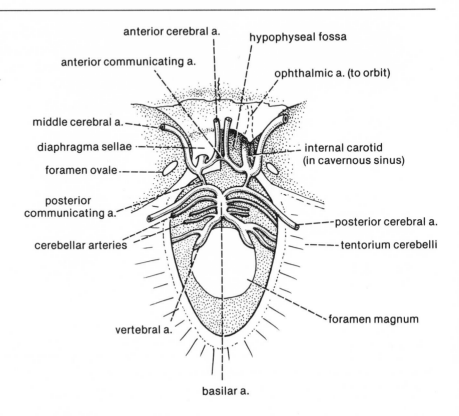

surface of the cortex usually anastomose with each other. But the deeper branches that plunge into the substance of the brain do not—so they can be fatally plugged up by a blood clot. Such a blockage, which may result in widespread cell death in the territory supplied by the plugged-up artery, is commonly known as a "stroke."

■ The Dural Venous Sinuses

Like the spinal cord, the brain is drained by superficial veins lying on the outside of the dura mater. When the new mammalian skull roof grew down around the brain, it trapped the brain's superficial veins between the dura mater and the inner periosteum of the skull roof. Because dura and periosteum fuse together everywhere else on the inside of the braincase, these venous channels are regarded as splitting the dura mater into "inner" and "outer" layers and lying in between the two. They are referred to as **dural venous sinuses.**

The dura follows the brain's major contours, dipping in and out of the clefts between the cerebral hemispheres and cerebellum. Most of the dural venous sinuses lie in the edges of these folds of dura (Fig. 19-10). Two of the folds are particularly large and important. The first is the midline fold that dips in between left and right hemispheres. It is called the **falx** (L., "sickle") **cerebri.** One venous sinus—the **inferior sagittal sinus**—hangs in the falx's free edge like the gut hanging from its dorsal mesentery. Above, the larger **superior sagittal sinus** runs along in the root of the falx, like the aorta in the root of the dorsal mesentery (Fig. 19-11).

The other major fold of dura is the **tentorium cerebelli,** which dips into the transverse cleft between the cerebellum and the cerebral hemispheres. It thus stretches horizontally over the cerebellum like a tent (hence its name), more or less perpendicular to the falx. The midline **straight sinus** runs back along the line where falx and tentorium meet. It receives the inferior sagittal sinus at its front end and has a variable communication with the superior sagittal sinus at the back. From that point in back, blood flows away to left and right

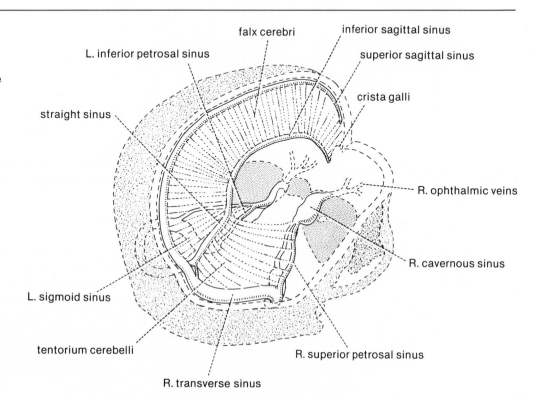

Fig. 19-10 The cranial venous sinuses and principal dural folds, seen looking downward and forward from the right. The stippling inside the braincase indicates the middle cranial fossa.

falx cerebri

inferior sagittal sinus

L. inferior petrosal sinus

superior sagittal sinus

crista galli

straight sinus

R. ophthalmic veins

R. cavernous sinus

L. sigmoid sinus

tentorium cerebelli

R. superior petrosal sinus

R. transverse sinus

Fig. 19-11   Cross section of the brain and its meninges, showing the spaces filled with venous blood and cerebrospinal fluid.

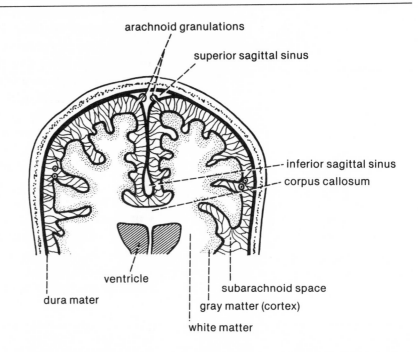

arachnoid granulations

superior sagittal sinus

inferior sagittal sinus

corpus callosum

ventricle

subarachnoid space

dura mater

gray matter (cortex)

white matter

through **transverse** sinuses running in the rear edge of the tentorium, where it is attached to the inner face of the occipital bone.

The tentorium is also attached (in front) to the upper edge of the petrous temporal. Its attachment there raises a sharp crest on the bone and encloses the backward-flowing **superior petrosal sinus.** The superior petrosal and transverse sinuses flow toward each other in the edge of the tentorium and join to form the **sigmoid sinus,** which is named for the S-shaped course it takes down the back edge of the petrous temporal toward the jugular foramen. As it leaves the skull through that foramen, the signoid sinus receives the small **inferior petrosal sinus** and becomes the internal jugular vein.

The superior and inferior petrosal sinuses on each side carry blood backward from two dural venous spaces lying on either side of the body of the sphenoid. These spaces are known as the **cavernous sinuses** because they are filled with connective-tissue strands that suggested the cavernous tissue of the penis to early anatomists. (It is surprising how many things looked like genitalia and breasts to early anatomists.) The **ophthalmic** veins that drain the eye and orbit pass back through the superior orbital fissure to enter the cavernous sinuses. Because these veins also transmit blood draining back from the upper part of the face, germs that get into facial veins (say, from a squeezed pimple) can wind up in the cavernous sinus. The connective-tissue strands there slow blood flow and furnish a hospitable surface for bacteria to grow on. Such infections in the cavernous sinus can be fatal unless treated with appropriate antibiotics. Avoid squeezing pimples.

The folds of dura mater dipping in between the brain's lobes and bulges not only enclose the brain's venous plumbing in their edges, but also provide the brain with support. The tentorium and falx cerebri are tough, taut structures, which serve as a sort of internal skeleton for the brain. (In some mammals, the tentorium lays down a rigid roof of bone over the cerebellum.) The whole outer surface of the dura acts as the skull's inner periosteum, and goes on depositing and resorbing bone throughout life to adjust the size and shape of the brain's bony enclosure.

The brain's most important protection from jars and bumps is the bath of cerebrospinal fluid in which it floats (Chapter 3). This lymphlike filtrate of blood plasma originates in the brain's central canal, which sports four large dilatations called **ventricles.** Vascular patches (**choroid plexuses**) in the ventricles' walls secrete the cerebrospinal fluid. It fills the ventricles and percolates out into the subarachnoid space through three small holes in the walls of the hindbrain. Cerebrospinal fluid returns to the general circulation through the superior sagittal sinus (Figs. 19-10 and 19-11). The subarachnoid space does not just open into the superior sagittal sinus directly; instead, outgrowths of the arachnoid mater protrude into the sinus through holes in the dura. The fluid inside these balloonlike **arachnoid granulations** diffuses through the arachnoid into the surrounding blood.

It is not clear how the cerebrospinal fluid surrounding the spinal cord fits into this picture. The spinal part of the subarachnoid space may just be a stagnant cul-de-sac of the cranial part, with no circulation of cerebrospinal fluid. But some experiments suggest that the spinal fluid gets drained off somehow at the bottom through vertebral veins and replenished by fresh brain-secreted fluid flowing in at the top.

In some infants, the cerebrospinal fluid is produced faster than it drains away. The accumulating fluid inflates the brain and the growing skull to abnormal size. This condition, which can result in brain damage and mental deficiency if not corrected, is called **hydrocephalus** (Gk., "water head").

Nose, Eye, and Ear

20

■ The Nasal Fossa and the Air Sinuses

The nasal passages start out as ectodermal pits. They grow deeper and deeper and soon pierce the roof of the mouth. In a frog, a turtle, or a human embryo, the internal nostrils are holes opening into the front of the mouth—behind and above where the front teeth would be if embryos, frogs, and turtles had any.

In the human fetus, a shelf of tissue grows in from the upper jaw on either side (Fig. 21-16A). These two shelves meet in the midline and ossify, thereby forming a bony roof over the mouth. This partition, the **hard palate,** separates the mouth below from the **nasal fossa** above. Most of it forms as an extension from the tooth-bearing upper jaw bone—the maxilla—but the back edge of the palate is formed by a pair of separate **palatine** bones (Fig. 21-16B). Another membrane bone—the **vomer** (Fig. 19-5)—grows upward from the midline of the palate and meets the vertical plate of the ethmoid. The two form a bony **nasal septum** in the midline between the left and right nasal passages (Fig. 20-1B).

The palate is characteristic of mammals. It allows us to breathe when our mouths are full of food or drink. What is more important is that it allows newborn mammals to suck milk from their mothers. We can see the palate's value most clearly when we look at babies with cleft palates, whose unfused palatine shelves have left them with a broad, reptilelike communication between mouth and nose. When they try to suckle, air rushes into the mouth through the nose and breaks the vacuum needed for sucking; and any milk they manage to press out erupts into their noses and makes them sneeze when they try to swallow. They usually manage to drink enough to survive, but they make a mess of it.

Walling off the nasal fossa from the mouth yielded some additional benefits for the early mammals. The organs inside their nasal passages could become far more elaborate and fragile once they became pro-

Fig. 20-1 The nasal fossa and its walls, displayed by sections through the head a little to the right (A) and left (B) of the midline nasal septum. White arrows in (A) show the connections of the frontal and sphenoid air sinuses with the nasal fossa. In (B), the mucous membrane covering the septum has been stripped off to display its constituent bones and cartilage.

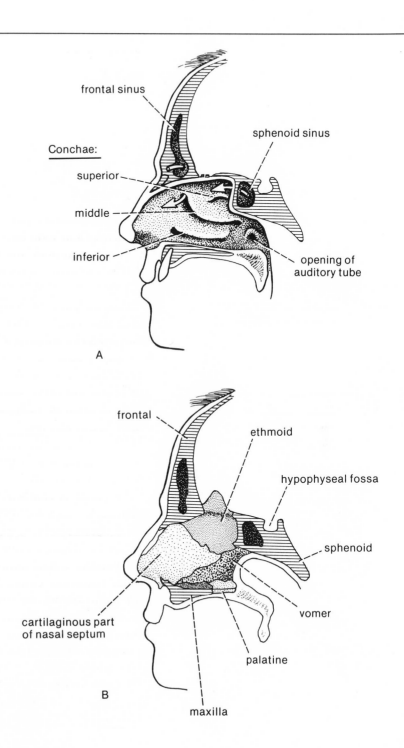

tected from all the crunching and slurping going on in the mouth. In most mammals today, the side walls of each nasal passage sprout delicate, branching scrolls of bone called **turbinals,** which fill the hollow tubular snout. The turbinals provide a vastly increased nasal surface, for detecting odors and for cooling the body by evaporation during panting.

Human beings have a rather feeble sense of smell and use the whole skin surface for cooling by evaporating sweat, so we no longer need such an elaborate nasal apparatus. Our turbinals are reduced to three little downward-curving bony shelves—the **conchae** (Fig. 20-1A), which just provide enough mucosal surface for warming and humidifying the air we inhale. The three spaces roofed over by the overhanging conchae are called the superior, middle, and inferior **meatuses of the nose.** Other cranial spaces open into the nasal fossa through holes in the lateral wall of each meatus. The nasolacrimal duct, through which tears drain into the nose (see below), opens into the inferior meatus. The other two meatuses contain the nasal openings of the air sacs that fill the hollow bones of the skull.

Why are many of the bones of the skull filled with air? The braincase stops enlarging early in childhood, but the bones of the face keep growing until well after puberty. As a result, the inner and outer surfaces of the skull become widely separated in the facial region. The intervening spaces could be filled with solid bone or fluid, but that would make the head needlessly heavy. Instead, as these cranial "waste spaces" develop, they are invaded by air-filled outpocketings of the nasal fossa. These air sacs are called the **paranasal air sinuses.** The principal sinuses and their openings into the nasal fossa are diagrammed in Figures 19-2 and 20-1. The mastoid process of the temporal bone is also filled with air cells, which communicate with the nasal fossa indirectly (via the middle-ear cavity and the auditory tube). A small maxillary sinus is present at birth, but the mastoid cells and other air sinuses do not appear until later on, when facial growth begins to run ahead of brain growth.

▪ The Eye

The eye forms as a photosensitive lobe of the brain lying just under the skin. During development, the lobe becomes indented to form a two-layered cup—the **retina**—connected with the rest of the brain through the optic nerve (Fig. 20-2). The inner layer of the retinal cup,

Fig. 20-2 The eye in a 10-mm human embryo (A), and its front (B) and back (C) ends in an adult. Diagrammatic horizontal sections.

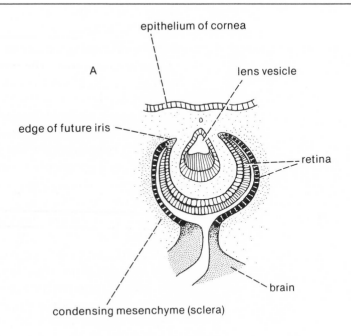

A

epithelium of cornea

lens vesicle

edge of future iris

retina

brain

condensing mesenchyme (sclera)

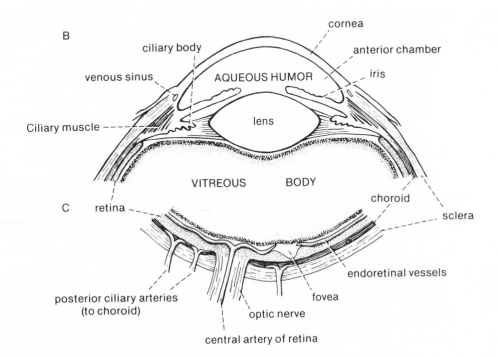

B

cornea

ciliary body

anterior chamber

venous sinus

AQUEOUS HUMOR

iris

Ciliary muscle

lens

VITREOUS   BODY

choroid

sclera

C   retina

endoretinal vessels

posterior ciliary arteries
(to choroid)

fovea

optic nerve

central artery of retina

onto which light falls after birth, gives rise to the retina's light-detecting receptor cells (rods and cones) as well as to the retinal neurons that relay visual information from the receptors to the brain. The outer layer of the retinal cup becomes a darkly pigmented sheet one cell thick. This cell layer absorbs light to keep it from bouncing around inside the eye and blurring the image. (Cameras are painted black on the inside for the same reason.)

As the lens vesicle invaginates and pinches off from the embryonic "skin" (Chapter 18), the rim of the retinal cup grows forward around it. The cup's opening narrows until only a small circular aperture—the **pupil**—remains. Retinal cells around the pupil's margin differentiate into smooth muscles that control the size of the aperture: a circular **Sphincter Pupillae** that shrinks the pupil and a radial **Dilator Pupillae** that opens it wide. The Sphincter contracts under parasympathetic impulses (via nerve III) that vary with the amount of light falling on the retina. But the Sphincter's antagonist, the Dilator muscle, contracts under *sympathetic* impulses—which originate down in the spinal cord and are not governed by retinal light levels. Our pupils therefore dilate briefly in response to any surge of excitement or interest. People read each other's pupils unconsciously to gauge emotional states. Artists and photographers use pupillary dilation more deliberately to produce cute or sexy facial expressions. The drug belladonna takes its name (It. *bella donna,* "beautiful woman") from a similar use by Italian courtesans of the Renaissance, who found that they could give themselves bedroom eyes by taking this stimulant to dilate their pupils.

The eye lies in the prechordal part of the head, so practically all its tissues develop from ectoderm of some sort. The retina derives from the dorsal nerve cord. So do the smooth muscles of the pupil(!). The lens forms as an invagination of the overlying "skin." Mesenchymal cells derived from neural-crest ectoderm condense around the retinal cup and differentiate into two concentric layers: (1) a vascular layer—the **choroid**—lying directly against the retina and (2) a more superficial, fibrous layer. This outermost fibrous layer forms the surface of the eyeball. It develops into the transparent **cornea** in front and the opaque, white **sclera** covering the rest of the eye. Pigment cells derived from neural crest also spread across the front of the pupillary muscles, producing the colored **iris** surrounding the pupil. The color of the iris depends on the amount of pigment in these cells: blue or green eyes have less pigment than brown ones.

Several important structures develop around the outer edge of the iris. Small blood vessels at the margin of the iris proliferate to form a ring-shaped mass of delicate vascular folds—the **ciliary body** (Fig. 20-2), which projects into the space between the iris and the lens. Like the analogous choroid plexuses of the brain, the ciliary body secretes a clear filtrate of blood plasma. This liquid, the **aqueous humor,** is the optic equivalent of cerebrospinal fluid. After bathing both sides of the iris and the inside of the cornea, aqueous humor drains off by osmosis into a tiny venous sinus that circles the sclerocorneal junction. If this drainage gets obstructed, aqueous humor accumulates and pressure builds up inside the eye. This condition, the optic equivalent of hydrocephalus, is called **glaucoma.** It can produce retinal damage and blindness.

The curved surface of the cornea does most of the job of bending incoming light to focus an image on the retina. All that the lens does is to make the finer adjustments that allow us to focus on objects at various distances. A camera's focus is changed by moving the lens forward and back, but we change the focus of our eye by changing the *shape* of the lens. This is accomplished by smooth **Ciliary muscles** lying behind the margin of the iris (Fig. 20-2). We might expect that these muscles would pull on the lens, flattening it out and thus increasing its focal distance, whenever we look at distant objects. Unfortunately, things work the other way: the lens is normally *held* flattened, by taut ligaments radiating from its rim. When we focus on things close at hand, the Ciliary muscles contract and relieve the tension on the ligaments, and the natural elasticity of the lens causes it to bulge. With age, the lens gets increasingly stiffer, and it eventually ceases to bulge when the tension is taken off—which is why most middle-aged people cannot focus on a book without using reading glasses. This shoddy focusing mechanism is an evolutionary makeshift. Reptiles and birds have a better setup (a belt of muscle around their lens *squeezes* it to make it bulge), but the small-eyed, nocturnal early mammals gave up focusing the eye altogether and lost this arrangement. When our monkeylike ancestors reinvented fine visual focus, they had to make do with leftover vestiges of the reptilian focusing apparatus.

The eye's light-transmitting tissues—the lens, the cornea, the aqueous humor, and the gelatinous **vitreous body** filling the center of the eyeball (Fig. 20-2B)—need to be perfectly transparent to avoid blurring of the retinal image. These tissues therefore contain no blood vessels. Whatever living cells they contain get nourished indirectly, by diffusion and by nutrients dissolved in the aqueous humor. Corneas can be freely transplanted without any danger of tissue rejection.

The other tissues of the eye contain blood capillaries. These are supplied via the **ophthalmic** branch of the internal carotid artery. After emerging from its canal in the petrous temporal bone, the internal carotid runs forward (inside the cavernous sinus) and then curves abruptly upward and backward to pierce the dura and enter the cerebral arterial circle. It gives off the ophthalmic artery at the apex of this hairpin curve (Fig. 19-9). The ophthalmic artery runs forward alongside the optic nerve into the eye socket, where it breaks up into a complex bush of branches (Fig. 20-3A). Its **ciliary** branches enter the eyeball and supply a network of capillaries in the choroid layer, on the outer surface of the retina. This network is a bit too far from the innermost layers of the retina to keep them alive, and it has to be supplemented with another capillary network on the inside of the retina. This second network is provided by another ophthalmic-artery branch—the **central artery of the retina,** which enters the eye within the optic nerve and branches out on the retina's inner surface (Fig. 20-2C). The blood in this endoretinal network of vessels does interfere with vision. We occasionally become aware of its shadow on the retina when a bright light is flashed in our eyes.

Because the endoretinal capillaries are absent from one central spot on the retina, we have a small field of extremely precise vision free of blood-vessel shadows. Enough food and oxygen diffuses in from the choroid to keep the receptor cells in this central patch alive. However, the retinal neurons that relay the receptors' impulses to the brain have to be shoved away from the patch in all directions so that they can be fed by the surrounding endoretinal capillaries. The central patch therefore takes the form of a pit inside a ring-shaped hump of displaced relay neurons. This pit is called the **fovea** (Fig. 20-2C). If the foveal receptors or their relay neurons are damaged by disease or injury (say, by looking too long at the sun), our fine central vision is irreparably lost and only a much fuzzier peripheral vision remains. Your ability to read this book depends on a two-square-millimeter patch of cells in the floor of each retinal fovea.

▪ The Orbit

The human eyeball sits in its conical bony socket, or **orbit,** like a small scoop of vanilla in a large ice cream cone. Practically every bone in

Fig. 20-3 The arteries of the right orbit (A) and corresponding branches of V₁ (B), exposed from above by removing the bony floor of the anterior cranial fossa. C, ciliary arteries; L, long ciliary nerves.

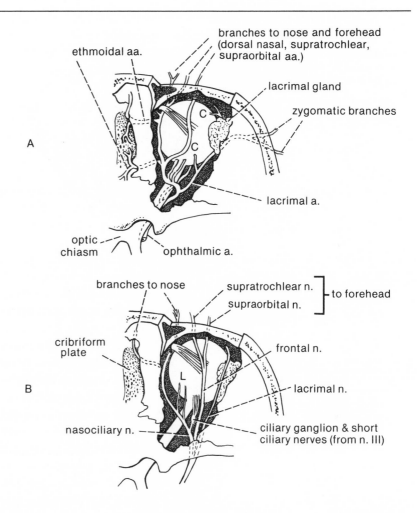

the region contributes to the orbit's walls (Fig. 19-2). The orbit encloses not only the eye, but also the eye's auxiliary apparatus, including the tear-secreting **lacrimal** gland and the little muscles that turn the eyeball this way and that.

There are six of these muscles (Fig. 20-4). The four **Rectus** muscles—superior and inferior, medial and lateral—arise back at the apex of the orbital cone, from a fibrous ring around the optic nerve. They run forward to attach to the eyeball at four equally spaced points around its equator (halfway between the front and back poles). There are also two **Oblique** muscles—a superior and an inferior. They run laterally away from the orbit's medial wall and wrap back-

Fig. 20-4 The extrinsic muscles of the right eye. A. View from above, with the orbit's bony roof removed. B. The two Oblique muscles seen from the front.

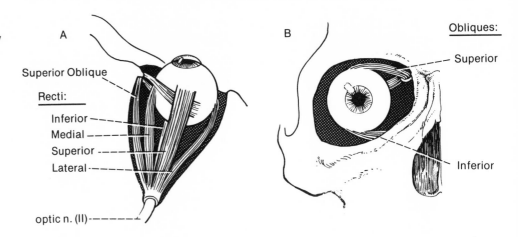

A

Superior Oblique

Recti:

Inferior
Medial
Superior
Lateral

optic n. (II)

B

Obliques:

Superior

Inferior

ward around the eyeball, inserting into its lateral side. The Inferior Oblique arises directly from the orbital wall; the Superior Oblique arises with the Recti and hooks through a fascial pulley high up on the medial wall of the orbit. From the pulley on, its course and attachments parallel those of the Inferior Oblique below it.

The actions of these muscles are not exactly what you might expect. Obviously each Rectus turns the eye in its own direction: the Superior Rectus swivels it upward, the Lateral Rectus abducts it (swings it laterally), and so on. Not so obviously, the Obliques and the upper and lower Recti act together to abduct and adduct the eye and hold it in certain positions—as shown in Figure 20-5.

All six muscles are innervated by primitive ventral roots. Two of the six have their own private cranial nerves. The **abducens** nerve (VI) innervates the Lateral Rectus, which *abducts* the eye. The **trochlear nerve (IV)** is so named because it supplies the Superior Oblique, which passes through a fascial **trochlea** (Gk., "pulley") on the medial wall of the orbit. The other four muscles are supplied by cranial nerve III, the **oculomotor** (L., "eye-moving") nerve.

The oculomotor nerve provides us with our first and simplest example of a cranial parasympathetic pathway. It carries the parasympathetic motor fibers that control the shape of the lens and pupil. Once inside the orbit, these fibers leave nerve III and synapse in the **ciliary ganglion,** a pinkish lump the size of a BB shot lying back near the orbit's apex (Fig. 20-3). Postsynaptic fibers from the ganglion run

oculomotur nerve also supplies the ciliary muscles

forward as a bundle of eight or so **short ciliary** nerves, and enter the eyeball in back to be distributed to the Ciliary and pupillary muscles.

The trigeminal's **ophthalmic** division (V_1) enters the orbit along with the oculomotor, trochlear, and abducens nerves. The ophthalmic nerve is the general sensory nerve to the orbit and its contents. Some of its sensory fibers reach the eyeball through the short ciliary nerves; others form separate *long* ciliary nerves that enter the eyeball near the edge of the cornea. In addition, the long ciliary nerves convey sympathetic fibers to the Dilator muscle of the pupil (Chapter 21).

The ophthalmic nerve also furnishes sensation to the nose and to the skin above the eye—from the upper eyelid up to the crown of the head—but not to the *lower* eyelid (Fig. 18-3). This difference between the two eyelids reflects the fundamental embryology of the face. The mouth of a five-week embryo (Fig. 20-6) is bounded by three rounded humps of tissue: the **frontonasal** process above, the **mandibular** process below, and a cheeklike **maxillary** process on each side. The

---

Fig. 20-5 The actions produced by the extrinsic muscles of the eye vary in abduction and adduction. The Oblique muscles raise and lower the adducted eyeball; but because they pass behind the eye's vertical axis (*black dot*), they can help the Lateral Rectus to hold the eye in an abducted position.

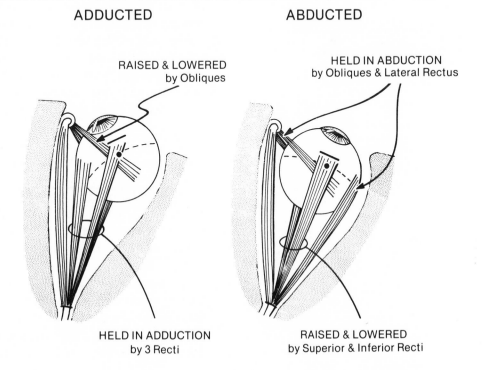

ADDUCTED

RAISED & LOWERED
by Obliques

HELD IN ADDUCTION
by 3 Recti

ABDUCTED

HELD IN ABDUCTION
by Obliques & Lateral Rectus

RAISED & LOWERED
by Superior & Inferior Recti

Fig. 20-6 How the ontogeny of the embryonic (A) and fetal (B) face correlates with its sensory innervation. The central part of the upper lip is secondarily invaded by fibers of V₂, after the nasolacrimal duct closes over; compare Fig. 18-3.

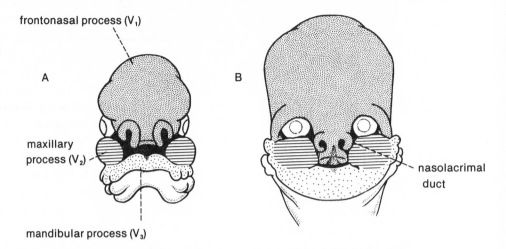

frontonasal process (V₁)

A

B

maxillary process (V₂)

nasolacrimal duct

mandibular process (V₃)

ophthalmic nerve (V₁) innervates the frontonasal process; the maxillary (V₂) and mandibular (V₃) divisions of the trigeminal innervate the correspondingly named processes. The eyeball is tucked into the cleft between frontonasal and maxillary processes, and so the two lids that grow over it are supplied by different trigeminal divisions.

The two eyelids fuse together briefly, enclosing the **conjunctival sac,** which is a flattened bag of specialized transparent "skin" (conjunctiva) applied to the front of the cornea. From the upper lateral margin of the sac, an invaginating pouch of ectoderm grows up and back into the orbit and forms the **lacrimal** gland (Fig. 20-3). After birth, when the eyelids are separated again and the sac is open to the air, tears secreted by the gland keep the conjunctiva from drying out. If we secrete too many tears, they spill out of the conjunctival sac and trickle down the face; but tears in normal amounts are carried away through little tubes in the edge of each eyelid (near the nose) and emptied into the inferior meatus of the nose. The **nasolacrimal duct** through which tears flow into the nose is simply the roofed-over groove between the embryo's frontonasal and maxillary processes (Fig. 20-6).

The lower eyelid is a more or less immobile flap of tissue, but the upper eyelid can be raised and lowered like a curtain, to wipe off the conjunctiva and shut out light. The upper eyelid is raised by a specialized slip of the Superior Rectus, called **Levator Palpebrae Superioris.** Like its parent muscle, it is innervated via nerve III. A wisp of smooth muscle in each eyelid (the tarsal muscle) pulls the eyelids farther apart under sympathetic stimulation, thus producing the staring expression seen in "fight-or-flight" situations.

■ The Inner Ear

The vesicle that forms the inner ear starts out as a simple sac of ectoderm, but growth and resorption change it into a maze of tiny ducts called the **membranous labyrinth** (Fig. 20-7A). Two complexes of ducts can be distinguished. An anterior outpouching of the sac called the **cochlear duct** houses the end organs of hearing. In mammals, it is so long (for detecting a broad range of pitches) that it has to be rolled into a helix to fit inside the petrous temporal. The three

Fig. 20-7 Labyrinths of the ear. A. Left membranous labyrinth seen from the left side. B. Diagram of membranous labyrinth inside bony labyrinth. Schematic horizontal section, seen from above.

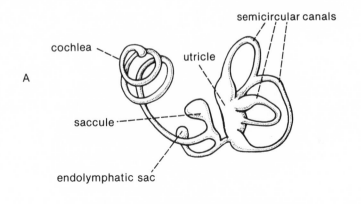

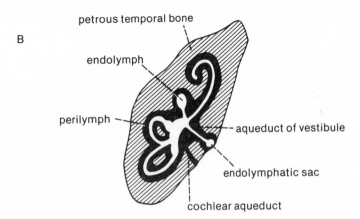

semicircular ducts develop from the posterior part of the inner-ear vesicle; a dilatation, or ampulla, at the base of each duct houses the receptors of our sense of balance.

The membranous labyrinth is suspended inside a similarly shaped but fatter cavity inside the petrous temporal bone (Fig. 20-7B). This cavity is the bony labyrinth. It is continuous with the subarachnoid space surrounding the brain (via a little duct called the cochlear aqueduct), and the perilymph that fills it is indistinguishable from cerebrospinal fluid. The endolymph that fills the inner, membranous labyrinth has a different composition and is presumably secreted somehow by the cells enclosing it. Sound striking the eardrum is converted into pressure waves in the perilymph, which in turn produce distortions in the membranous labyrinth. These distortions cause detector cells inside the membranous labyrinth to fire and send nerve impulses on to the brain—where they are perceived as sound.

21

The Pharyngeal Gut

In a primitive fish (Fig. 21-1), the pharyngeal arches form six U-shaped bands of voluntary muscle with little bones in them. These muscular slings suspend the pharynx from the overlying braincase. When the muscles contract, they squeeze the water out of the pharynx through slits between the arches. Feathery gills protruding into these slits pick up oxygen from the water and dump CO_2 into it as it rushes past.

In the human head, there are no gill slits. Gas exchange is handled by the lungs. Freed from their respiratory duties, the bones and muscles of our pharyngeal arches have been remodeled for doing things that fish do not need to do: speaking, transmitting airborne sound to the inner ear, chewing, sucking, blinking the eyelids, and so on. But some of the muscles of the posterior arches have preserved the old pharynx-squeezing function and have more or less primitive attachments. We will accordingly start this chapter with the tail end of the pharynx and work forward.

■ Vagal Territory: Arches 4 to 6

The last three pharyngeal arches get their innervation from the vagus nerve. (Most of these motor fibers emerge from the brain through the cranial root of nerve XI, which we will treat hereafter as part of the vagus.) To reach the pharynx, the vagal branches have to pass between the embryonic aortic arches. When the aortic arches slide down into the thorax, most of the vagal fibers to the posterior pharyngeal arches on each side get pulled into a loop that descends into the thorax and runs back up along the esophagus to the pharynx. This loop is the **recurrent laryngeal** nerve (Fig. 8-8). More anterior vagal fibers do not get dragged down into the thorax by the descent of the aortic arches. They form simple, direct **pharyngeal** and **superior**

Fig. 21-1 Superficial branchial muscles in a shark (A) and a reptile (B). The gray tint indicates the second-arch musculature.

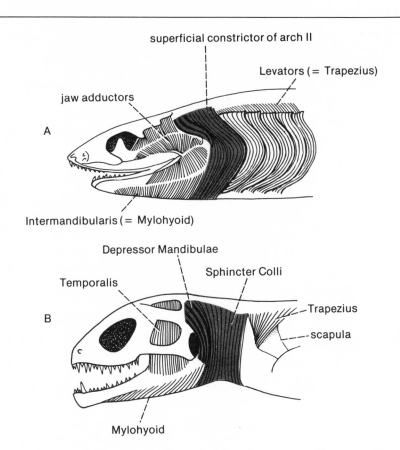

laryngeal nerves that run straight to the pharyngeal wall in the neck (Fig. 21-2).

The primitive arrangement of the fourth-arch muscles is seen in the **Inferior Constrictor of the pharynx.** This fan-shaped muscle has a long origin from a tendinous raphe that hangs down behind the gut and is fastened above to the underside of the occipital bone. From this raphe, the Inferior Constrictor's fibers sweep forward around either side of the gut tube and converge to attach to the remaining skeletal elements of the last three arches. In mammals these elements remain cartilaginous in the adult, forming the cartilages of the **larynx,** or voice box (Figs. 21-2 and 21-3). When the Inferior Constrictor contracts, it pulls the larynx back toward the tendinous raphe. Its contraction squeezes the contents of the pharynx down into the

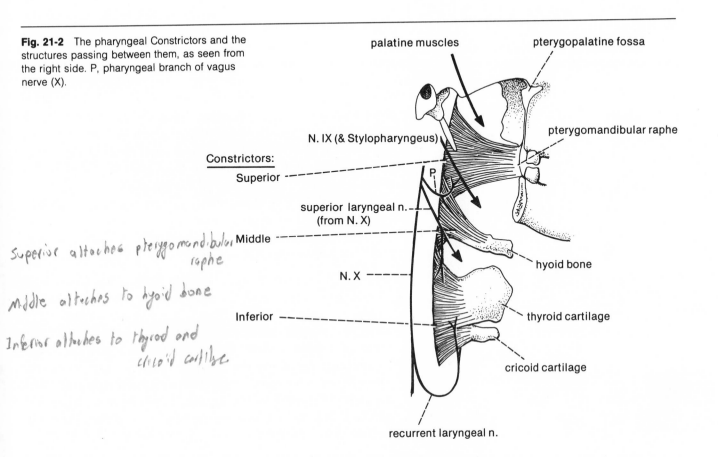

Fig. 21-2 The pharyngeal Constrictors and the structures passing between them, as seen from the right side. P, pharyngeal branch of vagus nerve (X).

palatine muscles

pterygopalatine fossa

N. IX (& Stylopharyngeus)

pterygomandibular raphe

Constrictors:

Superior

P

superior laryngeal n. (from N. X)

Middle

hyoid bone

N. X

thyroid cartilage

Inferior

cricoid cartilage

recurrent laryngeal n.

Superior attaches pterygomandibular raphe

Middle attaches to hyoid bone

Inferior attaches to thyroid and cricoid cartilage

esophagus when we swallow—or up into the mouth and nose, when we regurgitate.

Two more fourth-arch muscles, the **Superior** and **Middle Constrictors,** that embrace the pharynx further up. They have similar attachments to the midline raphe in back and likewise act to squeeze the pharynx, but they have shifted their ventral attachments up toward the mouth end of the gut tube. The Superior Constrictor now inserts into a fibrous **pterygomandibular raphe** in the wall of the cheek behind the teeth. The Middle Constrictor inserts on the **hyoid** bone. This little bone, attached to the rest of the skeleton only by muscles and ligaments, combines skeletal elements of arches 2 and 3. It looks like a horseshoe (third-arch cartilage) with two horns (second-arch cartilage) growing out of its back (Figs. 21-3 and 22-2).

The Inferior Constrictor is innervated by the recurrent and superior laryngeal nerves, but the fourth-arch muscles that have shifted their attachments upward are supplied by the pharyngeal branch of the vagus (Fig. 21-2). This little branch joins the third-arch nerve (IX) and forms a plexus with it in the walls of the pharynx. Fibers of IX in this **pharyngeal plexus** carry sensation to the third-arch territory on the inside of the gut (Fig. 21-6) and also innervate the one remaining third-arch muscle (Stylopharyngeus). The vagal fibers in the plexus are motor to the upper Constrictors and some other displaced fourth-arch muscles around the upper end of the gut tube.

The pharyngeal branch of the vagus actually pierces the Middle Constrictor (and innervates it) on its way to the pharyngeal plexus. Other structures entering the pharynx from either side pass through three gaps left between the Constrictor origins in front (Fig. 21-2):

1. Through the uppermost gap, between the Superior Constrictor and the base of the skull, pass the muscles that move the soft palate.
2. Between the upper two Constrictors passes cranial nerve IX, the nerve of the third arch. The lone third-arch muscle (Stylopharyngeus) also enters the pharynx here, alongside the nerve.
3. Through the gap between the lower two Constrictors, the **internal laryngeal** branch of the superior laryngeal nerve enters the pharynx. This branch supplies sensory innervation to the 4th- through 6th-arch territory, including the larynx (Fig. 21-6).

The lower end of the Inferior Constrictor muscle blends right into the upper end of the esophagus, which, like the Inferior Constrictor, is made of voluntary, striated muscle. The lower end of the esophagus is composed of smooth muscle, which begins to replace striated muscle about a third of the way down. The recurrent laryngeal nerve, running back up the esophagus out of the thorax, sends branchial-motor fibers to the striated esophageal muscles. The lower, involuntary part of the esophagus is innervated directly by the vagus nerves, which form a plexus on its surface.

■ The Larynx

The stiff, cartilaginous larynx acts as a valve. When its muscles relax, it holds the windpipe open without effort; contracting, its muscles shut off the windpipe and keep food from getting shoved down it when we swallow. Early mammals found that forcing air out through the closed larynx could produce a musical buzz, a sort of pharyngeal Bronx cheer. Later mammals have modified this buzz to produce various bleating, growling, yelping, and howling sounds used in communication. In human speech, the humming noise produced by the larynx is modulated by complex and delicately controlled movements of the tongue, teeth, lips, and palate. The larynx just produces the background tone that makes all these movements of the eating machinery easier to hear. Monotonous but intelligible speech can be produced by substituting a mechanical buzzer—for example, in a cancer victim whose diseased larynx has been removed.

The base of the laryngeal skeleton (Fig. 21-3) is the ring-shaped **cricoid** cartilage, which sits on top of the column of U-shaped tracheal "rings." The **thyroid** (Gk., "shield-shaped") cartilage rests

Fig. 21-3 The larynx. A. Exploded diagram of the laryngeal skeleton. B. Lateral view of the larynx and Cricothyroid muscle. C. Interior of hemisected larynx. All views from the left side.

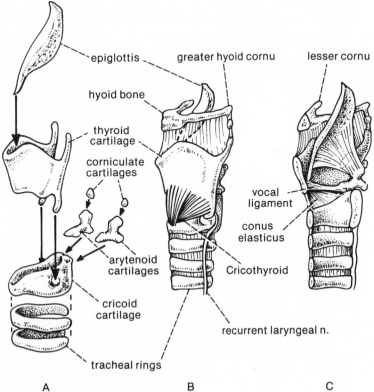

A   B   C

atop the cricoid. Like the tracheal cartilages, it is U-shaped and open behind. Its **inferior cornu** (L., "horn") on each side projects downward to a synovial facet on the cricoid ring. The whole thyroid cartilage can rock forward and backward on this pair of joints (Fig. 21-4). From two diminutive **arytenoid** cartilages perched on the back edge of the cricoid, inside the opening of the thyroid U, **vocal ligaments** stretch forward to the inside of the thyroid cartilage in front. When the thyroid rocks forward, these ligaments are drawn taut—making them vibrate audibly when air is forced between them. This produces the sound of the voice.

Most of the muscles of the larynx have names that reflect their attachments. They act on the skeleton of the larynx as follows:

Fig. 21-4 Actions of laryngeal muscles. A. Interior of hemisected larynx, showing how the Cricothyroid swings the thyroid cartilage forward and tightens the vocal ligaments (*dashed outlines*). B. Posterior view of cricoid and arytenoid cartilages and attached muscles: the left Posterior. Cricoarytenoid has been removed to expose the Lateral Cricoarytenoid in front of it. C and D. Diagrammatic views of the laryngeal opening (glottis) from above. The glottis is opened and the vocal folds swung apart by the Posterior Cricoarytenoids (C); Arytenoideus and the Lateral Cricoarytenoids have the opposite effect (D). SC, superior cornu of thyroid cartilage.

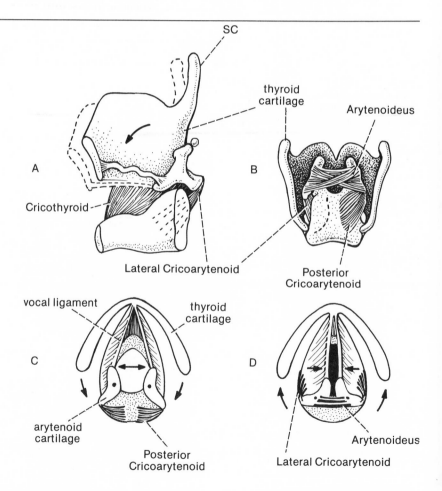

1. The **Cricothyroid** muscle (Fig. 21-3) swings the thyroid cartilage forward, thereby tensing the vocal ligaments and causing them to vibrate in the stream of air from the lungs. The harder the Cricothyroid contracts, the higher the pitch of the voice becomes.

2. The **Posterior Cricoarytenoid** muscle (Fig. 21-4) rotates the arytenoid cartilages laterally, thus widening the gap between the vocal ligaments. This has the effect of lowering the pitch of the voice.

3. The **Vocalis** muscles run alongside the vocal ligaments and share their attachments. They allow us to make delicate adjustments in the tension of the vocal ligaments.

The vocal ligament and Vocalis muscle on each side are covered with a single fold of mucous membrane, thereby producing the **vocal folds** or "vocal cords" that a doctor sees when he peers into your throat with a laryngoscope. These folds are continuous below with a cylinder of elastic connective tissue—the **conus elasticus** (Fig. 21-3), which is anchored around the rim of the cricoid ring.

4. The other laryngeal muscles (Lateral Cricoarytenoids, Arytenoideus, Thyroarytenoids, and so on) all act in one way or another to draw the vocal folds together and close the air passage, shutting off our wind. They contract in concert when we swallow.

All the laryngeal muscles are striated, gill-arch musculature and are derived from the last three branchial arches. The Cricothyroid is a specialized slip of the Inferior Constrictor; it has the same innervation (the superior laryngeal nerve's **external** branch) and similar attachments on the outside of the larynx. The other laryngeal muscles lie inside the larynx and are innervated by the recurrent laryngeal nerve—although their *sensory* innervation comes from the superior laryngeal nerve, via its **internal** branch.

■ The Third, Fourth, and Fifth "Gill Slits" and the Thyroid Gland

The gill slits in a human embryo never open. The outer clefts of the last three "gill slits" disappear without trace during fetal life, but the corresponding inner outpocketings (**pharyngeal pouches**) from the gut lining give rise to the thymus, thyroid, and parathyroid glands.

The **thymus** degenerates after puberty and is not detectable in most dissecting-room cadavers; but at birth, it is large and critically important in the establishment of the baby's immune system. It forms as a pair of saclike extensions of the third pharyngeal pouches. These sacs become attached to the outside of the pericardium while the developing heart still lies up in the cervical region. When the heart descends into the thorax, the paired sacs are drawn down with it and form a single thymus gland behind the sternum. In adult life, the thymus is gradually replaced by fat, but islands of its tissue persist and continue to play an important role in producing antibodies and lymphocytes.

A similar outpocketing of the last (fifth) pouch forms an accessory thymus in some mammals. Although this pouch is more or less vestigial in human beings, some of its tissues form a pair of blobs in the neck ("ultimobranchial bodies") that wind up as part of the **thyroid gland.**

Most of our thyroid gland develops from a separate midline invagination in the *floor* of the mouth. (A pit near the back of the tongue—the **foramen cecum** [Fig. 21-8]—marks the site of this invagination.) The invagination loses its connection with the mouth and becomes a two-lobed sac, which slides down the front of the neck. It winds up lying on the front of the trachea just below the larynx, deep to the "rectus cervicis" muscles. This sac fuses with the ultimobranchial bodies to become the definitive thyroid gland, which consists of two lobes joined by a narrow bridge, or **isthmus,** of thyroid tissue (Fig. 22-2). The path along which the sac descended from the mouth into the neck may be marked by a trail of accessory thyroid glands in the midline. Accessory thyroid glands have all the functions of the normal gland, and must be found and removed in performing a thyroidectomy.

The "tail" that the left and right halves of the thymus trail behind them also forms an endocrine gland, the **inferior parathyroid** gland. Similar outpocketings of the fourth pouches form a pair of **superior parathyroids.** (The third-pouch parathyroids start out above the fourth-pouch ones but wind up inferior because they get dragged further tailward by the descending thymus.) Both sets of parathyroids become embedded in the dorsal surface of the thyroid gland. A surgeon needs to avoid injuring them in removing a diseased thyroid; their secretions are vitally important in maintaining the calcium balance of the blood, and potentially fatal muscle spasms and convulsions (tetany) follow their removal.

▪ The Third Pharyngeal Arch and the Glossopharyngeal Nerve

Not much of the third pharyngeal arch remains in a human adult. Its skeletal elements are important, however, because they constitute most of the hyoid bone. This bone ties together several components of the neck. The larynx is suspended below it by ligaments attached to the upper "horns" (superior cornua) of the thyroid cartilage (Fig. 21-3). Some of the tongue muscles, some of the "rectus cervicis" hypaxial muscles, and some of the muscles of pharyngeal arches 1, 2, and 4 also attach to the hyoid bone. As all these muscles tug on it directly and indirectly during eating, drinking, and speaking, the hyoid bobs up and down under the mandible like a diminutive and highly mobile lower jaw. Although the hyoid is mostly third-arch skeleton, the only remaining third-arch muscle does not attach to it. This **Stylopharyngeus** muscle passes between the upper two Constrictors to contribute to an inner, longitudinal coat of pharyngeal muscles (Figs. 21-2 and 21-5).

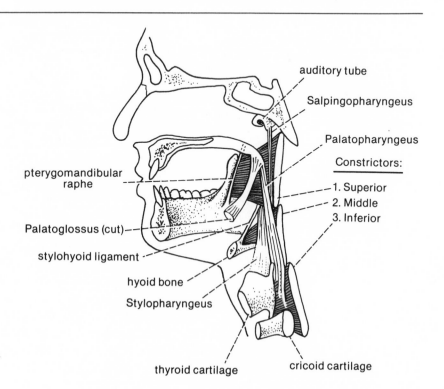

Fig. 21-5 Longitudinal muscles of the pharynx inside the Constrictors. Medial view of the hemisected head and neck (diagrammatic).

auditory tube

Salpingopharyngeus

Palatopharyngeus

Constrictors:

1. Superior
2. Middle
3. Inferior

pterygomandibular raphe

Palatoglossus (cut)

stylohyoid ligament

hyoid bone

Stylopharyngeus

thyroid cartilage

cricoid cartilage

The nerve of the third arch is the glossopharyngeal nerve (cranial nerve IX). Besides innervating Stylopharyngeus, it performs four important jobs:

1. Via the pharyngeal plexus, it furnishes general sensory innervation to the upper end of the pharynx (Fig. 21-6)—the third-arch territory on the gut tube's inner surface.

2. It provides taste fibers (as well as general sensory innervation) to the rear third of the tongue—which is also third-arch territory. (A few taste receptors at the back of the tongue fall in fourth-arch territory and are supplied by the vagus via the internal branch of the superior laryngeal nerve.)

3. Nerve IX sends sensory branches to the **carotid body.** The carotid body is a lentil-sized tangle of nerve fibers and blood sinusoids tucked into the fork of the common carotid artery. It monitors CO_2 levels in the blood. When these increase, afferent nerve impulses via cranial nerve IX (plus a few returning via X) prompt a speeding-up of

Fig. 21-6 General sensory innervation of the foregut. Schematic midline section.

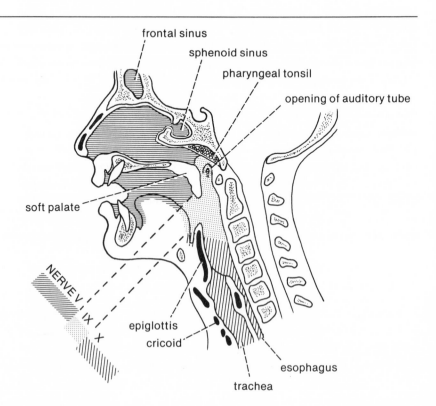

frontal sinus

sphenoid sinus

pharyngeal tonsil

opening of auditory tube

soft palate

NERVE V IX

epiglottis

cricoid

esophagus

trachea

breathing and heartbeats to bring more oxygen to the body's tissues. We are not consciously aware of this special "sense," so it probably does not have any projection to the cerebral cortex.

4. Nerve IX also contains parasympathetic fibers, which supply the **parotid** salivary gland (Fig. 21-7).

Salivary glands develop as branching outpocketings of the mouth lining. They are unique to mammals, which are the only animals that chew their food and need to moisten it with spittle. Three pairs of large salivary glands develop in the human embryo. The parotid gland is the largest of the three. It is about the size and shape of the external ear and lies beneath the skin just in front of the ear. Its duct curves forward across the underlying jaw muscle (Masseter) and then pierces the cheek muscle (Buccinator) to open into the mouth alongside the second upper molar tooth. This forward-pointing duct occasionally squirts saliva right out of the mouth, when we open up to bite into some especially tasty-looking morsel.

Like all other involuntary functions associated with eating, the secretion of saliva is prompted by parasympathetic impulses. The route by which those impulses reach the parotid gland is bizarrely convoluted (Fig. 21-7B). As nerve IX leaves the braincase, it sends a branch back into the skull through a little canal in the petrous temporal. This **tympanic** nerve carries sensory fibers to the tympanic (middle-ear) cavity, including the inner face of the eardrum (tympanum)—hence its name. It also contains presynaptic parasympathetics. These form a bundle—the **lesser petrosal** nerve—that *reenters the braincase* through the petrous temporal and runs along its inner surface toward foramen ovale (where V_3 comes out). The lesser petrosal nerve makes its final exit from the braincase through foramen ovale (or a separate little hole medial to it) and ends in the **otic ganglion** attached to V_3. Here its fibers synapse. The postsynaptic fibers are distributed to the parotid gland via branches of V_3.

▪ The Second "Gill Slit" and the Tonsils

The lining of the pouch between arches 2 and 3 develops into a mass of lymphoid tissue called the **palatine tonsil** (Fig. 21-8)—a sort of hatchery for white blood cells (lymphocytes), which multiply there and send their offspring forth into lymph vessels of the neck. The adult tonsil is shielded in front and in back by a couple of fourth-arch

Fig. 21-7 The parotid gland (A)—and its innervation, shown in a diagrammatic section to the left of the midline (B). Compare Fig. 21-12.

A

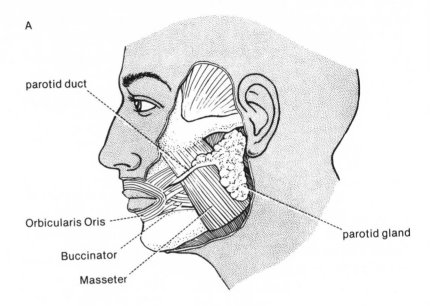

parotid duct

Orbicularis Oris

Buccinator

Masseter

parotid gland

B

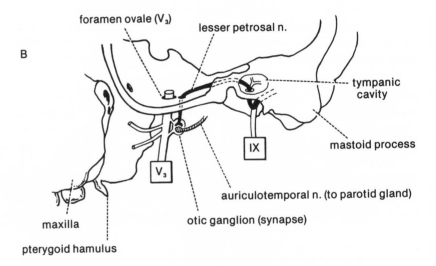

foramen ovale (V₃)

lesser petrosal n.

tympanic cavity

mastoid process

IX

V₃

auriculotemporal n. (to parotid gland)

otic ganglion (synapse)

maxilla

pterygoid hamulus

muscles (Palatoglossus, Palatopharyngeus) hanging down from the palate (Fig. 21-5). The glossopharyngeal nerve enters the pharynx just below the tonsil, and the internal carotid artery may rarely lie just on the other side of the thin pharyngeal wall—facts to bear in mind when performing a tonsillectomy.

A similar mass of lymphoid tissue—the **pharyngeal tonsil**—lies in the roof of the upper pharynx (nasopharynx), above and behind the soft palate (Fig. 21-6). When swollen by infection, this mass is called "adenoids," and may interfere with breathing through the nose. Little nodules of lymphoid tissue also lie just under the mucous membrane of the rear third of the tongue, giving it a lumpy appearance. These lumps are known collectively as the **lingual tonsil** (Fig. 21-8). The lingual, palatine, and pharyngeal tonsils form a **tonsillar ring** encircling the back of the mouth. Note that all the tonsils form in or adjacent to third-arch territory and are covered by gut lining innervated by the nerve of the third arch (IX). Like the thymus, the tonsils dwindle and regress after puberty.

■ The Second-Arch Skeleton and the Middle Ear

Quite a lot of the skeleton of the second or hyoid pharyngeal arch is left in *Homo sapiens*. It includes our styloid process and the lesser horn of the hyoid bone—and the **stylohyoid** ligament connecting the two. The human stylohyoid ligament may rarely develop into a chain

Fig. 21-8 Surface anatomy of the mouth and tongue. The anterior two-thirds of the tongue differs in texture and innervation from the rear third (which is supplied by nerve IX). The so-called arches framing the palatine tonsil are folds of mucous membrane covering similarly named fourth-arch muscles (Palatoglossus, Palatopharyngeus; compare Fig. 21-5).

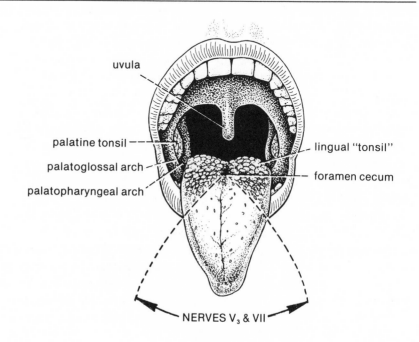

uvula

palatine tonsil

palatoglossal arch

palatopharyngeal arch

lingual "tonsil"

foramen cecum

NERVES V₃ & VII

of bones connected by synovial joints, producing a very fishlike second-arch skeleton (Fig. 19-8C).

When the first-arch skeleton gave rise to the primitive jaws (Fig.
19-8B), the uppermost bone in the second arch swung forward and
became a prop that braced the jaw joint against the bony ear capsule
(Fig. 19-8C). This forward rotation constricted the first gill slit into a
small **spiracle** in front of the second arch. In many fish, this vestigial
first gill slit disappears altogether (Fig. 6-2B). In air-breathing vertebrates, the endodermal part of the first gill slit developed into the air-
filled middle-ear cavity, as part of a solution to the problem of
detecting sound waves in air.

Airborne sound is not absorbed easily by water; it gets reflected
from the water surface. A vertebrate's head is essentially a bony box
full of water, so sound waves in air mostly bounce off it. Land-
dwelling vertebrates remained deaf to airborne sound until mechanisms evolved for converting it into pressure waves in the inner-ear
fluid.

The second-arch bone that swung forward behind the spiracle to
prop up the jaw joint is called the **stapes.** Because it touched the ear
capsule, the stapes could carry sound vibrations from the skin back to
the petrous temporal, thus setting up waves in the perilymph. In air-
breathing vertebrates, the stapes is specialized for doing just that. The
stapes of a frog, bird, or lizard is a slender rod fastened to a **tympanic
membrane,** or eardrum, stretched across the opening of the spiracle.
The other end of the stapes is a tiny piston that fits into a membrane-
covered window (**fenestra vestibuli**) in the ear capsule. When sound
waves push the eardrum in and out, the stapes focuses all the energy
of the vibrating eardrum on the much smaller window—and thus
converts low-energy, airborne sound waves into higher-energy waves
in the perilymph. The air-filled middle-ear cavity surrounding the
stapes is needed to make this setup work. If the stapes were surrounded by liquid, the eardrum would just be another air–water
interface; and sound waves would bounce off it.

Mammals improved on this arrangement in several ways. In mammals, the old first-arch bones that formed the reptilian jaw joint have
become tiny bony levers that intervene between the eardrum and
stapes (Fig. 21-9). These first-arch elements—the **malleus** (lower jaw)
and **incus** (upper jaw)—form a mechanical linkage that amplifies the
vibration of the eardrum. The mammalian eardrum itself is sunken

Fig. 21-9 The middle-ear cavity. Diagrammatic cross section of the left ear, seen from the front.

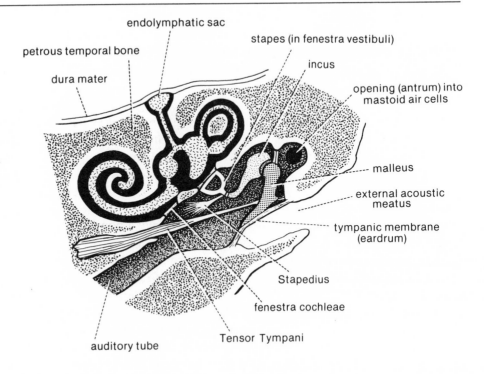

endolymphatic sac

stapes (in fenestra vestibuli)

petrous temporal bone

incus

dura mater

opening (antrum) into mastoid air cells

malleus

external acoustic meatus

tympanic membrane (eardrum)

Stapedius

fenestra cochleae

auditory tube

Tensor Tympani

into the side of the head and lies at the bottom of a skin-lined ear hole, the **external acoustic meatus.** The eardrum's withdrawal from the body surface has allowed it to become extremely delicate and fragile—and therefore responsive to the slightest sound. A cartilaginous tube surrounds the meatus and spreads out at the body surface to form a sound-directing funnel of cartilage—the external ear, or **auricle.** Most mammals have large, mobile auricles that can be swung this way and that to locate sources of sound. It is not clear why our external ears have lost this mobility.

All these improvements, plus the elongation of the cochlea (Chapter 20), make the mammalian ear more sensitive than the ears of most birds or reptiles, especially to high-frequency sounds. Human beings, who have ears of roughly average acuteness for mammals, can detect sound waves carrying as little energy as one ten-millionth of a microwatt per square centimeter.

■ The Second-Arch Muscles and the Facial Nerve

The facial nerve is mainly a branchial-motor nerve to the muscles that develop from the second pharyngeal arch. Those muscles are complex and varied. Their primitive attachment to the second-arch skeletal elements is preserved in our **Stylohyoid** muscle (Fig. 21-10), which runs alongside the stylohyoid ligament and has the same attachments (from the styloid process to the second-arch part of the hyoid bone).

The Stylohyoid muscle is pierced by the tendon of the **Digastric** muscle. As its name implies, the Digastric has two bellies: an anterior belly attached to the lower jawbone below the chin and a posterior belly arising from the medial surface of the mastoid process (Fig. 21-10). The two are connected by a shared tendon. When either belly contracts, it pulls the front of the mandible downward and backward and opens the mouth.

The Digastric is unique to mammals. A reptile's jaw-opening muscle—the Depressor Mandibulae (Fig. 21-1)—is a second-arch slip that inserts into a separate dermal bone on the back edge of the lower jaw. In mammals, this bone has become the bony frame around the eardrum (the tympanic part of the temporal bone) and the Depressor Mandibulae has been lost. A new jaw-opening muscle has been produced by pasting a second-arch slip onto a slip of the first-arch musculature that forms the floor of the mouth. The resulting Digastric muscle has a dual innervation: the anterior, first-arch belly is supplied by the first-arch nerve (V_3) and the posterior, second-arch belly is supplied by the second-arch nerve (VII).

Almost all the rest of a mammalian embryo's second-arch musculature spreads forward from the ear region across the face, differentiating into **facial muscles** attached to the skin. They drag their motor branches from nerve VII behind them, thus producing a fan of facial-nerve fibers that radiate from the stylomastoid foramen into the face (Fig. 21-11).

The facial muscles are another mammalian peculiarity. Although the most conspicuous function of our facial muscles is twitching the skin of the face to express emotions, they probably evolved to facilitate suckling. A newborn mammal cannot have a rigid face like a bird or a turtle; it needs mobile lips and cheeks that can press and suck on the mother's nipple. Suckling is made possible by two facial muscles: **Orbicularis Oris,** which puckers the lips, and **Buccinator** (Fig. 21-7A), which tenses the cheeks against the suction exerted by

Fig. 21-10   The submandibular region. A. View from the right side. B. Cross section through the point indicated by the arrow in A. Gray tone indicates pharynx (A) and tongue muscles (B).

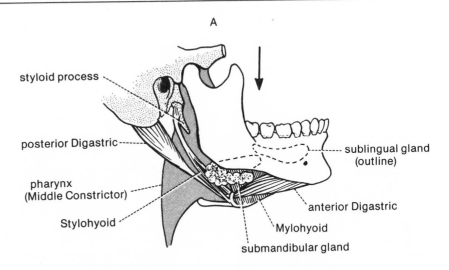

A

styloid process

posterior Digastric

pharynx
(Middle Constrictor)

Stylohyoid

sublingual gland
(outline)

anterior Digastric

Mylohyoid

submandibular gland

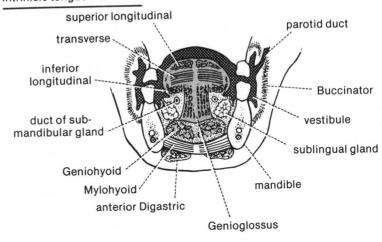

Intrinisic tongue muscles:

superior longitudinal

transverse

inferior
longitudinal

duct of sub-
mandibular gland

Geniohyoid

Mylohyoid

anterior Digastric

Genioglossus

parotid duct

Buccinator

vestibule

sublingual gland

mandible

B

the tongue. (Whales and dolphins, which have birdlike beaks, do not really suckle; the mother actively squirts milk down the baby's throat.)

The **Orbicularis Oculi** is another functionally important facial muscle. It forms a flat, disklike sphincter inside the eyelids, just as Orbicularis Oris does in the lips. When it contracts, it brings the upper and lower lids together and draws them a bit toward the bridge of the

Fig. 21-11 The facial muscles and their nerve supply (N. VII).

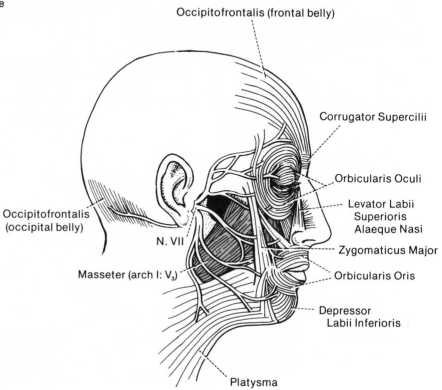

Occipitofrontalis (frontal belly)

Corrugator Supercilii

Orbicularis Oculi

Levator Labii Superioris Alaeque Nasi

Zygomaticus Major

Orbicularis Oris

Depressor Labii Inferioris

Occipitofrontalis (occipital belly)

N. VII

Masseter (arch I: V₃)

Platysma

nose. A short burst of contraction produces a blink; more powerful contraction closes the eyes in a tight squint. Because periodic blinking and squinting are needed to keep the eye's surface clean and moist, any facial-nerve injuries that paralyze Orbicularis Oculi may result in ulceration of the cornea.

Other serious effects of facial-nerve injury can include perpetual drooling (owing to paralysis of Orbicularis Oris) and bite wounds inside the cheeks (because the paralyzed Buccinator cannot draw the cheek out of the way of the teeth during chewing). Paralysis of the facial nerve also immobilizes all the purely expressive little muscle slips diagrammed in Figure 21-11, making it impossible to scowl (Corrugator Supercilii), smile (Zygomaticus Major), pout (Depressor Labii Inferioris), flare the nostrils (Levator Labii Superioris Alaeque Nasi), and so on. Because the temporal bone of a newborn baby has no mastoid process, the stylomastoid foramen lies directly beneath the skin, and injury to nerve VII at this point—say, by an obstetrician's forceps—can paralyze the facial muscles and interfere with suckling.

■ Parasympathetic Branches of Nerve VII

Two peculiar branches of the facial nerve—the greater petrosal nerve and the chorda tympani (Fig. 21-12)—split off from it inside the petrous temporal before it comes out of the stylomastoid foramen. These branches carry nerve VII's parasympathetic outflow, which supplies glands in the face. They also bring back taste sensations from the tongue and palate.

GREATER PETROSAL NERVE

The **greater petrosal** nerve (Fig. 21-12) emerges from the petrous temporal's upper surface and runs forward below the temporal lobes of the brain. As it nears the foramen lacerum, the greater petrosal nerve is joined by a bundle of postsynaptic sympathetic fibers (the **deep petrosal** nerve) from the sympathetic plexus around the internal carotid artery. The two petrosal nerves merge to form the **nerve of the pterygoid canal,** which runs forward inside the root of the pterygoid process of the sphenoid bone (Fig. 19-4). It emerges in the pterygopalatine fossa, alongside the maxillary division of the trigeminal (V_2). Here it enters a parasympathetic ganglion hanging below V_2 (the **pterygopalatine ganglion**), and its parasympathetic fibers synapse. The postsynaptic autonomic fibers are distributed, via branches of V_2, to the glands of the nasal cavity and the roof of the mouth. Some of them enter the orbit (in the zygomatic branch of V_2; see below), where they jump across to V_1's lacrimal branch (Fig. 20-3) and run forward to innervate the lacrimal gland.

CHORDA TYMPANI

The **chorda tympani** (Fig. 21-12) branches from the facial nerve inside the petrous temporal and emerges into the rear of the middle-ear cavity. It runs right across the inner surface of the eardrum (hence its name) and leaves the skull through a crack between the petrous and tympanic parts of the temporal bone. Emerging on the inner side of the jaw joint, it joins the nearby lingual nerve (from V_3), which is the sensory nerve to the front two-thirds of the tongue. Its parasympathetic fibers synapse in the **submandibular ganglion** hanging from the

Fig. 21-12 The parasympathetic component of the facial nerve (VII). A. Diagrammatic section to the left of the midline, showing the named nerves involved and their connections. B and C. Dispositions of preganglionic (*black*) and post-ganglionic (*hatched*) parasympathetic axons supplying the lower salivary glands (B) and lacrimal gland (C).

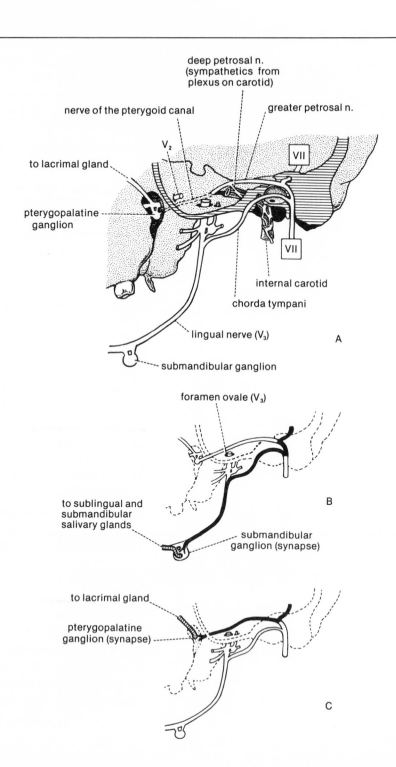

lingual nerve. Postsynaptic fibers go on from there to innervate the salivary glands beneath the tongue (sublingual and submandibular glands; see below).

Taste sensations from the anterior two-thirds of the tongue return to the brain via the chorda tympani. The greater petrosal nerve has a similar but smaller sensory component, which supplies a few taste buds on the palate.

■ The First "Gill Slit": Auditory Tube and Middle Ear

The "gill slit" between our first and second arches is closed only by the eardrum. Poking a hole in the eardrum would restore the old spiracle and allow you to blow air out through your ears. The demonstration is not worth the attendant loss of hearing.

The endodermal pouch of this first "gill slit" expands into the air-filled spaces of the middle ear (Fig. 21-9). Those spaces remain connected to the pharynx through the **auditory tube,** which is known as the Eustachian tube to everybody but anatomists. This persistent connection of the middle ear to the outside world allows germs to enter and cause middle-ear infections, but it is needed to keep air pressure the same on both sides of the eardrum (so that our eardrums do not tend to burst whenever the barometer falls or we climb a mountain). Although the tube is normally held closed by its cartilaginous walls, palate muscles arising from the cartilage (Fig. 21-17) open the tube and let air in or out when we swallow.

A very different function is served by the little **Tensor Tympani** muscle, which also arises from the tubal cartilage. This muscle runs backward into the middle ear and attaches to the malleus (Fig. 21-9). It contracts reflexically in noisy surroundings, damping the vibrations of the eardrum and reducing the energy input to the inner ear. A similar **Stapedius** muscle running forward from the posterior wall of the middle-ear cavity has a similar attachment to the stapes. Together, these two muscles provide a sort of volume control that prevents loud sounds from damaging the sensitive inner-ear apparatus. Inasmuch as the malleus and stapes are derived from the first and second arches respectively, Tensor Tympani and Stapedius are respectively innervated by nerves V (first arch) and VII (second arch).

If the middle-ear cavity develops from the first pouch, between arches 1 and 2, why does it get its sensory innervation from nerve IX (third arch)? The growing first pouch expands backward to incorporate most of the second pouch as well. Nerve IX's sensory branch to that pouch thus gets drawn into the back of the cavity and becomes the tympanic nerve (see Third Pharyngeal Arch, above). Its branches eventually spread into all the air-filled spaces of the middle ear, including the auditory tube. (Note that the auditory tube opens into nerve IX's territory at the top of the pharynx; cf. Fig. 21-6.) The external ear hole is innervated in front by the first-arch nerve, as you might expect—but its rear surface, for reasons too complex to bother with here, is supplied by the vagus.

▪ The Trigeminal Nerve and the First Arch

Practically nothing is left of our first-arch skeleton except the malleus and incus in the middle ear. However, the first-arch muscles that snap the jaws of a shark shut (Fig. 21-1) have shifted their attachments over to other bones in the human skull and retain their old function and importance. Together with the first-arch muscles that form the floor of the mouth, they form a U-shaped sling wrapped around the underside of the gut tube and attached to the mandible (Fig. 21-13)—the standard pharyngeal-arch arrangement, but with a dermal bone substituting for the gill-arch skeleton.

The trigeminal nerve (V) is the nerve of the first pharyngeal arch and the largest of the twelve cranial nerves. It leaves the brain and runs forward within the dura, thus splitting the dura into "inner" and "outer" layers just as a dural venous sinus does. A large, crescent-shaped, dorsal-root (sensory) ganglion lying on the trigeminal in this dural "cave" contains the cell bodies of the trigeminal's sensory neurons. (Similar but smaller sensory ganglia occur on the other gill-arch nerves, reminding us that these are all primitive dorsal roots.) Just anterior to this ganglion, the trigeminal splits up into the three major divisions for which it is named. These comprise a branch to the orbit and forehead (V_1), a branch to the upper jaw (V_2), and a branch to the lower jaw (V_3). We will describe them in that order.

V_1: THE OPHTHALMIC NERVE

The **ophthalmic nerve** (V_1) is a strictly sensory nerve to the most ancient part of the face: the tissues of the eye, orbit, and nose, lying above the secondarily acquired jaws. It enters the orbit via the superior orbital fissure and splits into three main branches: a **frontal** branch to the forehead, a **lacrimal** branch to the conjunctiva and upper eyelid (carrying parasympathetic fibers from VII to the lacrimal

Fig. 21-13 The first-arch muscles surrounding the mouth. A. Superficial view. B. Deeper dissection; the Masseter and the center of the zygomatic arch have been removed to show the Temporalis attachments. C. The two Pterygoids.

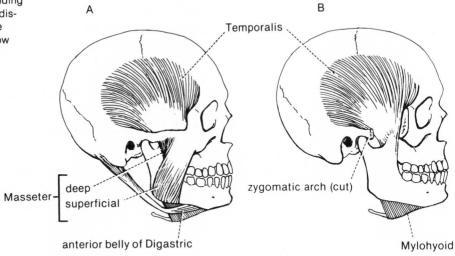

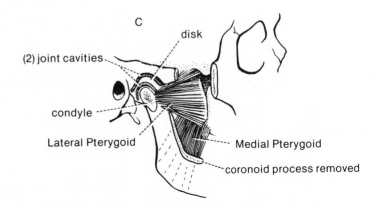

gland), and a **nasociliary** branch. This last innervates the eyeball and the nose. The branches of V_1 are accompanied by roughly corresponding branches of the ophthalmic artery (Fig. 20-3); and sympathetic fibers from the plexus around the internal carotid (Chapter 22) enter the orbit with the ophthalmic artery and pass into the nasociliary nerve to reach the Dilator Pupillae muscle (Chapter 20).

V_2: THE MAXILLARY NERVE

The **maxillary nerve** (V_2) is also strictly a sensory nerve. It supplies the derivatives of the embryonic maxillary process (Chapter 20). The

[handwritten margin note: continues into the orbit, forming the infraorbital nerve when it enters through the inferior orbital fissure, from there, it exits]

maxillary nerve emerges through the foramen rotundum (Figs. 19-3 and 19-4), into the pterygopalatine fossa (Fig. 21-14). Most of its fibers continue forward underneath the greater wing of the sphenoid into the orbit, forming the **infraorbital** nerve. The gap through which they pass is called the **inferior orbital fissure** (Fig. 19-2). The infraorbital nerve runs forward under the **periorbita,** the periosteum of the eye socket. The groove in which it runs grows deeper anteriorly and is roofed over there by periorbital bone, forming an **infraorbital canal.** The nerve emerges through the **infraorbital foramen** below the orbit (Fig. 19-5A) and sends sensory branches in all directions to the overlying skin (Figs. 18-3 and 21-14). While in the orbit, it gives off branches (**anterior superior alveolar** nerves) to the upper front teeth—a territory it annexes from V_1 after the nasolacrimal duct closes over (Fig. 20-6).

Other branches of V_2 radiate from the pterygopalatine fossa. A little **zygomatic** branch follows the infraorbital nerve through the inferior orbital fissure and supplies the skin lateral to the orbit. **Palatine** and **nasal** branches of V_2 run downward and medially through various holes and canals in the palatine bone (Fig. 21-14B), innervating the roof of the mouth and the inside of the nasal passages. **Posterior superior alveolar** branches enter tiny canals in the maxilla and supply the back teeth in the upper jaw.

The pterygopalatine ganglion, one of the four peripheral parasympathetic ganglia, is attached to V_2 just outside the skull. Parasympathetic fibers of VII from the nerve of the pterygoid canal (Fig. 21-12) enter this ganglion and synapse. Some of the postganglionic fibers are distributed with branches of V_2 to the nasal passages and palate. Others join the zygomatic nerve and enter the orbit to supply the lacrimal gland.

V_3: THE MANDIBULAR NERVE

The **mandibular** nerve (V_3) contains the trigeminal's motor fibers, all of which innervate first-arch muscles. Most of them go into the **masticatory** muscles that run from cranium to lower jaw. There are four of these muscles—the superficial Temporalis and Masseter muscles, and the deeper-lying Medial and Lateral Pterygoids.

The **Temporalis,** the mammalian equivalent of the old reptilian jaw adductor (Figs. 19-7 and 21-1), stretches from the skull roof to the **coronoid process** of the mandible (Fig. 19-5A). It fills up the space enclosed by the zygomatic arch. The **Masseter** represents a detached

Fig. 21-14   The pterygopalatine fossa. Fore-and-aft section of skull through left orbit. A. Entry of maxillary nerve (V₂) and artery into fossa. B. Their branches leave the fossa by running up through the infraorbital canal (1), down through the palatine and superior alveolar canals (2), or medially (3) through the sphenopalatine foramen into the nasal fossa.

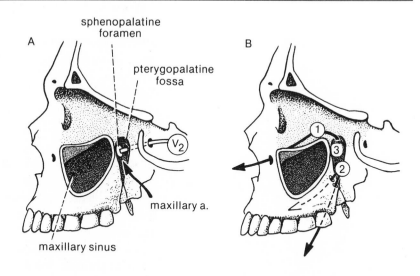

superficial layer of the Temporalis mass that originates from the zygomatic arch itself (Fig. 21-13). It runs downward and backward between the mandible and the skin, inserting into the mandible's back lower corner (or angle).

The Pterygoid muscles (Fig. 21-13) originate from (and are named after) the dangling pterygoid "talons" of the sphenoid bone (Fig. 19-4). The Medial and Lateral Pterygoids arise respectively from the medial and lateral surfaces of the **lateral pterygoid plate**, directly in front of foramen ovale (Fig. 19-5). The **Medial Pterygoid** inserts into the angle of the mandible, on its deep aspect. It thus parallels the Masseter, but on the inner rather than the outer surface of the lower jaw. The **Lateral Pterygoid** inserts further up on the mandible. Its fibers converge on a tendon that attaches to the front of the mandible's condylar **neck**, just below the mandibular **condyle** that fits into the jaw socket on the squamous part of the temporal bone. Its uppermost fibers, arising from the greater wing of the sphenoid, insert into an articular **disk** interposed between the condyle and its socket. When the Lateral Pterygoid contracts, it pulls the condyle and disk forward. This forward tug at the top of the mandible acts (in concert with the Digastric's backward pull under the chin) to open the mouth. The other three masticatory muscles all act to pull the jaw back upward, bringing the teeth together in biting or chewing.

As nerve V_3 emerges through foramen ovale, it passes between the two Pterygoid muscles where they arise from opposite surfaces of the lateral pterygoid plate. It sends motor branches into them (and into the adjoining "Tensor" muscles; see below). Its motor branches to the two superficial masticatory muscles (Temporalis and Masseter) pass laterally over the Lateral Pterygoid; its sensory **auriculotemporal** branch (to the scalp behind and above the jaw joint) loops under the Lateral Pterygoid's lower edge.

A few motor fibers of V_3 accompany V_3's sensory branch to the lower teeth, the **inferior alveolar** nerve. This nerve enters the mandible on its inner side and traverses a canal in the bone, supplying the roots of the teeth and then emerging as a cutaneous nerve through the **mental foramen** (Fig. 19-5) alongside the chin (L. *mentum,* "chin"). The accompanying motor fibers leave the inferior alveolar nerve before it enters the canal in the mandible; they supply the first-arch muscles (Mylohyoid and anterior Digastric belly) in the floor of the mouth (Figs. 21-10 and 21-13).

The remaining branches of V_3 are sensory nerves to the tongue (**lingual** nerve) and the inside of the cheek (**buccal** nerve). They run down toward the mouth around opposite sides of the lateral Pterygoid. As might be expected, the nerve to the tongue runs on the tongue side of the muscle, and the nerve to the cheek runs on the cheek side (following the buccal artery; Fig. 21-15).

■ The Upper Pharynx and the Soft Palate

The bony **hard palate** between nose and mouth does not extend back beyond the upper teeth (Fig. 21-16). Behind that, the nasal fossa is separated from the mouth by a movable aponeurotic flap—the **soft palate,** which hangs down from the back edge of the hard palate (Fig. 21-6). Muscles attached to the base of the skull reach the soft palate by passing through the uppermost gap in the Constrictor muscles (Fig. 21-2). They tense the soft palate and pull it upward, thus shutting off the nasal fossa from the pharynx and keeping the mouth contents from erupting into the nose when we swallow. There are two of these muscles (Fig. 21-17). The **Levator Veli Palatini** (L., "lifter of the palatine veil") lifts the palate upward toward the petrous temporal bone, where it originates. The **Tensor Veli Palatini** originates more laterally, from the side of the auditory tube's cartilage and the surrounding structures. It hooks around a bony pulley (the **hamulus**)

Fig. 21-15 The maxillary artery and its principal branches. Branches of the mandibular nerve (*white*) radiate from foramen ovale and follow the arterial branches to the lower jaw and first-arch muscles.

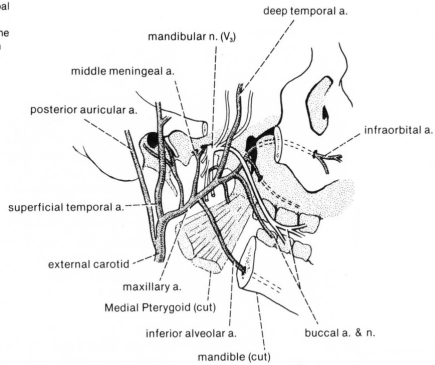

deep temporal a.

mandibular n. (V₃)

middle meningeal a.

infraorbital a.

posterior auricular a.

superficial temporal a.

external carotid

maxillary a.

Medial Pterygoid (cut)

inferior alveolar a.

buccal a. & n.

mandible (cut)

Fig. 21-16 Formation of the palate (A) and its anatomy in the adult (B). The mucous membrane on the right half of the palate is removed in B to expose the bones and the Tensor muscle.

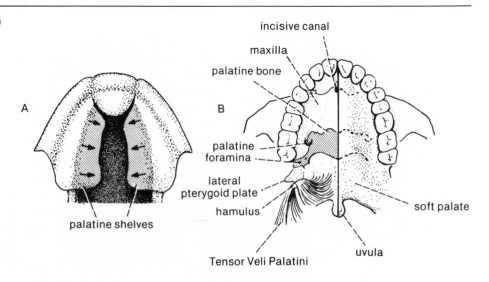

incisive canal

maxilla

palatine bone

palatine foramina

lateral pterygoid plate

hamulus

A

B

palatine shelves

soft palate

Tensor Veli Palatini

uvula

Fig. 21-17 The Levator and Tensor of the soft palate. Diagrammatic view from behind. The right Levator has been removed to expose the Tensor and the pterygoid hamulus.

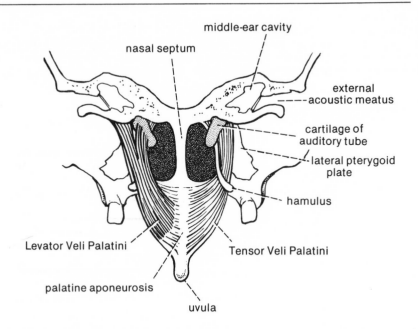

middle-ear cavity

nasal septum

external acoustic meatus

cartilage of auditory tube

lateral pterygoid plate

hamulus

Levator Veli Palatini

Tensor Veli Palatini

palatine aponeurosis

uvula

sticking out from the medial pterygoid plate (Fig. 21-16) and inserts into the whole aponeurosis of the soft palate. When the Tensor contracts, it pulls sideways on its lower attachments (thus drawing the palatine aponeurosis taut) and downward on its upper attachments (thus opening the auditory tube and making the ears "pop" when we swallow).

Two other muscles, the feeble **Palatoglossus** and the more substantial **Palatopharyngeus,** run downward from the palatine aponeurosis to the tongue and the walls of the pharynx respectively (Fig. 21-5). They produce the palatoglossal and palatopharyngeal "arches" on either side of the back of the tongue. These mucous-membrane-covered folds delimit the mouth cavity in back and enclose the palatine tonsil between them (Fig. 21-8). When the enclosed muscles contract, they draw the halves of each arch together like a curtain. With a little help from the back of the tongue, this plugs the mouth's opening into the pharynx, thereby preventing food in the pharynx from erupting back into the mouth when the Constrictors contract. The Palatopharyngeus merges with Stylopharyngeus inside the pharynx, thus forming an inner layer of longitudinal muscles (Fig. 21-5) that lift the pharynx upward during swallowing.

Tensor Veli Palatini is a first-arch muscle, innervated by V_3. (It shares some fibers with Tensor Tympani, the other first-arch "tensor" muscle that comes off the auditory tube.) Stylopharyngeus is the lone third-arch muscle (nerve IX). The remaining muscles of the palate and upper pharynx are fourth-arch muscles with the usual vagal innervation.

▪ The Mouth and the Tongue

When the upper and lower teeth are brought together, they divide the cavity of the mouth into the **vestibule** (between the teeth and the cheek) and the **oral cavity** proper (where the tongue sits). Mucous and salivary glands empty into both divisions of the mouth. The parotid gland (and many small mucous glands inside the cheeks and lips) empty into the vestibule; the **submandibular** and **sublingual** salivary glands (and many small mucous glands on the palate) empty into the oral cavity proper (Fig. 21-10). A fold of mucous membrane runs around the base of the tongue. Onto the summit of this fold, the submandibular gland opens into the mouth through a single big duct in front, and the sublingual gland opens through several small ones further back.

The floor of the mouth is formed by two layers of muscle: a deep hypaxial strip and a more superficial first-arch layer wrapped around the hypaxial strip's underside. The hypaxial strip—the **Geniohyoid** muscle—is the head end of our "rectus cervicis" complex (the cervical equivalent of Rectus Abdominis; Fig. 5-2). The Geniohyoid stretches from the hyoid bone to the jaw near the midline. It is covered beneath by two superficial muscles of the first arch—the transversely running **Mylohyoid** attached to jaw and hyoid (Fig. 21-13B) and the anterior belly of the Digastric (Fig. 21-10). Being hypaxial, the Geniohyoid is innervated by ventral rami (cervical plexus); the two first-arch muscles are supplied by the first-arch nerve (V_3).

The muscles that make up the flesh of the tongue are derived from the occipital somites back near the foramen magnum. During development, they creep forward around the pharyngeal Constrictors and their nerves, passing deep to the overlying derivatives of arches 1 and 2. Arriving in the floor of the mouth, they push up the gut lining to form the **tongue**—a lump of somitic muscle covered with mucous membrane. The hypoglossal nerve (XII) that innervates these migrating muscles gets dragged along behind them. In the adult, it marks the trail they followed as they moved forward (Fig. 21-18B).

The tongue muscles can be divided into an **extrinsic** group of three muscles (attached to bones in the neighborhood) that pull the whole tongue this way and that and an **intrinsic** group of three muscles that are not attached to any bones and act mainly to change the tongue's shape. The three extrinsic muscles (Fig. 21-18) consist of the **Genioglossus** (Gk., "chin" + "tongue"), which arises from the inside of the bony chin and fans out backward to provide a muscular core for the tongue; the **Hyoglossus,** which is a square, flat muscle that runs up from the whole greater horn of the hyoid and inserts into the side of the tongue; and the **Styloglossus,** which fans out from the styloid process and runs down to interdigitate with the Hyoglossus. (The feeble Palatoglossus descending to the tongue from the palate is a fourth-arch derivative, innervated by X rather than XII.)

The tongue's intrinsic muscle fibers (Fig. 21-10), which are interwoven with each other and with the extrinsic muscles, can be divided into longitudinal, transverse, and vertical groups. The longitudinal group has separate upper and lower bands. The upper band curves the tongue tip upward, the lower band curves it downward, and the two acting together shorten the tongue. Contracting unilaterally, these muscles bend the tongue to the left or right. The transverse group of intrinsic muscles makes the tongue long and thin; the vertical group makes it flat and broad. Because the tongue is essentially a bag of water, it has a constant volume, so it cannot get shorter in one dimension without growing longer in some other dimension.

The tongue muscles are innervated by the primitive ventral-root nerve XII. But because the mucous membrane that covers the tongue derives from the gut lining of the first four pharyngeal arches, the tongue gets its *sensory* innervation from the four gill-arch nerves (Fig. 21-6). Nerves V and VII cover the same territory (the front two-thirds of the tongue) but carry different sorts of sensation (touch via V, taste via VII); the nerves of arches 3 and 4 (nerves IX and X) carry both touch and taste back from their discrete territories.

▪ Chewing and Swallowing

Chewing and swallowing are complicated, partly reflexical acts that involve most of the voluntary muscles in the head. While you read this section, try eating some tough food—celery, a raw carrot, dried

Fig. 21-18   The extrinsic tongue muscles (A)
and their relationships (B).

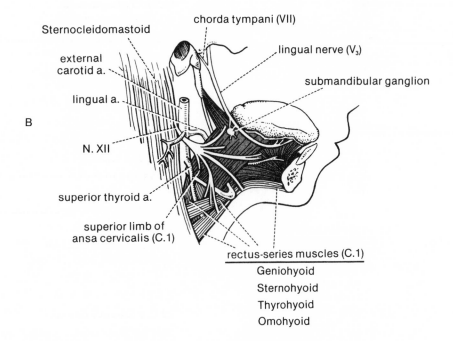

EXTRINSIC TONGUE MUSCLES:

A

mastoid process

styloid process

stylohyoid ligament

hyoid

1. Styloglossus
2. Hyoglossus
3. Genioglossus

mandible

B

Sternocleidomastoid

external
carotid a.

lingual a.

N. XII

superior thyroid a.

superior limb of
ansa cervicalis (C.1)

chorda tympani (VII)

lingual nerve (V₃)

submandibular ganglion

rectus-series muscles (C.1)
Geniohyoid
Sternohyoid
Thyrohyoid
Omohyoid

meat, or some such. Notice that you bite off chunks with your front
teeth and chew them mostly on one side in back, occasionally shifting sides. Put a fingertip in front of one ear and feel the condyle of the
lower jaw sliding back and forth as you chew. The condyle moves
backward when the jaw closes or swings toward the condyle's side
and moves forward when the opposite movements occur. As you

chew, your tongue and your cheek muscles (Buccinator) nimbly pitch lumps of half-chewed food in and out of the vestibule and oral cavity, darting in to shove food between the teeth when the jaw swings down and (usually) getting out of the way as the teeth come together again—and again and again, between one and two times every second. The whole performance is a marvel of agility and coordination, although you should remember that a rat can do it much faster than you can.

Once the food has been reduced to semiliquid pap that can be shoved down the esophagus, the urge to chew vanishes, and the tongue scoops up the mouth contents and thrusts them back between the arches at the back of the mouth. Simultaneously, the floor of the mouth and the hyoid bone are elevated. An involuntary swallowing reflex now takes over: the soft palate rises and shuts off the nose, the larynx closes to keep food out of the windpipe, and the longitudinal muscles of the pharynx lift the pharynx and larynx upward. The wad of chewed food passes backward and down into the elevated pharynx. The **epiglottis**, a spoon-shaped cartilage draped in mucosa and wisps of fourth-arch muscle (Fig. 21-3), sticks up from the thyroid cartilage behind the tongue; the passing food bends it backward, covering the larynx like a lid and providing some extra protection against thrusting food into the lungs. The pharyngeal Constrictors contract in serial order from top to bottom, milking the food downward into the esophagus. This wave of contraction continues down the esophagus until the food is propelled into the stomach. Although all these muscles are striated and under voluntary control (except for the lower third or so of the esophagus), most of the act of swallowing is an involuntary reflex. Anything that the tongue stuffs into the oral part of the pharynx will ordinarily wind up in the stomach—unless the swallowing reflex gets overridden at the last second by a gagging reflex that causes us to spit up the contents of the pharynx.

■ The External Carotid and Its Branches

The common carotid artery ends on the esophagus just behind the thyroid cartilage, where it splits into the internal and external carotid (Fig. 21-19). The internal carotid gives off no branches before it enters the skull, but the external carotid branches copiously. It supplies almost all the tissues of the head outside the braincase and quite a bit of the upper neck as well. Its main stem runs up the neck under

Fig. 21-19 Branches of the external carotid and subclavian arteries.

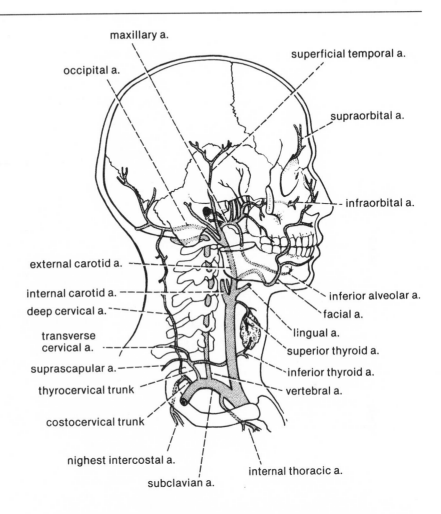

maxillary a.

occipital a.

superficial temporal a.

supraorbital a.

infraorbital a.

external carotid a.

internal carotid a.

deep cervical a.

transverse cervical a.

suprascapular a.

thyrocervical trunk

costocervical trunk

nighest intercostal a.

subclavian a.

inferior alveolar a.

facial a.

lingual a.

superior thyroid a.

inferior thyroid a.

vertebral a.

internal thoracic a.

cover of the Sternocleidomastoid, deep to the second-arch muscles (Stylohyoid, posterior Digastric). It ends by emerging as the **superficial temporal** artery between the outer ear and the condylar neck of the mandible (Fig. 21-15).

Three of the external carotid's lower branches (superior thyroid, ascending pharyngeal, and occipital arteries) will be dealt with as part of the neck (Chapter 22). Of the remaining branches (Fig. 21-19), the following are the most important.

1. The **lingual** artery runs forward parallel to the hypoglossal nerve (XII) and enters the tongue, which it supplies. Note that the tongue's

Branches of external carotids:

artery and motor nerve are separated in the middle of their course by the Hyoglossus (Fig. 21-18); nerve XII runs lateral to this and the other muscles it innervates.

2. The **facial** artery usually arises from the external carotid a bit higher up than the lingual artery, although the two occasionally have a common stem. It hooks around the lower edge of the mandible (just in front of Masseter) and snakes up the face, sending branches to the surrounding skin and muscles. Back near its origin, the facial artery gives off an **ascending palatine** artery that runs up the pharynx to supply the palate. (A **transverse facial** branch of the superficial temporal artery provides an additional route of blood supply to the face.)

3. The **maxillary** artery is the external carotid's largest and most widely distributed branch. It plunges in behind the condylar neck of the mandible, entering the fascial plane between the Medial and Lateral Pterygoids. The mandibular nerve (V$_3$) enters this same space as it leaves the skull (Fig. 21-15), and branches of the artery accompany those of the nerve: up into the temporal fossa (**deep temporal** artery) and down to the jaw and cheek (**inferior alveolar** and **buccal** arteries). Other arterial branches supply the surrounding masticatory muscles. Further back, the maxillary artery sends branches up to the meninges of the brain (**middle meningeal** artery) and to the ear.

The main stem of the maxillary artery runs forward around the Lateral Pterygoid (sometimes medial to it, sometimes lateral) and enters the pterygopalatine fossa. Here it joins the maxillary nerve (V$_2$) and is distributed with the branches of that nerve—to the infraorbital canal and face, the upper teeth, and the palate and nasal fossa (Fig. 21-14).

22

The Cervical Segments

▪ The Neck: A Transitional Region

The neck joins the head to the trunk. It resembles both in different ways. Like the trunk (but not the head), the neck has vertebrae, mixed spinal nerves, and separate epaxial and hypaxial muscle masses. But the hypaxial muscles in the neck are discontinuous and do not form a complete body wall—and do not need to, because the neck (like the head) lacks a celom.

In the trunk, the gut is enclosed in smooth muscles derived from unsegmented mesoderm. In the neck (as in the head), striated branchial-arch muscles surround the gut tube. Other branchial muscles spread down the neck beneath the skin. The neck's incomplete "body wall" thus lies between two layers of branchial-arch muscles: an inner, gut-enclosing layer (the muscles of pharynx and larynx) derived from the last three arches, and a superficial layer derived from arch 2 (facial muscles) and the old gill levators (Trapezius and Sternocleidomastoid).

Finally, the neck has some peculiarities of its own. The first two vertebrae (Chapter 2) are uniquely specialized. The cervical segments of the spinal cord are the only ones with a branchial-motor outflow; this outflow forms the spinal root of the accessory nerve (Fig. 18-4) and innervates the Trapezius (gill-levator) muscle group. The neck's major differences from the typical body segment are diagrammed in Figure 22-1.

▪ Hypaxial Muscles in the Neck

Like all hypaxial muscles, those of the neck are innervated by ventral rami of spinal nerves. They can be divided into four groups. The first three groups are cervical equivalents of Rectus Abdominis, the Intercostals, and Serratus Anterior. The neck's fourth hypaxial group—

Fig. 22-1 Schematic cross sections of the typical body segment (*left*) and neck (*right*). A, artery; S, sympathetic trunk; U-G, urogenital organs; V, vein. The heavy dashed line on the right (surrounding the common carotid, internal jugular vein, and vagus nerve) represents the carotid sheath.

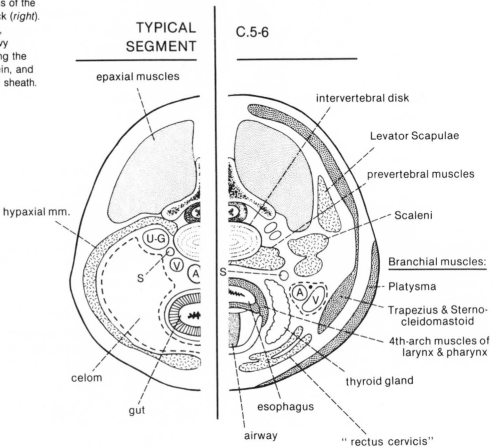

the prevertebral muscles—does not have an obvious equivalent elsewhere in the human body.

Rectus Series Five short longitudinal muscles, serial homologs of the Rectus Abdominis, stretch between the sternum and the lower border of the mandible. None of them goes the whole distance; each is attached in between to the thyroid cartilage or the hyoid bone or both. Four of these five "rectus cervicis" muscles lie below the hyoid bone and are sometimes called the infrahyoid muscles. There are two layers of them: a deep layer (Fig. 22-2) attached to the thyroid cartilage (**Sternothyroid, Thyrohyoid**), and a longer, more superficial layer

(Fig. 5-2) running from the hyoid bone down to the sternum (**Sternohyoid**) and scapula (**Omohyoid**). The Omohyoid has two bellies, held at an angle to each other by a fascial sling. Far too feeble to lift our scapula, the Omohyoid acts rather to depress or to stabilize the hyoid bone. The fifth "rectus cervicis" muscle is the **Geniohyoid,** which forms an incomplete floor for the mouth (Chapter 21). The names of these five muscles reveal their attachments—if you can remember that *genio-* means "chin" and *omo-* means "shoulder" in Greek.

 Lateral "Body Wall" From the cervical transverse processes, the three Scalene muscles (Fig. 22-3) run down to the first two ribs. They

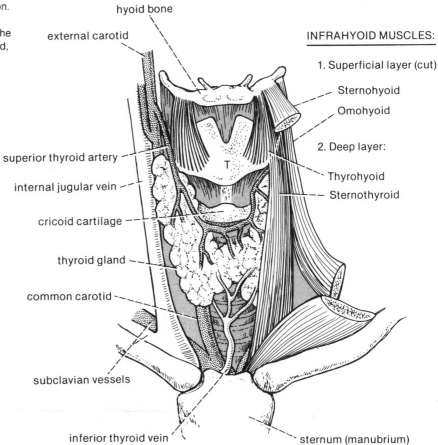

Fig. 22-2 Anterior view of the infrahyoid region. T, thyroid cartilage. The superficial infrahyoid muscles have been cut and pushed aside on the left—and removed, along with the Sternothyroid, on the right—to expose underlying structures. Compare Fig. 5-2.

hyoid bone

external carotid

superior thyroid artery

internal jugular vein

cricoid cartilage

thyroid gland

common carotid

subclavian vessels

inferior thyroid vein

INFRAHYOID MUSCLES:

1. Superficial layer (cut)

Sternohyoid

Omohyoid

2. Deep layer:

Thyrohyoid

Sternothyroid

T

sternum (manubrium)

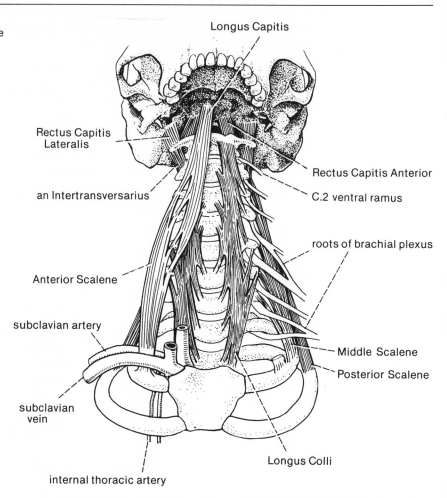

Fig. 22-3 Prevertebral muscles and Scaleni. Longus Capitis and the Anterior Scalene muscle have been removed on the left side.

Longus Capitis

Rectus Capitis Lateralis

Rectus Capitis Anterior

an Intertransversarius

C.2 ventral ramus

roots of brachial plexus

Anterior Scalene

subclavian artery

Middle Scalene

Posterior Scalene

subclavian vein

Longus Colli

internal thoracic artery

correspond to the dorsal parts of the Intercostal muscles and the abdominal Obliques. The Scalenes' action in breathing was noted in Chapter 8.

Serratus Layer   In the thorax, a special outer layer of lateral body-wall muscles stretches from the ribs to the scapula, forming the Serratus Anterior (Fig. 13-6). A separate cervical slip of this layer—the **Levator Scapulae**—arises from the upper three or four cervical transverse processes (the neck's vestigial ribs; cf. Fig. 2-3). It attaches to the upper medial corner of the scapula, and pulls the scapula upward and medially when it contracts. Like the other hypaxial limb muscles on the back, it lies deep to the Trapezius sheet (Figs. 13-4 and 22-1).

Prevertebral Muscles   In the embryo, the hypaxial muscles form on the sides of the vertebral column (Fig. 1-9). Most of them migrate ventrally to form the body wall and limb muscles. But in the cervical and lumbar segments, some hypaxial muscles stay put alongside the vertebrae to flex and support those backward-curving parts of the vertebral column. These vertebra-hugging muscles constitute the prevertebral musculature. *Two major ones are!*

In the lumbar segments, most of the prevertebral musculature gets incorporated into Psoas Major, and only a few little Intertransversarii are left as independent muscles. The neck's prevertebral muscles are more distinct. They, too, include a series of Lateral and Anterior Intertransversarii. The Intertransversarii joining the atlas (C.1) to the skull have special names—**Rectus Capitis Lateralis** and **Rectus Capitis Anterior** (Fig. 22-3). (Compare the *epaxial* Rectus Capitis *Posterior* muscles, Chapter 4.) Ventral to these lie two longer prevertebral muscles—**Longus Capitis** and **Longus Colli.** Longus Capitis runs from the upper cervical transverse processes to the base of the skull, an arrangement something like that of the epaxial muscle Semispinalis Capitis around on the other side of the vertebral column. Longus Colli ties the cervical vertebral bodies together. Both muscles flex the neck, acting in opposition to their epaxial counterparts. A layer of elastic **prevertebral fascia** separates the prevertebral muscles from the back wall of the pharynx, allowing the mobile pharynx to slide up and down freely in front of them.

■ The Branches of the Subclavian Artery

The biggest artery in the neck—the common carotid—does not give off any branches below the larynx. The lower part of the neck gets its blood via branches of the subclavian artery that come up from below. Down at the root of the neck, the subclavian artery arches over the dome of the pleura and out through the cervical "body wall" (between the Anterior and Middle Scaleni) into the upper limb. As it runs across the pleura, the subclavian artery gives off four branches (Fig. 21-19): the vertebral artery, the internal thoracic artery, the costocervical trunk, and the thyrocervical trunk.

1. The **vertebral** artery runs upward and backward from the sub-clavian artery to the cervical transverse processes and climbs up the neck through the **transverse foramina** of the upper six cervical verte-brae. The front rim of each of these foramina represents a fused vestigial rib (Fig. 2-3). The vertebral artery forms as a longitudinal anastomosis between the neck's intersegmental arteries. These disap-pear before birth, leaving only the anastomotic channel running up from the enlarged seventh intersegmental artery (the subclavian; Fig. 6-4B). The two vertebral arteries enter the foramen magnum and merge to form the brain's basilar artery, which we have already ex-amined inside the braincase (Fig. 19-9).

2. The **internal thoracic** artery is another longitudinal anastomosis between intersegmental arteries—in this case, between the intercostal arteries in front. It runs tailward along the inside of the body wall all the way down to the abdomen (Fig. 5-5), where it enters the rectus sheath and becomes the superior epigastric artery.

3. The small **costocervical** trunk runs from the subclavian back over the pleura to the neck of the first rib. There it splits into (1) a **deep cervical** branch to the epaxial muscles and (2) the **highest inter-costal** artery. The highest intercostal is yet another of those longitudi-nal anastomoses between intersegmental arteries. It replaces the direct aortic branches to the first two intercostal spaces. (Compare the venous drainage of those spaces; Fig. 7-11.)

4. The larger **thyrocervical** trunk has three branches. Two of these—the transverse cervical and suprascapular arteries—run back to the scapula (Fig. 13-16) and supply blood to limb muscles. The third branch—the **inferior thyroid** artery—runs medially to reach the thyroid gland and ramifies on its back side. The inferior thyroid artery supplies the parathyroids and part of the esophagus as well as the lower and rear parts of the thyroid. It also gives off **inferior laryngeal** branches, which follow the recurrent laryngeal nerve be-hind the synovial cricothyroid joint and into the larynx.

As might be expected, the vertebral artery sends branches to the cervical part of the spinal cord. So does the inferior thyroid artery, via its **ascending cervical** branch. This little artery runs up the neck be-tween the scalene and prevertebral muscles, supplying both—and sending spinal branches in through the intervertebral foramina as it runs along.

The thyrocervical trunk and its branches spread out along the sur-face of the Scaleni, in the plane of the dorsal part of the body wall. Accordingly, the structures that are morphologically inside the body wall—the common carotid artery, internal jugular vein, sympathetic trunk, thoracic duct, and so on—all lie ventral to the thyrocervical trunk and its branches.

▪ The Carotid Arteries in the Neck

The common carotid artery develops inside the body wall; so it runs behind the "rectus cervicis" muscles as it ascends the neck (Fig. 22-2). As an aortic arch should, it wraps dorsally upward around the gut (Fig. 9-6), running from the front of the trachea (at the root of the neck) around to the dorsal "body wall" in back (the Scaleni and prevertebral muscles). As it travels up the neck in the cleft between the pharynx and the prevertebral muscles, the common carotid is enclosed in a fascial tube called the **carotid sheath** (Fig. 22-1). The sheath also contains the internal jugular vein—and the stem of the vagus nerve, here pulled away from the gut by the descent of the aortic arches. The sympathetic trunk ascends the neck on the front of the cervical "body wall," too; but it remains behind and outside of the carotid sheath.

Of the common carotid's two branches, only the external carotid artery (Fig. 21-19) has branches that enter the neck. Three of them are worth noting:

1. The **superior thyroid** artery is the lowest branch of the external carotid. It curves downward to the front of the thyroid gland (Fig. 22-2), supplying it and giving off branches to neighboring muscles and the larynx on the way down.
2. A little **ascending pharyngeal** branch of the external carotid runs up the back side of the pharynx and helps to supply it with blood.
3. The **occipital artery** arises further up, above the facial and lingual arteries. It runs back up across the internal carotid, deep to the gill-arch muscles (Trapezius sheet, posterior Digastric), and enters the epaxial region. There, it ramifies beneath the superficial layer of epaxial muscles (Erector Spinae + Splenius) and sends branches up the back of the scalp.

▪ The Sympathetic Trunk

The sympathetic trunk runs up the neck from the thorax, sending gray rami communicantes to all the cervical ventral rami. In the typical body segment, the sympathetic trunk lies on the sides of the vertebral bodies; but in the neck, the prevertebral muscles intervene, and the trunk is embedded in the prevertebral fascia (Fig. 22-1). Near the top of the neck, the sympathetic trunk dissolves into a spray of postsynaptic fibers that form a plexus around the adjacent internal carotid artery and follow its branches.

The trunk's ganglia in the neck tend to fuse with each other during development. There are normally only three sympathetic ganglia—the **superior, middle,** and **inferior cervical ganglia**—on each side in an adult's neck. The superior, which is the largest, is a spindle-shaped conglomeration of the upper four segmental ganglia. The variable middle ganglion forms from segmental sympathetic ganglia C.5–C.6. When present, it lies at about the level of vertebra C.6. The inferior cervical ganglion incorporates the remaining paravertebral ganglia in the neck; sometimes it takes in the first thoracic ganglion as well and is then called the cervicothoracic or **stellate** ganglion. Medially running **cardiac** nerves carry postsynaptic motor fibers from all these ganglia down to the heart and lungs (Figs. 8-9 and 9-16).

■ The Veins of the Neck

The **internal jugular** vein drains the blood from the brain via the jugular foramen. Its tributaries outside the skull correspond fairly closely to the branches of the external carotid. Nearly all the territory supplied by the carotid arteries is drained by the internal jugular vein alone.

The much smaller **external jugular** vein (Fig. 22-4) is not equivalent to the external carotid, but rather to the thyrocervical trunk (described earlier as a branch of the subclavian artery). Like that trunk, the external jugular vein is a branch of a subclavian vessel, and it has scapular tributaries that correspond to the thyrocervical trunk's branches to the scapula.

There are two important differences between the external jugular and the thyrocervical trunk. The first is that the vein does not have an inferior thyroid tributary. (There is an inferior thyroid vein, but it lies deeper and empties directly into the brachiocephalic vein in front; see Fig. 22-4.) The second difference is that the external jugular vein extends up the neck to anastomose with the facial and temporal vessels. The **retromandibular** vein, which is the venous equivalent of the superficial temporal artery, empties primarily into the internal

Fig. 22-4 The principal veins of the neck. The external jugular and its tributaries are stippled.

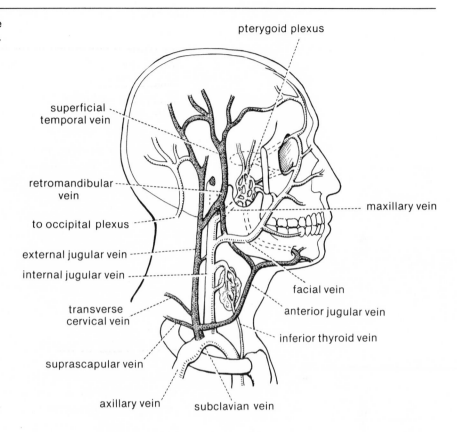

pterygoid plexus

superficial temporal vein

retromandibular vein

to occipital plexus

external jugular vein

internal jugular vein

transverse cervical vein

suprascapular vein

axillary vein

subclavian vein

inferior thyroid vein

anterior jugular vein

facial vein

maxillary vein

jugular (via the facial artery's companion vein); but some of the retromandibular blood passes into an anastomosis with the external jugular below the ear (Fig. 22-4). The **anterior jugular** vein, a superficial tributary of the external jugular in front, has a more direct anastomosis with the facial vein behind the angle of the mandible.

Note that the internal jugular vein runs lateral to the common carotid artery (Fig. 22-2). The subclavian vein ends by joining the internal jugular (to form the brachiocephalic vein), so it does not extend as far medially as the subclavian artery. As a result, the veins that correspond to the subclavian artery's most medial branches (the vertebral and internal thoracic vessels) do not empty into the subclavian vein. They end in the brachiocephalic vein instead.

▪ The Lymphatics of the Neck

All the lymph of the head and neck eventually drains into **deep cervical nodes** studding the outside of the carotid sheath. The uppermost of these nodes lies just behind the hyoid bone, where it may be palpable when inflamed. Lymphatic vessels leaving the deep cervical nodes form a **jugular trunk,** which usually empties into the thoracic duct (on the left) or the beginning of the brachiocephalic vein (on the right) (Fig. 7-12).

The upper end of the thoracic duct, which carries lymph returning from most of the rest of the body, lies in the root of the neck. Running up the ventral surfaces of the thoracic vertebrae, the duct curves to the left across the prevertebral muscles and ends by opening through one or more channels into the tributaries of the left brachiocephalic vein. This course takes it over the top of the subclavian artery.

▪ The Cervical Plexus

The cervical plexus (Fig. 22-5) is formed from the first four cervical ventral rami—that is, from the rami that do not join the nerve plexus of the upper limb. (The brachial plexus does, however, receive a variable contribution from C.4.) All eight cervical ventral rami run laterally from their intervertebral foramina, passing in front of the hypaxial Intertransversarii. The lower six or seven rami run across the front surface of the Middle Scalene, and they innervate it and the other Scalenes as they go by. Ventral rami C.5 through C.8 continue on into the axilla (Fig. 22-3). The C.4 ventral ramus gives off the phrenic nerve to the diaphragm (usually with some contributions from C.3 and C.5) and a branch to Levator Scapulae, and then breaks up into cutaneous **supraclavicular** branches (Fig. 22-6). The ventral rami of C.2 and C.3 give off similar branches—the **lesser occipital** nerve from C.2 and the **transverse cervical** and **great auricular** nerves from both C.2 and C.3. All these sensory nerves correspond to the lateral cutaneous branch of a typical spinal nerve's ventral ramus (Fig. 1-12).

A delicate loop of ventral-ramus motor fibers innervates the five "rectus cervicis" muscles. The lower end of this **ansa cervicalis** is formed by branches from C.2 and C.3; C.1 fibers coming down from above complete the loop.

Most of C.1's ventral ramus joins the hypoglossal nerve (XII) be-

Fig. 22-5 The cervical plexus (simplified). Cutaneous, purely sensory nerves are stippled. Some chiefly sensory branches to the Trapezius sheet and motor twigs to the prevertebral muscles and Scaleni have been left out of this picture.

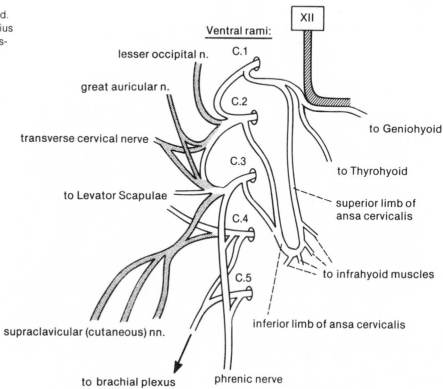

low the skull. Some older texts will tell you that the hypoglossal nerve itself innervates the Geniohyoid and Thyrohyoid and sends off the superior limb of the ansa cervicalis. Things looked that way to the early dissectors; but in fact, these "hypoglossal" branches contain only C.1 fibers. The old description is not far off, however, because C.1 is often a primitive ventral-root nerve like XII, with no sensory component. The main difference between them is that C.1 has a dorsal ramus. The two nerves are otherwise very similar and closely associated (Fig. 18-4).

▪ The Cranial Nerves in the Neck

Because there are gill-arch muscles in the neck, most of the gill-arch nerves have cervical branches. The last two of these nerves (X and XI) run down through the neck on the way to their target organs.

Fig. 22-6 Cutaneous nerves, corresponding to the lateral cutaneous branch of a typical spinal nerve, radiate through the gap between Trapezius and Sternocleidomastoid.

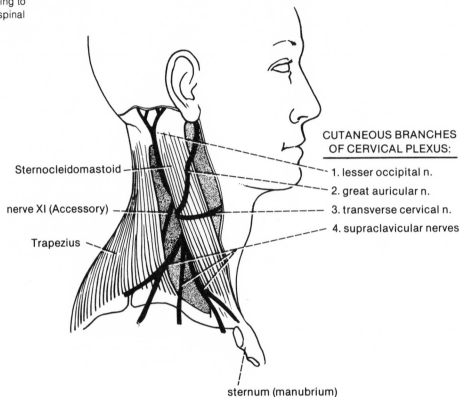

Sternocleidomastoid

nerve XI (Accessory)

Trapezius

CUTANEOUS BRANCHES OF CERVICAL PLEXUS:
1. lesser occipital n.
2. great auricular n.
3. transverse cervical n.
4. supraclavicular nerves

sternum (manubrium)

You are already familiar with the course that the vagus nerve (X) follows down the neck inside the carotid sheath. The spinal root of the accessory nerve (XI) traverses the upper part of the neck twice—once on its way up through the vertebral canal into the braincase and again as it runs back down underneath the old gill-levator muscles, sending motor fibers into them. There are two of these muscles: the Trapezius and the more ventral **Sternocleidomastoideus** (Fig. 22-6), a stout cylindrical muscle running from the mastoid process down to the sternum and medial end of the clavicle. The two muscles have a common embryonic origin, which is reflected in their shared innervation, their continuous attachment to the skull, and the common sheet of dense fascia enclosing them. The actions of the Trapezius were described in Chapter 13 (Fig. 13-5). (If you have forgotten them, just shrug your shoulders and think about it.) The Sternocleidomastoid's job is flexing the cervical vertebrae. You can feel it contracting power-fully if you lie face up on the floor and then lift your head. When it contracts on one side only, it turns the head toward the opposite side.

The Trapezius and Sternocleidomastoid are almost, but not quite, the most superficial muscles in the neck. They are overlain by **Platysma**, a thin facial muscle that runs down from the corners of the mouth and attaches to the skin on the front of the upper thorax (Fig. 21-11). It produces a distinctive down-in-the-mouth grimace when it contracts and raises a fan of thin ridges in the skin on the front of the neck. These ridges are conspicuous in old people with loose neck skin (or in young people making hideous faces).

Being a facial muscle, Platysma is innervated by motor branches of VII. So are the less specialized second-arch muscles that lie deeper in the neck (posterior Digastric and Stylohyoid). Cervical branches of the vagus supply the pharynx and larynx. A few motor fibers of the third-arch nerve (IX) descend into the neck with the Stylopharyngeus muscle on the inside of the pharynx (Fig. 21-2). The first gill-arch nerve—the trigeminal—has no cervical branches of any sort.

Index

JNC pt 20374.75

	need	actual
Bill	18793.25	19718.25
stipend	10043.5	10043.5
Total expense	28836.75	29761.75
School Sch	8183	8183
Should-be JNC	20653.75	21578.75
Actual	20374.75	20374.75
Diff	279	1204

As of now 9764.5   (975 included)
Should be 10043.5   (279 included)

Call Registrar

8452
8183
269

8183